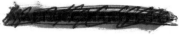

CURRENT NEURO-OPHTHALMOLOGY®
Volume 3

CURRENT

NEURO-
OPHTHALMOLOGY®

VOLUME 3

Edited by

Simmons Lessell, M.D.
Professor of Ophthalmology
Harvard Medical School
Director of Neuro-Ophthalmology
Department of Ophthalmology
Massachusetts Eye and Ear Infirmary
Boston, Massachusetts

and

J. T. W. van Dalen, M.D., Ph.D.
Associate Professor of Ophthalmology
Department of Ophthalmology
The University of Arizona Health Sciences Center
Tucson, Arizona

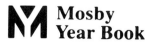
Mosby
Year Book

St. Louis   Baltimore   Boston   Chicago   London   Philadelphia   Sydney   Toronto

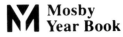
Mosby
Year Book

Dedicated to Publishing Excellence

Sponsoring Editor: Amy L. Reynaldo
Associate Managing Editor, Manuscript Services: Denise Dungey
Assistant Director, Manuscript Services: Frances M. Perveiler
Production Coordinator: Max Perez
Proofroom Manager: Barbara M. Kelly

Editorial Office:
Mosby–Year Book, Inc.
200 North LaSalle St.
Chicago, IL 60601

International Standard Serial Number: 0893-0147
International Standard Book Number: 0-8151-5390-2

Contributors

Martin L. Albert, M.D., Ph.D.
Professor of Neurology
Boston University School of Medicine
Director, Behavioral Neuroscience
Department of Neurology
Boston University School of Medicine and Boston Veterans Administration
Medical Center
Boston, Massachusetts

Myles M. Behrens, M.D.
Professor of Clinical Ophthalmology
Columbia-Presbyterian Medical Center
New York, New York

Raymond F. Carmody, M.D.
Associate Professor of Radiology
University of Arizona College of Medicine
University of Arizona Health Sciences Center
Attending Neuroradiologist
University Medical Center
Tucson, Arizona

Jon Currie, M.B., B.S., F.R.A.C.P.
The Mental Health Research Institute of Victoria
Parkville, Victoria, Australia
The Save Sight and Eye Health Institute
University of Sydney
Sydney, New South Wales, Australia

L.F. Dell'Osso, Ph.D.
Professor, Departments of Neurology and Biomedical Engineering
Case Western Reserve University School of Medicine
Director, Ocular Motor Neurophysiology Laboratory
Veterans Administration Medical Center
Cleveland, Ohio

Carl Ellenberger, Jr., M.D.
Medical Director
Lebanon Magnetic Imaging
Lebanon, Pennsylvania

John W. Gittinger, Jr., M.D.
Professor of Surgery and Neurology
University of Massachusetts Medical School
Worcester, Massachusetts

Joel S. Glaser, M.D.
Professor, Ophthalmology, Neurology, and Neurologic Surgery
Bascom Palmer Eye Institute
Department of Ophthalmology
University of Miami School of Medicine
Miami, Florida

Randy H. Kardon, M.D., Ph.D.
Assistant Professor of Ophthalmology
University of Iowa College of Medicine
Neuro-ophthalmology Service
Iowa City, Iowa

Michael Kazim, M.D.
Instructor in Clinical Ophthalmology
Columbia University College of Physicians and Surgeons
Assistant Attending
Columbia-Presbyterian Medical Center
Edward S. Harkness Eye Institute
New York, New York

John S. Kennerdell, M.D.
Clinical Professor of Ophthalmology
University of Pittsburgh School of Medicine
Adjunct Professor of Surgery (Ophthalmology)
Medical College of Pennsylvania
Director, Department of Ophthalmology
Allegheny General Hospital
Pittsburgh, Pennsylvania

Martin L. Leib, M.D.
Assistant Clinical Professor of Ophthalmology
Columbia University College of Physicians and Surgeons
Director, Orbit and Ophthalmic Plastic Surgery Service
The Edward S. Harkness Eye Institute
Columbia-Presbyterian Medical Center
New York, New York

Michael S. Mega, M.D.
Teaching Fellow in Neurology
Department of Neurology
Boston University School of Medicine
Resident in Neurology
Boston Veterans Administration Medical Center
Boston, Massachusetts

Ekkehard Mehdorn, M.D.
Marienhospital Aachen
Aachen, Federal Republic of Germany

Peter Michalos, M.D.
Teaching Fellow
Columbia University College of Physicians and Surgeons
Clinical Fellow
Orbit and Ophthalmic Plastic Surgery
The Edward S. Harkness Eye Institute
Columbia-Presbyterian Medical Center
New York, New York

Jeffrey G. Odel, M.D.
Assistant Professor of Clinical Ophthalmology
Columbia-Presbyterian Medical Center
New York, New York

Joseph F. Rizzo, III, M.D.
Assistant Professor of Ophthalmology
Department of Ophthalmology
Harvard Medical School
Massachusetts Eye and Ear Infirmary
Boston, Massachusetts

Peter J. Savino, M.D.
Director, Neuro-Ophthalmology Service
Wills Eye Hospital
Philadelphia, Pennsylvania

Robert Jan Schimsheimer, M.D., Ph.D.
Erasmus University
Academic Hospital Dijkzigt
Department of Clinical Neurophysiology
Rotterdam, The Netherlands

Dieter Schmidt, M.D.
Professor, Universitäts-Augenklinik
Freiburg, Germany

Patrick A. Sibony, M.D.
Associate Professor of Ophthalmology
Department of Ophthalmology
State University of New York at Stony Brook Health Sciences Center School
    of Medicine
Stony Brook, New York

H. Stanley Thompson, M.D.
Professor of Ophthalmology
Director of Neuro-ophthalmology Service
University of Iowa College of Medicine
Iowa City, Iowa

Jonathan D. Trobe, M.D.
Professor of Ophthalmology
Associate Professor of Neurology
W.K. Kellogg Eye Center
Department of Ophthalmology and Neurology
University of Michigan Medical School
University of Michigan Medical Center
Ann Arbor, Michigan

B. Todd Troost, M.D.
Professor and Chairman
Department of Neurology
Bowman Gray School of Medicine
Wake Forest University
Winston-Salem, North Carolina

Ronald J. Tusa, M.D., Ph.D.
Assistant Professor
Departments of Neurology and Ophthalmology
The Johns Hopkins University School of Medicine
Baltimore, Maryland

J.T.W. van Dalen, M.D., Ph.D.
Associate Professor
Department of Ophthalmology
University of Arizona College of Medicine
University of Arizona Health Sciences Center
Tucson, Arizona

Wim I.M. Verhagen, M.D., Ph.D.
Department of Neurology and Clinical Neurophysiology
Canisius Wilhelmina Hospital
Nijmegen, The Netherlands

Michael Wall, M.D.
Associate Professor of Neurology
University of Iowa College of Medicine
Iowa City, Iowa

Jon Erik Ween, M.D.
Teaching Fellow in Neurology
Department of Neurology
Boston University School of Medicine
Resident in Neurology
Boston Veterans Administration Medical Center
Boston, Massachusetts

Mark T. Yoshino, M.D.
Assistant Clinical Professor of Radiology
Section of Neuroradiology
University of Arizona College of Medicine
University of Arizona Health Sciences Center
Tucson, Arizona

David S. Zee, M.D.
Professor, Departments of Neurology and Ophthalmology
The Johns Hopkins University School of Medicine
Baltimore, Maryland

Preface

This volume of *Current Neuro-ophthalmology®* is the ninth in a series of critical reviews of neuro-ophthalmology since 1980. Neuro-ophthalmology is not only a subspecialty field in neurology and ophthalmology, but it also encompasses aspects of neurosurgery, radiology, pediatrics and internal medicine. As a consequence of this, the neuro-ophthalmological literature is not just to be found in a few specialty journals but in many areas of medicine. It is therefore difficult and perhaps impossible to stay abreast and fully informed about the newest developments in the field of neuro-ophthalmology.

With these considerations in mind, a series was created to critically review the neuro-ophthalmology literature over the preceding 2 years. Each author has reviewed the literature in his field and condensed the information into a concise and readable chapter.

The field of neuro-ophthalmology has seen tremendous changes during the last few years. For instance, a decade ago, neuro-ophthalmologists were still discussing CT scan modalities. It has become clear, as demonstrated in the section on neuroradiology, that MR imagery has virtually overtaken CT scanning, in a period of approximately 10 years.

Dr. Currie discussed the subject of optic neuritis, and one of the articles he reviewed showed an unexpected clustering of conversion to MS among the patients with optic neuritis treated with high dose IV methylprednisolone. Other authors interested in the disease of the optic nerve/chiasm are Drs. Glaser, Kennerdell, and Behrens. Dr. Behrens discussed the newest findings in Leber's hereditary optic neuropathy, in addition to optic nerve sheath decompression in papilledema and its newly suggested use in progressive anterior ischemic optic neuropathy.

Ocular motility was discussed by Drs. Dell'Osso (nystagmus); Tusa and Zee (ocular alignment); Mehdorn (nuclear and supranuclear disorders); Gittinger (non-myasthenic ophthalmoplegia); and Schmidt (myasthenia gravis).

The subjects of transient monocular blindness and stroke were reviewed by Drs. Rizzo and Trobe.

Dr. Troost surveyed the subject of migraine for which an exact pathogenesis has yet to be found. He quoted Dr. W. Gowers, who, almost 100 years ago (!), wrote: "When all has been said that can be, mystery still envelops the mechanism of migraine."

True to the tradition of *Current Neuro-ophthalmology*®, the chapters have extensive bibliographies for the reader who is interested in studying the reviewed subjects in more detail.

J.T.W. van Dalen, M.D., Ph.D.
Simmons Lessell, M.D.

Contents

xiii

PART ONE

THE VISUAL SYSTEM

CHAPTER 1

Optic Neuritis

Jon Currie, M.B., B.S., F.R.A.C.P.

The Mental Health Research Institute of Victoria, Parkville, Victoria, Australia; The Save Sight and Eye Health Institute, University of Sydney, Sydney, New South Wales, Australia

DIFFERENTIAL DIAGNOSIS

Infective Optic Neuritis

A number of case reports[1-5] confirm that unilateral or bilateral optic neuritis (ON) can arise as a complication of Lyme disease *(Borrelia burgdorferi)*, usually during stages II (meningitis) or III (late disease).[4] Occasionally ON may present as an isolated manifestation of Lyme disease,[5] but in most cases it occurs in association with other manifestations of either ocular inflammation (e.g., uveitis, retinal vasculitis) or systemic or neurologic involvement, including cranial nerve palsies (especially cranial nerves VI or VII), meningitis, or radiculopathy.[3-5] The clustering of other neurologic signs with ON may make clinical differentiation from multiple sclerosis (MS) difficult, and this difficulty is heightened by recent reports that Lyme disease may also cause multiple periventricular and subcortical white matter lesions on magnetic resonance imaging (MRI)[2,5] and oligoclonal bands in the cerebrospinal fluid (CSF).[5] Neuroretinitis can also occur.[2, 5]

Effective treatment often requires intravenous (IV) antibiotics, and patients may still relapse and require prolonged treatment with oral antibiotics.[4, 5] If Lyme disease is not recognized, and initial treatment of visual loss is only with oral or IV corticosteroids, visual acuity can progressively worsen.[4] As with syphilis, seronegative Lyme disease may occur,[4–6] and Winward et al.[4] described one patient with ON in whom serologic assays for Lyme disease with both indirect immuno-fluorescence assay (IFA) and enzyme-linked immunosorbent assay (ELISA) were negative on two occasions. Clinical diagnosis was finally confirmed with Western blot analysis.

There were surprisingly few reports of ON occurring in the setting of human immunodeficiency virus (HIV) infection,[7–11] and no reports suggesting that ON can arise from direct HIV infection of the optic nerve. Mansour[7] found two cases of ON caused by cytomegalovirus (CMV) infection among 177 patients with the acquired immunodeficiency syndrome (AIDS) who underwent neuro-ophthalmic examination. Gross et al.[8] described two patterns of ON associated with CMV infection in ten patients with AIDS. Seven cases involved spread of a limited CMV retinitis to the optic disk margin. Vision was relatively well preserved, with arcuate or altitudinal field defects and paracentral scotomata, which generally did not resolve despite treatment. These field defects were similar to those that occur in glaucoma or anterior ischemic optic neuropathy (AION) and may have been caused by microinfarction of the optic nerve head or focal infection of the peripapillary nerve fiber layer. In contrast, three patients had isolated CMV papillitis, presumably as a primary infection of the optic nerve. The initial visual acuity was usually excellent, but rapidly deteriorated despite prompt and aggressive treatment with IV ganciclovir. In comparison with the cases of peripapillary CMV retinitis, visual loss progressed to no light perception in two of these three patients.

In four case reports, Winward et al.[9] illustrated the spectrum of HIV-associated ON. These cases included bilateral syphilitic optic perineuritis, a CMV papillitis that also progressed to visual acuity of no light perception, cryptococcal retrobulbar ON, and herpes zoster ON where visual acuity improved from hand motions to 20/60 with IV acyclovir. In patients with HIV infection, optic nerve disease may be one of the initial presentations, and investigation for a specific underlying cause is important since some are responsive to therapy. However, Litoff and Catalano[10] reported a case of herpes zoster ON in a patient with HIV infection in whom visual acuity progressed to no light perception despite aggressive treatment with acyclovir and steroids. Becerra et al.[11] noted that in patients who are HIV seropositive, infection with syphilis may lead to more extensive and aggressive eye disease that is more frequently bilateral.

Spalton et al.[12] described bilateral ON following a systemic illness and aseptic meningitis caused by coxsackie B5 virus. Right eye acuity was 6/5 and the left eye had hand motion perception, accompanied by pain on eye movement, vitritis, marked bilateral optic disk swelling with peripapillary nerve fiber layer hemorrhages and a left eye macular star figure. Following treatment with high-dose oral prednisolone, left eye acuity recovered from hand motion to 6/9. The authors suggest that this treatment may account for the better visual outcome than that previously reported. Bilateral ON and bilateral reversible sixth cranial nerve palsies complicated a case of acute meningoencephalitis caused by Q fever (*Coxiella burnetti*).[13] Many of the neuro-ophthalmic features of this case are similar to those described by Schuil et al.[14] Chrousos et al.[15] documented another case of neuro-retinitis caused by cat-scratch disease, confirmed in this patient with positive skin antigen testing.

Several reports reemphasize paranasal sinusitis as an uncommon but important and treatable cause of ON.[16-18] The pathophysiologic mechanisms by which sinusitis can cause ON remain uncertain, but include both direct spread of inflammation (e.g., ethmoid sinus) and indirect immuno-inflammatory effects from other sinuses that do not have a contiguous relationship with the optic nerve (e.g., maxillary sinus). Aggressive therapy including antibiotics and/or surgical drainage may be necessary to save sight. Plain sinus x-rays may be normal and conventional CT scans often incompletely image the sinuses unless coronal views are obtained. MRI is likely to prove the most sensitive technique for exclusion of sinusitis-induced ON.[18] Sphenoidal sinus mucocele can also cause a reversible ON that may mimic demyelinating ON.[19]

A very interesting report from South Africa[20] identified six cases of neuromyelitis optica (NMO; Devic's disease: bilateral optic neuropathy and acute myelopathy) and one case of unilateral ON that were associated with pulmonary tuberculosis (TB). In the same 11-year period, only five other cases of idiopathic NMO were seen, suggesting that the close temporal relationship to pulmonary TB was not coincidental. The pattern of the clinical features in these cases was fairly consistant, usually with the onset of optic neuropathy occurring relatively soon after the onset of TB symptoms (mean, 2 months) and preceding myelopathy by up to 3 months. Visual loss was usually bilateral and severe with little recovery. In four of the 167 cases, neurologic symptoms preceded the onset of anti-tuberculous drug therapy and suggested that these medications were not implicated in the pathogenesis of this syndrome. There was also no evidence of direct central nervous system (CNS) infection with TB. Pathologic findings included extensive demyelination of the optic nerves and spinal cord in keeping with an autoimmune basis for this syndrome. Recognition of the association of NMO and TB is clinically important in areas where TB is endemic and may also have considerable relevance since an increasing number of cases of TB are seen in patients with HIV infection.

Autoimmune ON and Systemic Lupus Erythematosis

Kupersmith et al.[21] provide further support and a valuable review of the concept of autoimmune ON in a report of 14 patients (12 women). Clinical features included severe visual loss (often 20/200 or less) and progressive or recurrent disease despite conventional doses of oral corticosteroids. Laboratory evidence of autoimmune abnormality was usually present, although often insufficient to allow diagnosis of a specific illness such as systemic lupus erythematosus (SLE). Of interest, skin biopsy specimens were abnormal in 6 of 7 cases and may prove to be a valuable tool in the diagnosis of autoimmune ON. Treatment with high-dose IV corticosteroids improved vision in 11 of 12 patients, but 9 patients needed continued treatment with oral prednisolone and cytotoxic agents to maintain visual function. The authors emphasize the importance of recognizing and treating this special subgroup of patients with ON, since spontaneous recovery is uncommon and residual visual loss can be severe. Several reports[22-25] again document that ON may occur with SLE, although this appears to be a very rare complication.[24] If SLE causes bilateral ON in combination with transverse myelitis, it may mimic Devic's disease or MS,[25] although serologic indicators of SLE are usually, but not always, present.[22]

Inflammatory, Metabolic, and Malignant ON

Perioptic neuritis or optic perineuritis are terms used to describe inflammatory disorders of the optic nerve sheaths. A variety of causes have been reported, including syphilis, but in many cases the cause remains obscure. Margo et al.[26] described an unusual case of bilateral idiopathic perioptic neuritis with the histologic finding of necrobiotic granulomas in the optic nerve sheaths of a 68-year-old woman with progressive bilateral vision loss over 4 months. Galetta et al.[27] reported an instructive case of sarcoid optic neuropathy in which the clinical course mimicked that of typical idiopathic or demyelinating ON, with acute and severe visual loss in one eye, followed by spontaneous resolution over 3 weeks. The other eye had optic disk swelling and inflammatory vitreal cells without visual loss, retinal lesions, or periphlebitis. Diagnosis of sarcoidosis was established on the basis of an elevated angiotensin converting enzyme level, hilar lymphadenopathy on chest X-ray, and biopsy from a papular skin rash. This report again emphasizes the importance of careful clinical and laboratory workup in all cases of ON, even when they present as a seemingly straightforward idiopathic/demyelinating ON.

Visual loss that mimics idiopathic ON can also occur from delayed damage to the optic nerves or chiasm following external beam radiation therapy.[28, 29] Visual loss is usually gradual over a period of less than 3 weeks but is not accompanied by ocular pain or pain on eye movement. Achromatopsia is common, and optic disk swelling may be present. Onset of visual loss is usually between 4 months and 3 years after radiation therapy (mean, 1 year) and requires total radiation doses above 4,500 cGy, but it can occur with daily fractions of less than 200 cGy to the anterior visual pathway. Hyperbaric oxygen therapy and/or high-dose corticosteroid therapy does not appear to improve the visual outcome.[28]

An important report by Ducker et al.[30] documented five cases of ON accompanied by secondary impairment of retinal venous outflow, producing the clinical appearance of impending or actual central retinal vein occlusion. Clinical features included reduced visual acuity, acquired dyschromatopsia, relative afferent pupil defect, central scotomata or arcuate visual field defects, optic disk edema, poste rior vitreous cells, and tortuous, dilated retinal veins with or without peripapillary and posterior pole nerve fiber layer hemorrhages. Visual loss was entirely attributable to optic nerve involvement because the clinical and fluorescein angiographic examinations showed no evidence of macular edema or hemorrhage and no evidence of capillary nonperfusion. This clinical picture could be distinguished from ischemic or nonischemic central retinal vein occlusion and papillophlebitis, optic disk vasculitis or retinal vasculitis, and this differentiation was important for both diagnosis and management.

Several masses, tumors, and malignancies were associated with optic neuropathies that resembled demyelinating ON to varying degrees. These included an optic nerve glioma,[31] a giant aneurysm of the anterior communicating artery,[32] angioimmunoblastic lymphadenopathy,[33] nonHodgkin's lymphoma,[34] and one case associated with extracranial, intraarterial cisplatin infusion for a carcinoma of the tonsillar fossa.[35]

Saini et al.[36] reported a case of bilateral optic neuropathy as the initial presentation of uremia and renal failure. Visual loss was rapid and severe and unresponsive to steroid therapy but resolved markedly after hemodialysis. This case was very similar to several cases reported previously by Knox et al.[37] Winward[38] added another case of uremic optic neuropathy resembling ON in a patient well controlled with hemodialysis who had only unilateral involvement for several months before the second eye became involved and in whom the visual response to further hemodialysis was poor. ON can also occur with chronic inflammatory polyradiculopathy[39] as well as with the more acute forms of the Guillain-Barré syndrome.[40]

TREATMENT

The controversial question of the role of corticosteroids in the treatment of ON remains unresolved. Spoor and Rockwell[41] had previously suggested a role for high-dose IV methylprednisolone in the treatment of ON. Cox[42] was less than enthusiastic about this therapy and castigated the editors who published the article. Wall[43] provided control data from 26 untreated patients with idiopathic ON to show that their outcome, as measured with Snellen visual acuity, did not differ significantly from that in Spoor and Rockwell's treated patients. However, as indicated in their original publication[41] and reiterated in their subsequent reply,[44] Spoor and Rockwell did not advocate high-dose corticosteroid therapy for patients with typical idiopathic/demyelinating ON but for a selected subgroup of patients with atypical ON and progressive visual loss, usually of the autoimmune ON subgroup[21] first described by Dutton et al.[45]

Use of high-dose IV methylprednisolone in treating various forms of ON was documented in a number of other case reports.[8, 10, 21, 28, 30] A cautionary note was sounded by Herishanu et al.,[46] who found an unexpected clustering of conversion to MS among those patients with ON treated with methylprednisolone. In a small study of 26 patients with ON, 6 were untreated, 14 received oral prednisolone for 4 to 6 weeks, and 6 were treated for 3 days with IV methylprednisolone but without subsequent oral steroids. Improvement in visual acuity was greater in both treated groups compared with the untreated group, and recovery of vision was significantly faster in patients treated with methylprednisolone. However, both recurrent ON and conversion to MS were significantly more frequent in patients treated with methylprednisolone (4 of 6 with recurrent ON; 5 of 6 with conversion to MS) than in untreated patients (2 of 6 with recurrence; 0 of 6 with MS) or patients treated with oral prednisolone (2 of 14 with recurrence; 1 of 14 with MS). The authors emphasize their small sample size and the need to verify these findings in a larger population, but certainly this possible adverse outcome needs to be addressed in future studies. The Optic Neuritis Treatment Trial[47] is a multicenter study in the United States, developed to answer the following questions: (1) does treatment of optic neuritis with either oral or intravenous steroids reduce permanent optic nerve damage? (2) does either treatment speed recovery? (3) are the complications of steroid treatment insignificant in relation to the magnitude of the treatment effect? Randomized treatment arms include: (1) oral prednisolone (1 mg/kg/day for 14 days); (2) IV methylprednisolone (1,000 mg/day for 3 days followed by oral prednisolone for 11 days); and (3) oral placebo for 14 days. Outcome measurements include contrast sensitivity, static and kinetic perimetry, visual acuity, and color vision assessed during the first month and at 6 months after onset of ON. At least 435 patients will be enrolled, and recruitment is likely to be completed early in 1991. With more than 75% of the required patients already recruited, no treatment arm has so far produced outcomes that differ enough to warrant cessation of the trial for ethical reasons.[48]

OPTIC NEURITIS AND MULTIPLE SCLEROSIS

Rate of Conversion of ON to MS

There were few clinical studies examining the rate of progression of isolated ON to MS,[49-54] and little dispute[55] of the methods or findings of the recent study by Rizzo and Lessell,[56] which remained the benchmark for clinical reference. Over a 0.5- to 3.5-year follow-up, Sanders and Van Lith[49] found that 29 (60%) of 48 patients with isolated ON developed MS. They attributed this relatively high progression rate to improved diagnostic criteria for ON that included not only clinical history, but also visual field defects and abnormal pattern visual-evoked responses (pVER) and suggested that these were the most useful of the auxiliary diagnostic tests available in patients presenting with ON. A report from Chile[50] suggested that in Latin America the rate of progression of isolated ON to MS was very low, with only 1 (4%) of 23 patients developing MS during a follow-up period of 2 to 18 years (mean, 10 years). However, some caution is needed in interpreting the results of this retrospective study, since 82 (78%) of the original cohort of 105 patients with ON were excluded, frequently for lack of available initial or follow-up information, and of the final 23 cases analyzed, 8 were children aged 7 years or less.

Conversely, a study from Sardinia[51] suggests that Italy has a medium-to-high risk rate for progression to MS. In the arctic region of the two northernmost counties of Norway, the rate of progression to MS was 42% (15/36) at a mean of 2 years follow-up,[52] while in central Norway, the rate over 2 to 11 years was 57% (17/30), with the majority of cases occurring within the first 3 years after onset of ON.[53] Of interest in this study, the rate rose to 79% if the CSF at the time of onset of ON contained oligoclonal bands (OCBs) but was only 10% if no OCBs were present.

Wilson and Smith[57] questioned the contention of Parmley et al.[58] that patients with neuroretinitis (optic disk swelling and a macular star figure) do not have the same risk of developing MS as do patients with ON without a star figure. However, the differentiation of these two clinical pictures does seem prognostically valid, and Parmley et al. have not subsequently received reports documenting MS in association with neuroretinitis.[59]

Sandberg-Wollheim et al.[54] provided long-term follow-up data (median, 12.9 years) and MS risk factors from an important prospective study of 86 patients presenting with isolated ON. Thirty-three (38%) of the 86 patients developed clinically definite MS, with the rate of progression predicted by actuarial analysis as 45% at 15 years. At follow-up, the only diagnostic category for MS included in this study was clinically definite MS. The results are very similar to those of Rizzo and Lessell[56] for this diagnostic category (35% definite MS at 14.9 years), but in that study an additional 23% of their patients had probable or possible MS. Sandberg-Wollheim et al. found that the risk of progression to MS was significantly greater in those patients who were less than 25 years of age at the onset of ON, and also in those with recurrent ON (57% progression vs. 35% progression without recurrent ON). Of the 16% of patients with recurrent ON, the recurrence occurred earlier in those who subsequently developed MS (median, 7.5 months vs. 33 months for recurrent ON without progression). MS occurred more frequently in women (44% of women, 28% of men), but this trend did not reach statistical significance. There was no seasonal variation in the time of onset of ON in general, nor in those progressing to MS. The frequency of HLA D/DR2 was increased in patients with ON compared with control subjects, but did not differentiate which patients with ON subsequently developed MS. Patients with abnormal CSF at the onset of ON (pleocytosis, OCBs) had a significantly increased risk of developing MS (47% vs. 23% with normal CSF). Twenty-five patients with ON without progression to MS underwent MRI 7 to 18 years after the onset of ON. Eleven (44%) of these images had abnormal white matter lesions consistent with MS, and 82% of the abnormal images were in patients with abnormal CSF at the onset of ON.

Thus younger age and abnormal CSF at onset of ON, and early recurrence of ON were the significant risk factors for progression to MS following presentation with isolated ON.

MAGNETIC RESONANCE IMAGING

A number of new studies have been published reporting MRI use in patients presenting with ON to detect additional white matter lesions in the brain (Table 1).[60-66] Previous studies[67-71] had shown that 40% to 70% of patients with clinically isolated, unilateral ON had multifocal white matter brain lesions at the time of presentation. Miller et al.[60] argued that since the MRI abnormalities that occur in MS correspond to plaques of demyelination, the development of new but clinically silent MRI lesions in patients with isolated ON is a valid criterion for the diagnsosis of MS. The difference between the clinical and MRI criteria for the diagnosis of MS is then simply whether the location of the new lesion(s) is in a region in which damage leads to symptoms. In 53 patients with clinically isolated ON, Miller et al.[60] found that 64% had multifocal white matter lesions on MRI at the time of presentation with ON. In a mean follow-up period of 12.3 months, 34% (12/34) of those with abnormal MRI images developed clinically diagnosed MS, increasing to 56% (19/34) if either clinical criteria or MRI criteria of new white matter lesions were used (7 subjects with clinical events, 7 with new MRI lesions, 5 with both clinical and MRI lesions). In comparison, none of the 19 patients with ON and normal MRI images at presentation developed clincially diagnosed MS, and only 3 (16%) developed new MRI brain lesions (relative risk, 6.8).

TABLE 1.
White Matter Abnormalities on MRI: Progression to MS in Acute Isolated Optic Neuritis

| | | Rate of Progression to MS | | |
| | | --- | --- | |
Study Group	Percent With Abnormal Initial MRI (number)	Percent With Initial MRI Abnormal (number)	Percent With Initial MRI Normal (number)	Length of Follow-up, mo
Staedt et al.[62]	79% (19/24)			
Guthoff et al.[63]	53% (18/23)			
Frederiksen et al.[61]	62% (31/50)	23% (7/31)*	0	11 (median)
Miller et al.[60]				12 (mean)
All ON	64% (34/53)	56% (19/34)†	16% (3/19)	
	35% (12/34)*		0	
Unilateral ON	71% (29/41)	52% (15/29)†	17% (2/12)	
Bilateral simultaneous ON	20% (1/5)	100% (1/1)†	20% (1/4)	
Bilateral consecutive ON	57% (4/7)	75% (3/4)†	0	

*Progression to MS defined by clinical diagnostic criteria only.
†Progression to MS defined by clinical diagnostic criteria and/or new MRI lesions.

Frederiksen et al.[61] studied 50 consecutive patients at the time of their initial attack of isolated ON prior to any treatment. All patients with a history of MS or previous ON were excluded as were all patients with any current neurologic signs or symptoms other than ON. Seventy-two percent were women and ages ranged from 12 to 53 years (median, 30 years). Six patients had bilateral simultaneous ON. MRI was performed from 3 to 49 days (median, 16 days) after the onset of symptoms. Sixty-two percent of the patients had multiple asymptomatic lesions in the white matter of the central nervous system and the morphology and pattern of distribution was similar to those found in patients with definite MS. The majority of lesions were located in the cerebral white matter, predominantly in the periventricular areas. Lesions in the brain stem and cerebellum were rare. The number of lesions ranged from 1 to 30 and the size ranged from 2 to 20 mm. There was no correlation between the presence of white matter lesions and patient age, sex, or severity of visual loss. During a follow-up period of 1 to 20 months (median, 11 months), 7 (14%) of the 50 patients developed clinical signs and/or symptoms of multiple sclerosis 1 to 9 months (median, 3 months) after the onset of ON. As in the study of Miller et al.,[60] all of these patients had abnormal initial MRI images, while no patient with a normal initial MRI image progressed to clinical MS. The results of these two studies are in accordance with those of previous studies[67-71] and suggest that MRI may be of prognostic value in acute, monosymptomatic ON.

Frederiksen et al.[61] have also suggested that the majority of white matter lesions present on MRI 1 or 2 days after the initial onset of an attack of ON are not part of a shower of recent simultaneous lesions but have developed silently over a period of time. Staedt et al.[62] examined 24 patients with isolated ON from 0 to 176 weeks (median, 5 weeks) after the onset of symptoms. White matter lesions were present in 79% of patients, and the number of lesions ranged from 1 to 38 (median, 2). All patients with more than two lesions on MRI had CSF abnormalities (pleocytosis, elevated protein, or OCBs). Guthoff et al.[63] found subclinical MRI brain lesions in 53% of 34 patients with isolated ON. Again the distribution of the lesions was similar to that in MS, and neither the severity of visual loss nor the course of visual recovery correlated with the MRI findings. In 3 patients with ON and persistent visual loss, Wiegand[64] found MRI evidence of inflammatory lesions in the intracanalicular portion of the optic nerve, when he used a short time inversion recovery (STIR) sequence. Larger studies are needed to determine the frequency with which poor visual recovery in ON is associated with lesions in this unfavorable location and whether early detection and treatment would be of benefit. Weintraub[72] noted that if orbital surface coils are used to image the optic nerve with MRI, they may generate sufficient local heat to cause transient worsening of visual function, an effect similar to the hot bath test for MS.

Guy et al.[73, 74] provided two studies examining the use of gadolinium-DTPA (Gd-DTPA) enhancement in MRI of ON. In animal studies of ON associated with experimental allergic encephalomyelitis (EAE),[73] increased permeability of the blood-optic nerve barrier was an early event in autoimmune demyelination and was similar to that seen in patients with acute ON. In 13 patients with acute ON,[74]

Gd-DTPA enhancement of the optic nerve was seen in only 7 (54%) patients imaged within 2 weeks of the onset of ON. Five of these patients had enhancement of the intracranial optic nerve and two had involvement of the optic nerve at the orbital apex. Surprisingly, none of the five patients with optic disk swelling showed enhancement of the intraorbital optic nerve, but two did have enhancement of the intracranial portion of the nerve. Only 1 of the 11 patients with isolated ON had enhancement of other regions of the brain.

These results vary somewhat from those of Miller et al.,[75] who found high signal regions in 84% of the affected optic nerves when he used the STIR MRI technique for fat suppression, and no additional lesions with Gd-DTPA enhancement. In contrast, Guy et al. reported that the STIR sequence reduced the signal from Gd-DTPA. Klein[76] provided a useful discussion of the differences between these two articles and suggested that MRI technique must be varied for examination of different segments of the optic nerve. For the intraorbital portion, a surface coil, coronal sections, and a fat suppression technique (STIR) should be used. For the intracanalicular and intracranial segments, a head coil is used with axial and coronal sections and intravenous Gd-DTPA. Gd-DTPA-enhanced MRI is of particular use in differentiating new demyelinating lesions from old CNS plaques and is also of value in the differential diagnosis of radiation-induced optic neuropathy.

In patients with Leber's optic neuropathy, the STIR MRI sequence showed optic nerve abnormalities in all patients.[77] The lesions were usually more extensive than those in idiopathic ON and were located more posteriorly in the intraorbital portions of the nerve. Importantly, no subjects with Leber's optic neuropathy had any additional brain lesions, in clear contrast to the majority of patients with idiopathic ON.

Miller et al.[66] performed MRI in 12 children presenting with clinically isolated ON. In comparison with the adult cohorts, 75% of the children were boys and 33% had bilateral ON. Brain white matter lesions were found in only 2 (17%) of the 12 patients, and in both of these patients, the clinical history and MRI abnormalities were atypical. One patient had developed bilateral ON following chickenpox, and on MRI, he had bilateral extensive asymptomatic confluent parietal lobe white matter abnormalities. The second patient had subsequent remitting episodes of encephalopathy at 1 and 3 months with both cortical and subcortical MRI lesions. In contrast, the MRI appearances in children with definite MS, rather than isolated ON, were essentially the same as those in adults[66, 78] and clearly differed from these two cases. This MRI study[66] further supports the contention that isolated ON in children appears clinically distinct from its adult counterpart.

CHILDHOOD ON

ON in childhood is usually bilateral and often associated with a febrile illness that is frequently presumed to be of viral origin. Visual symptoms tend to improve rapidly, especially with steroid therapy, and visual acuities are often normal within 4 to 6 weeks of onset. A study from the United Kingdom[79] presented 39 children with isolated ON followed up for a period of 3 months to 29 years (mean, 8.8 years). Age ranged from 3 to 15 years (mean, 8.6 years), and 74% of subjects were female. There appeared to be a seasonal peak for onset of ON, with twice as many cases presenting in April as in any other month. In 46% of cases, there was an associated febrile prodrome. Seventy-four percent of subjects had bilateral ON (25/39 simultaneous, 4/39 sequential). Seventy-four percent had swollen optic disks at onset. Twenty-three percent had other neurologic signs or symptoms within 6 weeks of onset of ON.

At follow-up, acuity was 6/6 or better in 78% of the examined eyes, and only 18% had visual field defects or dyschromatopsia, although 88% had optic disk pallor. Only 45% of the patients had abnormal visual-evoked responses (VERs) at follow-up (including all 4 cases with unilateral ON), in comparison with adult rates of 90% to 95%. Multiple sclerosis developed in only 15% of cases (7% for those with bilateral ON), and only 10% had recurrent ON. No reliable risk factors for the development of MS could be identified, including unilateral or bilateral ON, HLA type, or associated neurologic signs during the initial episode. Farris and Pickard[80] reported 6 further cases of bilateral ON in childhood, 5 of which were associated with a proven episode of infection. All cases were treated with intravenous corticosteroids because of very severe visual loss (10/800-no light perception). Their clinical findings and rates of recovery were very similar to those of Kriss et al.,[79] although surprisingly this large study was not cited. These studies contrast strongly with the findings of Riikonen et al.,[81] where 9 (43%) of 21 children with idiopathic ON developed MS. However, this cohort was atypical in the large number of cases of unilateral ON (8/21), other specific etiologies (5/21), and previous evidence of MS (3/21). In fact, although MS developed in 7 (88%) of the 8 patients with unilateral ON, only 2 (15%) of 13 patients with bilateral ON developed MS. This is more in agreement with the other childhood studies, as were most of the clinical features in the bilateral ON group.

CLINICAL ASPECTS

Celesia et al.[82] provided a useful prospective study of visual outcome at 12 months in 20 patients with an initial attack of isolated ON. Their results were similar to those of several other recent studies.[83-85] Color vision, visual fields, and VERs at 15-minute check size were initially abnormal in all patients, while visual acuity (90%) and contrast sensitivity (95%) were also usually impaired. Optic disk swelling was present in 50% of cases. Seventy percent of subjects had severe visual impairment (acuity <20/200) on a graded visual impairment scale (GVIS) that incorporated a variety of clinical and psychophysical measures of visual function. In the 12-month follow-up period, the recurrence rate for ON was 10% and only 1 patient (5%) developed clinical MS, although 59% of patients had additional central white matter lesions on MRI. The time for visual recovery varied for different visual functions in different patients, with slow recovery continuing in some cases for up to 12 months after the onset of ON. No single visual measure satisfactorily defined a patient's residual impairment, nor was any measure predictive of the visual outcome at 12 months, no matter how severe its initial abnormality. For clinical assessment and follow-up of ON, the authors therefore advocate the use of a GVIS rather than any *single* measure of visual function. The GVIS at the onset of ON was significantly correlated with the final GVIS at 12 months and also correlated well with the patients' symptoms of visual impairment. Overall, 35% of subjects had some residual deficit on GVIS at 1 year follow-up, although in 80% of cases, individual measures of visual acuity, fields, color vision, and contrast sensitivity had returned to normal. In comparison, 95% of VERs and 60% of pupil responses remained abnormal. Of those initially classified as having total or severe blindness (<20/1000), 60% were left with residual visual impairment.

In most clinical aspects, idiopathic ON in the elderly (>50 years) did not differ from the typical disorder that occurs in younger age groups.[86] The incidence of simultaneous bilateral ON was slightly higher (28% vs. 20% in younger age groups) and only 5% of affected eyes had optic disk edema (vs. 50% in younger cases). In a follow-up period of 38 to 90 months (mean, 57 months), only 21% of cases developed clinically definite MS. The authors emphasized the importance of extensive investigation for alternative causes of visual loss before making a diagnosis of ON in the elderly. They speculated that the lower rate of progression to MS in their cases may reflect inclusion of unsuspected cases of ischemic optic neuropathy. An interesting study by Birk et al.[87] prospectively monitored eight women with MS during pregnancy and for the first 6 months postpartum. Seven of the eight women had either no change or clinical improvement of MS during pregnancy, while one woman had mild worsening of her symptoms. In contrast, six (75%) of the eight women experienced relapse or worsening of their MS in the early postpartum period, including one case of bilateral ON. Relapse severity ranged from mild to severe, and most relapses occurred within the first 6 weeks after delivery. Annual relapse rates fell from 0.66 prior to pregnancy to 0.17 during pregnancy and then rose 17.7 times in the first 3 postpartum months to 1.74. Measurements of T-cell subsets and immunoactive pregnancy associated proteins did not predict clinical disease activity.

In a somewhat cumbersome paper, Honan et al.[88] assessed visual function in 58 patients with MS and a range of clinical severity using a variety of psychophysical measures. Not surprisingly, they found that the clinical MS classification was an important variable in predicting the occurrence of abnormal visual function in MS. Only 31% of patients in the suspected MS group had abnormal visual function, compared with 75% to 100% of patients in the early probable, clinically definite, and optic neuritis groups! Abnormal visual function did not increase with duration of MS unless the disease severity increased.

IMMUNOPATHOLOGY

An interesting paper by Kinnunen et al.[89] compared immunologic function in six patients with active, progressive MS and in six patients with isolated ON that had not progressed to MS after 10 to 15 years follow-up. Both groups of patients had similar abnormalities of immunologic function that distinguished them from healthy control subjects. The authors concluded that immunologic factors could not explain the neuropathologic confinement of the lesions in isolated ON. They speculated that protection against progression to MS may be by some as yet undefined genetic influence, or that isolated ON may actually be an etiologically different disease.

In patients with MS, reduced suppressor T-cell (CD8) activity and increased CD4/CD8 ratios may occur with the appearance of new lesions on MRI.[90] However, in patients with isolated acute unilateral ON, Guy et al.[91] found that this periodic alteration of circulating T-cell subpopulations did not occur and the T-cell profile did not differ from that in control subjects. A characteristic elevation of the CD4/CD8 ratio did subsequently occur in one patient 5 weeks after he developed ON, at the time of onset of additional neurologic deficits suggesting MS. These findings are similar to those of Riikonen and Von Willebrand[92] in children with isolated ON, where CD4/CD8 ratios were also usually normal.

A provocative study by Riikonen[93] examined the role of infections, vaccination, and events that impaired the blood-brain barrier (BBB) in the development of ON and MS in a group of 18 children presenting with ON. The age of onset of measles was much later in children with ON who developed MS than in control subjects, and increased intrathecal synthesis of IgG or viral antibodies occurred at the time of onset of ON or MS. In the period preceding the onset of ON or MS, there was an increased rate of common bacterial or viral infections, vaccination with live or live-attenuated vacines (polio: Salk, Sabin, or booster; rubella), and events that may have caused a temporary impairment of the BBB function (e.g., convulsions, meningitis/encephalitis, head trauma). Riikonen suggested that these events may all be independent factors associated with an increased risk of developing ON or MS. Their close temporal correlation with the onset of ON/MS suggests a causal association, and each event may be involved in the sequence of events leading to demyelination. For example, temporary impairment of the BBB may allow entry of lymphocytes into the brain that had been committed to specific antibody synthesis outside the brain. Riikonen also suggested that vaccination with live or live-attenuated viruses cannot be recommended for children with MS nor during at least the first year after the onset of an attack of ON. One reservation that must be expressed about these results is that the patient cohort may have been somewhat atypical, in that 11 (61%) of the 18 children had unilateral ON, and 10 (56%) of 18 subsequently developed MS.

Guy et al.[94] also speculated that an alteration of the BBB may be of primary importance in the pathogenesis of optic nerve demyelination. In experimental ON associated with EAE, the specific detoxifying actions of catalase and glutathione peroxidase in detoxifying hydrogen peroxide suggest a role for oxygen metabolites in the pathogenesis of increased microvascular permeability in experimental ON.

ELECTROPHYSIOLOGY AND PSYCHOPHYSIOLOGY

A number of studies utilized electrophysiologic and psychophysical techniques in attempts to improve the diagnosis of ON or to investigate its pathophysiology.[95–113] Heinrichs and McLean[95] found that abnormalities of VER latency were the same in patients with ON due to MS and in patients with isolated ON. Abnormal VERs at the time of acute ON returned to normal in 35% of the patients, and this normalization was not related to the severity of the initial VER abnormality. These results are somewhat at variance with previous VER studies that suggest that 90% to 95% of patients with ON have abnormal VERs at follow-up.

Several studies compared VERs and automated static field perimetry testing in ON.[96–99] Not surprisingly, there was considerable correlation of VER abnormalities with the central visual field defects detected with static perimetry.[97, 99] In patients with idiopathic ON, static visual field loss may be most dense in the central 10 degrees, while in patients with ON/MS, the visual field is lost more diffusely over the central 30 degrees.[100] Berninger and Heider[98] suggested that static perimetry may be as sensitive or more sensitive than VER in detecting residual visual pathway abnormalities in ON. In patients with MS, combining measurement of VER latencies with measurements of retinal nerve fiber layer (RNFL) defects and an abnormally small neuroretinal rim area increased the detection of optic nerve abnormalities to 86%, compared with 63% using VER alone.[101] The RNFL defects suggested that in addition to plaques of demyelination, extensive and diffuse axonal loss commonly occurs in the optic nerves of patients with MS. Kaufman et al.[102] found that pattern reversal VER was superior to pattern electroretinography (PERG) in the diagnosis of acute and chronic ON. However, a significant reduction in the PERG b wave with three separate stimulus check sizes correlated closely with failure of visual recovery and the eventual development of severe optic atrophy, suggesting that PERG may be of prognostic value in the assessment of ON. The early and selective attenuation of the PERG b wave in patients with demyelinating ON is consistent with localized retinal damage that is independent of the optic nerve pathologic condition and may reflect vascular abnormalities in the retina that precede optic nerve demyelination, possibly affecting the Müller cells.[103]

Accornero et al.[104] showed that in healthy subjects the critical fusion frequency (CFF) of a flickering light increased when body temperature was raised by 0.5° C, but CFF decreased in patients with ON, the equivalent of the MS hot bath test. CFF was also adapted to measure automated flicker perimetry,[105] which may represent a specific functional test of the retinal Y (or M) ganglion cells. Considerable interest was also shown in the Tübingen or Aulhorn flicker test,[34, 106–109] and

Trauzettel-Klosinski[109] reported a diagnostic sensitivity in ON of 85.5%, similar to that of VER, but with much higher specificity (98%) than VER for inflammatory/demyelinating ON. Using the Aulhorn flicker test, she was also able to divide the course of ON into five stages and to accurately determine the duration of the active phase of inflammation and to distinguish between active ON, resolved ON, and chronic, low-grade inflammation. Results of the Aulhorn flicker test depend on the activity of inflammation present in the optic nerve and not on the extent of impairment of other visual functions. The test is therefore useful in determining the prognosis for outcome in inflammatory ON, since there is little chance of improvement in visual function once the flicker test is normalized.[109]

Using the Cambridge Low Contrast Gratings (CLCG), Fahy et al.[110] found abnormalities in 33% of patients with definite MS, compared with 82% of patients with abnormal VERs. There was no correlation between the degree of abnormality in contrast sensitivity and VER. The authors concluded that although a proportion of patients with MS have abnormal contrast sensitivity, its detection is not clinically useful and it is insensitive as a measure of subclinical ON. However, this is more likely to reflect inadequacies in the CLCG test than in contrast sensitivity testing as a whole. Using the measurement of temporal modulation sensitivity in patients with recovered ON, Edgar et al.[111] found a general loss to all temporal frequencies at 0 and 2.5 degrees of visual field eccentricity, loss to medium temporal frequencies at 5 degrees eccentricity, and no loss to any frequency at 10 degrees eccentricity. The authors concluded that in ON, smaller diameter fibers were most affected by demyelination. Similarly, Wall[112] found greater involvement of P(X) than M(Y) ganglion cell axons in resolved ON, with impaired detection of high spatial frequency pattern and movement. In comparison, using measurements of loss of chromatic, spatial, and temporal sensitivity, Dain et al.[113] found that most patients with recovered ON showed losses in sensitivity that were nonselective, indicating involvement of both larger and smaller axons, and involvement of both foveal and peripheral axons.

REFERENCES

1. Gustafson R, Svenungsson B, Unosson-Hallnas K: Optic neuropathy in Borrelia infection. *J Infect* 1988;17:187–188.

2. Bialasiewicz AA, Huk W, Druschky KF, et al: *Borrelia burgdorferi* infection with bilateral optic neuritis and intracerebral demyelinization lesions. *Klin Monatsbl Asugenheilkd* 1989; 195:91–94.

3. Del Sette M, Caponnetto C, Fumarola D, et al: Unusual neurological manifestations of Lyme disease: A case report. *Ital J Neurol Sci* 1989; 10:455–456.

4. Winward KE, Smith JL, Culbertson WW, et al: Ocular Lyme borreliosis. *Am J Ophthalmol* 1989; 108:651–657.

5. Lesser RL, Kornmehl EW, Pachner AR, et al: Neuro-ophthalmologic manifestations of Lyme disease. *Ophthalmology* 1990; 97:699–706.

6. Dattwyler RJ, Volkman DJ, Luft BJ, et al: Seronegative Lyme disease: Dissociation of specific T and B-lymphocyte responses to *Borrelia burgdorferi*. *N Engl J Med* 1988; 319:1441–1446.

7. Mansour AM: Neuro-ophthalmic findings in acquired immunodeficiency syndrome. *J Clin Neuro Ophthalmol* 1990; 10:167–174.

8. Gross JG, Sadun AA, Wiley CA, et al: Severe visual loss related to isolated peripapillary retinal and optic nerve head cytomegalovirus infection. *Am J Ophthalmol* 1989; 108:691–698.

9. Winward KE, Hamed LM, Glaser JS: The spectrum of optic nerve disease in human immunodeficiency virus infection. *Am J Ophthalmol* 1989; 107:373–380.

10. Litoff D, Catalano RA: Herpes zoster optic neuritis in human immunodeficiency virus infection. *Arch Ophthalmol* 1990; 108:782–783.

11. Becerra LI, Ksiazek SM, Savino PJ, et al: Syphilitic uveitis in human immunodeficiency virus—infected and noninfected patients. *Ophthalmology* 1989; 96:1727–1730.

12. Spalton DJ, Murdoch I, Holder GE: Coxsackie B5 papillitis. *J Neurol Neurosurg Psychiatry* 1989; 52:1310–1311.

13. Shaked Y, Samra Y: Q fever meningoencephalitis associated with bilateral abducens nerve paralysis, bilateral optic neuritis and abnormal cerebrospinal fluid findings. *Infection* 1989; 17:394–395.

14. Schuil J, Richardus JH, Baarsma GS, et al: Q fever as a possible cause of bilateral optic neuritis. *Br J Ophthalmol* 1985; 69:580–583.

15. Chrousos GA, Drack AV, Young M, et al: Neuroretinitis in cat scratch disease. *J Clin Neuro Ophthalmol* 1990; 10:92–94.

16. Zavgorodniaia VP, Rogozhin VA, Moiseeva NI: A case of odontogenic sinusitis with infiltration of the orbit and optic nerve. *Oftalmol Zh* 1988; 2:126–127.

17. Khlystov IuA, Iamshechikov SI, Razumnyi VP, et al: Retrobulbar neuritis and inflammatory processes of the paranasal sinuses. *Med Sestra* 1988; 47:24–26.

18. Awerbuch G, Labadie EL, Van Dalen JTW: Reversible optic neuritis secondary to paranasal sinusitis. *Eur Neurol* 1989; 29:189–193.

19. Da Paepe E, Dewever M, Parisse J: Retrobulbar neuritis in an isolated sphenoidal mucocele. *Acta Otorhinolaryngol (Belg)* 1989; 43:169–175.

20. Silber MH, Wilcox PA, Bowen RM, et al: Neuromyelitis optica (Devic's syndrome) and pulmonary tuberculosis. *Neurology* 1990; 40:934–938.

21. Kupersmith MJ, Burde RM, Warren FA, et al: Autoimmune optic neuropathy: Evaluation and treatment. *J Neurol Neurosurg Psychiatry* 1988; 51:1381–1386.

22. Deutsch TA, Corwin HL: Lupus optic neuritis with negative serology. *Ann Ophthalmol* 1988; 20:383–384.

23. Lahoz RC, Arribas L Jr, Monereo A, et al: Optic neuritis and systemic lupus erythematosus. *Rev Clin Esp* 1989; 184:216.

24. Drosos AA, Petris CA, Petroutsos GM, et al: Unusual eye manifestations in systemic lupus erythematosus patients. *Clin Rheumatol* 1989; 8:49–53.

25. Ichiki S, Ohfu M, Niimi K, et al: A case of systemic lupus erythematosus associated with meningitis, myelitis, and bilateral optic neuritis. *Ryumachi* 1989; 29:126–133.

26. Margo CE, Levy MH, Beck RW: Bilateral idiopathic inflammation of the optic nerve sheaths. *Ophthalmology* 1989; 96:200–206.

27. Galetta S, Schatz NJ, Glaser JS: Acute sarcoid optic neuropathy with spontaneous recovery. *J Clin Neuro Ophthalmol* 1989; 9:27–32.

28. Roden D, Bosley TM, Fowble B, et al: Delayed radiation injury to the retrobulbar optic nerves and chiasm. *Ophthalmology* 1990; 97:346–351.

29. Zimmerman CF, Schatz NJ, Glaser JS: Magnetic resonance imaging of radiation optic neuropathy. *Am J Ophthalmol* 1990; 110:389–394.

30. Duker JS, Sergott RC, Savino PJ, et al: Optic neuritis with secondary retinal venous stasis. *Ophthalmology* 1989; 96:475–480.

31. Ramani A, Raja A, Lakshmaiah V, et al: Optic glioma masquerading as optic neuritis. *J Assoc Physicians India* 1988; 36:335–337.

32. Sjaastad O, Saunte C, Fredriksen TA, et al: Cluster headache-like headache, Hagman trait deficiency, retrobulbar neuritis and giant aneurysm. Autonomic function studies. *Cephalalgia* 1988; 8:111–120.

33. Matthews JH, Smith NA, Foroni L: A case of angioimmunoblastic lymphadenopathy associated with a long spontaneous remission, retrobulbar neuritis, a clonal rearrangement of the T-cell receptor gamma chain gene and an unusual marrow infiltration. *Eur J Haematol* 1988; 41:295–301.

34. Pittke EC, Thill-Schwaniger M: The Aulhorn flicker test. I: Concomitant neuritis in malignant non-Hodgkin's lymphoma and leukodystrophy. *Klin Monatsbl Augenheilk* 1988; 193:157–164.

35. Urba S, Forastiere A: Retrobulbar neuritis in a patient treated with intraarterial cisplatin for head and neck cancer. *Cancer* 1988; 62:2094–2097.

36. Saini JS, Jain IS, Dhar S, et al: Uremic optic neuropathy. *J Clin Neuro Ophthalmol* 1989; 9:131–133.

37. Knox DL, Hanneken AM, Hollows FC, et al: Uremic optic neuropathy. *Arch Ophthalmol* 1988; 106:50–54.

38. Winward KE: Optic neuropathy in uremia. *J Clin Neuro Ophthalmol* 1989; 9:134–135.

39. Taniwaki T, Kira J, Tashima S, et al: Chronic inflammatory demyelinating polyradiculoneuropathy (CIDP) associated with acute optic neuritis. *Rinsho Shinkeigaku* 1988; 28:798–792.

40. Pall HS, Williams AC: Subacute polyradiculopathy with optic and auditory nerve involvement. *Arch Neurol* 1987; 44:885–887.

41. Spoor TC, Rockwell DL: Treatment of optic neuritis with intravenous megadose corticosteroids. *Ophthalmology* 1988; 95:131–134.

42. Cox TA: Megadose corticosteroids for optic neuritis. *Ophthalmology* 1988; 95:1005–1006.

43. Wall M: Megadose corticosteroids for optic neuritis. *Ophthalmology* 1988; 95:1006.

44. Rockwell DL, Spoor TC: Megadose corticosteroids for optic neuritis. *Ophthalmology* 1988; 95:1006–1007.

45. Dutton JJ, Burde RM, Klingele TG: Autoimmune optic neuritis. *Am J Ophthalmol* 1982; 94:11–17.

46. Herishanu YO, Badarna S, Sarov B, et al: A possible harmful late effect of methylprednisolone therapy on a time cluster of optic neuritis. *Acta Neurol Scand* 1989; 80:569–574.

47. Beck RW: The optic neuritis treatment trial. *Arch Ophthalmol* 1988; 106:1051–1052.

48. Miller NR: Personal communication, September 1990.

49. Sanders EA, Van Lith GH: Optic neuritis, confirmed by visual evoked response, and the risk for multiple sclerosis: A prospective study. *J Clin Neurosurg Psychiatry* 1989; 52:799–800.

50. Alvarez G, Cardenas M: Multiple sclerosis following optic neuritis in Chile. *J Neurol Neurosurg Psychiatry* 1989; 52:115–117.

51. Congia S, Vacca MA, Tronci S: Epidemiologic and clinical features of optic neuritis in the 20th and 21st sanitary districts of the Sardinia (Italy). *Acta Neurol (Napoli)* 1989; 11:10–14.

52. Cheding M, Mellgren SI, Schive K: Optic neuritis in the two northernmost counties of Norway. A study of incidence and the prospect of later development of multiple sclerosis. *Arctic Med Res* 1989; 48:117–121.

53. Anmarkrud N, Slettnes ON: Uncomplicated retrobulbar neuritis and the development of multiple sclerosis. *Acta Ophthalmol (Copenh)* 1989; 67:306–309.

54. Sandberg-Wollheim M, Bynke H, Cronqvist S, et al: A long-term prospective study of optic neuritis: Evaluation of risk factors. *Ann Neurol* 1990; 27:386–393.

55. Weintraub MI: Optic neuritis and MS. *Neurology* 1988; 38:1660–1661.

56. Rizzo JF, Lessell S: Risk of developing multiple sclerosis after uncomplicated optic neuritis: A long term prospective study. *Neurology* 1988; 38:185–190.

57. Wilson WB, Smith DB: Does neuroretinitis rule out multiple sclerosis? *Arch Neurol* 1989; 46:358.

58. Parmley VC, Schiffman JS, Maitland CG, et al: Does neuroretinitis rule out multiple sclerosis? *Arch Neurol* 1987; 44:1045–1048.

59. Parmley VC: Does neuroretinitis rule out multiple sclerosis? *Arch Neurol* 1989; 46:358.

60. Miller DH, Ormerod IE, McDonald WI, et al: The early risk of multiple sclerosis after optic neuritis. *J Neurol Neurosurg Psychiatry* 1988; 51:1569–1571.

61. Frederiksen JL, Larsson HB, Henriksen O, et al: Magnetic resonance imaging of the brain in patients with acute monosymptomatic optic neuritis. *Acta Neurol Scand* 1989; 80:512–517.

62. Staedt D, Kappos L, Rohrbach E, et al: Contributions of magnetic resonance imaging to the diagnosis of MS in isolated optic neuritis. *Psychiatry Res* 1989; 29:295–296.

63. Guthoff R, Terwey B, Bragelmann L: Role of nuclear magnetic resonance imaging in the diagnosis of monosymptomatic optic neuritis. *Klin Monatsbl Augenheilkd* 1988; 192:311–316.

64. Wiegand W: Neutron spin tomography of the optic nerve in retrobulbar neuritis and optic nerve atrophy: demonstration of inflammation and demyelination. *Ophthalmologica* 1988; 197:193–201.

65. Kakisu Y, Adachi-Usami E, Kojima S, et al: Magnetic resonance imaging (MRI) in the diagnosis of optic neuritis and neuropathy. *Nippon Ganka Gakkai Zasshi* 1989; 93:281–286.

66. Miller DH, Robb SA, Ormerod IEC, et al: Magnetic resonance imaging of inflammatory and demyelinating white-matter diseases of childhood. *Dev Med Child Neurol* 1990; 32:97–107.

67. Omerod IEC, McDonald WI, duBoulay DH, et al: Disseminated lesions at presentation in patients with optic neuritis. *J Neurol Neurosurg Psychiatry* 1986; 49:124–172.

68. Johns K, Lavin P, Elliot JH, et al: Magnetic resonance imaging of the brain in isolated optic neuritis. *Arch Ophthalmol* 1986; 104:1486–1488.

69. Jacobs L, Kinkel PR, Kinkel WR: Silent brain lesions in patients with isolated idiopathic optic neuritis. *Arch Neurol* 1986; 43:452–455.

70. Kinnunen E, Larsen A, Ketonen L, et al: Evaluation of central nervous system involvement in uncomplicated optic neuritis after prolonged follow-up. *Acta Neurol Scand* 1987; 76:147–151.

71. Ormerod IEC, Miller DH, McDonald WI, et al: The role of NMR imaging in the assessment of multiple sclerosis and isolated neurological lesions. *Brain* 1987; 110:1579–1616.

72. Weintraub MI: Surface-coil heat concentration in MR as a possible exacerbating factor in retrobulbar neuritis: Is this a local "hot bath test?" *AJNR* 1989; 10:207–208.

73. Guy J, Fitzsimmons J, Ellis A, et al: Gadolinium-DTPA-enhanced magnetic resonance imaging in experimental optic neuritis. *Ophthalmology* 1990; 97:601–607.

74. Guy J, Mancuso A, Quisling RG, et al: Gadolinium-DTPA-enhanced magnetic resonance imaging in optic neuropathies. *Ophthalmology* 1990; 97:592–599.

75. Miller DH, Newton MR, Van de Poel JC, et al: Magnetic resonance imaging of the optic nerve in optic neuritis. *Neurology* 1988; 38:175–179.

76. Klein LB: Gadolinium-DTPA-enhanced magnetic resonance imaging in optic neuropathies (discussion). *Ophthalmology* 1990; 97:599–600.

77. Kermode AG, Moseley IF, Kendall BE, et al: Magnetic resonance imaging in Leber's optic neuropathy. *J Neurol Neurosurg Psychiatry* 1989; 52:671–674.

78. Millner MM, Ebner F, Justich E, et al: Multiple sclerosis in childhood: Contribution of serial MRI to earlier diagnosis. *Dev Med Child Neurol* 1990; 32:769–777.

79. Kriss A, Francis DA, Cuendet F, et al: Recovery after optic neuritis in childhood. *J Neurol Neurosurg Psychiatry* 1988; 51:1253–1258.

80. Farris BK, Pickard DJ: Bilateral postinfectious optic neuritis and intravenous steroid therapy in children. *Ophthalmology* 1990; 97:339–345.

81. Riikonen R, Donner M, Erkkila H: Optic neuritis in children and its relationship to multiple sclerosis: A clinical study of 21 children. *Dev Med Child Neurol* 1988; 30:349–359.

82. Celesia GG, Kaufman DI, Brigell M, et al: Optic neuritis: A prospective study. *Neurology* 1990; 40:919–923.

83. Sanders EA, Volkers AC, van der Poel JC, et al: Estimation of visual function after optic neuritis: A comparison of clinical tests. *Br J Ophthalmol* 1986; 70:918–924.

84. Sanders EA, Volkers AC, van der Poel JC, et al: Visual function and pattern visual evoked response in optic neuritis. *Br J Ophthalmol* 1987; 71:602–608.

85. Fleishman JA, Beck RW, Linares DA, et al: Deficits in visual function after resolution of optic neuritis. *Ophthalmology* 1987; 94:1029–1035.

86. Jacobson DM, Thompson HS, Corbett JJ: Optic neuritis in the elderly: Prognosis for visual recovery and long-term follow-up. *Neurology* 1988; 38:1834–1837.

87. Birk K, Ford C, Smeltzer S, et al: The clinical course of multiple sclerosis during pregnancy and the puerperium. *Arch Neurol* 1990; 47:738–742.

88. Honan WP, Heron JR, Foster DH, et al: Visual loss in multiple sclerosis and its relation to previous optic neuritis, disease duration and clinical classification. *Brain* 1990; 113:975–987.

89. Kinnunen E, Konttinen YT, Bergroth V, et al: Immunological studies on patients with optic neuritis without evidence of multiple sclerosis. *J Neurol Sci* 1989; 90:43–52.

90. Oger J, O'Gorman M, Willoughby E, et al: Changes in immune function in relapsing MS correlate with disease activity as assessed by magnetic resonance imaging. *Ann NY Acad Sci* 1988; 540:597–601.

91. Guy JR, Feldberg NT, Savino PJ, et al: T-lymphocyte subpopulations in acute unilateral optic neuritis. *Ophthalmology* 1989; 96:1054–1057.

92. Riikonen R, von Willebrandt E: Lymphocyte subclasses and function in patients with optic neuritis in childhood with special reference to multiple sclerosis. *Acta Neurol Scand* 1988; 78:58–64.

93. Riikonen R: The role of infection and vaccination in the genesis of optic neuritis and multiple sclerosis in children. *Acta Neurol Scand* 1989; 80:425–431.

94. Guy J, Ellis EA, Hope GM, et al: Antioxidant enzymes reduce loss of blood-brain barrier integrity in experimental optic neuritis. *Arch Ophthalmol* 1989; 107:1359–1363.

95. Heinrichs IH, McLean DR: Evolution of visual evoked potentials in optic neuritis. *Can J Neurol Sci* 1988; 15:394–396.

96. Grochowicki M, Vighetto A: Evaluation of the central visual field by the Friedmann Mark I analyzer and color vision in 85 patients with multiple sclerosis. Correlation with visual evoked potentials in 50 cases. *J Fr Ophthalmol* 1988; 11:61–65.

97. Fujimoto N, Adachi-Usami E: Comparison of automated perimetry and pattern visually evoked cortical potentials in optic neuritis. *Doc Ophthalmol* 1988; 69:263–269.

98. Berninger TA, Heider W: Electrophysiology and perimetry in acute retrobulbar neuritis. *Doc Ophthalmol* 1989; 71:293–305.

99. Fujimoto N, Adachi-Usami E: Relationship between central visual field and pattern VECP in optic neuritis. *Nippon Ganka Gakkai Zasshi* 1989; 93:646–650.

100. Fujimoto N: A comparison of central visual field measurement by automated perimetry in optic neuritis due to multiple sclerosis and of unknown etiology. *Nippon Ganka Gakkai Zasshi* 1989; 93:581–586.

101. Macfayden DJ, Drance SM, Douglas GR, et al: The retinal nerve fiber layer, neuroretinal rim area, and visual evoked potentials in MS. *Neurology* 1988; 38:1353–1358.

102. Kaufman DI, Lorance RW, Woods M, et al: The pattern electroretinogram: A long-term study in acute optic neuropathy. *Neurology* 1988; 38:1767–1774.

103. Papakostopoulos D, Fotiou F, Hart JC, et al: The electroretinogram in multiple sclerosis and demyelinating optic neuritis. *Electroencephalogr Clin Neurophysiol* 1989; 74:1–10.

104. Accornero N, De Vito G, Rotunno A, et al: Critical fusion frequency in MS during mild induced hyperthermia. *Acta Neurol Scand* 1989; 79:510–514.

105. Lachenmayr B, Gleissner M, Rothbacher H: Automated flicker perimetry. *Fortschr Ophthalmol* 1989; 86:695–701.

106. Pittke EC, Thill-Schwaninger M: Contributions to the Aulhorn flicker test. II: The flicker test and the Pulfrich phenomenon in clinical diagnosis. *Klin Monatsbl Augenheilkd* 1988;193:382–387.

107. Trauzettel-Klosinski S, Aulhorn E: Significance of the Tubingen flicker test in the differential diagnosis of optic neuritis. *Fortschr Ophthalmol* 1988; 85:557–561.

108. Trauzettel-Klosinski S, Schupbach M, Aulhorn E: Standardization of the Tubingen flicker test. *Graefes Arch Clin Exp Ophthalmol* 1989; 227:221–229.

109. Trauzettel-Klosinski S: Various stages of optic neuritis assessed by subjective brightness of flicker. *Arch Ophthalmol* 1989; 107:63–68.

110. Fahy J, Glynn D, Hutchinson M: Contrast sensitivity in multiple sclerosis measured by Cambridge low contrast gratings: A useful clinical test? *J Neurol Neurosurg Psychiatry* 1989; 52:786–787.

111. Edgar GK, Foster DH, Honan WP, et al: Optic neuritis: Variations in temporal modulation sensitivity with retinal eccentricity. *Brain* 1990; 113:487–496.

112. Wall M: Loss of P retinal ganglion cell function in resolved optic neuritis. *Neurology* 1990; 40:649–653.

113. Dain SJ, Rammohan KW, Benes SC, et al: Chromatic, spatial, and temporal losses of sensitivity in multiple sclerosis. *Invest Ophthalmol Vis Sci* 1990; 31:548–558.

CHAPTER 2

Tumors of the Optic Nerve

John S. Kennerdell, M.D.

Clinical Professor of Ophthalmology, University of Pittsburgh School of Medicine; Adjunct Professor of Surgery (Ophthalmology), Medical College of Pennsylvania; Director, Department of Ophthalmology, Allegheny General Hospital, Pittsburgh, Pennsylvania

Michael Kazim, M.D.

Instructor in Clinical Ophthalmology, Columbia University College of Physicians and Surgeons; Assistant Attending Columbia-Presbyterian Medical Center, Edward S. Harkness Eye Institute, New York, New York

The most common intrinsic optic nerve tumors are gliomas and meningiomas. The management of these tumors continues to evolve as our collective experience broadens and the tools of diagnostic imaging improve. The use of radiation therapy and chemotherapy as primary therapy as well as adjunctive therapy also has expanded.

DIAGNOSTIC IMAGING

The computed tomography (CT) characteristics of optic nerve tumors have been extensively described with the newest generation high-resolution scanners. Of great interest to us is the rapid evolution of the resolving power of magnetic resonance imaging (MRI). Imaging with MRI is based on the differential behavior of tissues in a magnetic field. The magnetic fields currently used are generally 1.0 to

1.5 tesla units. The most active molecule in the field is water, since it contains two hydrogen molecules, each with an unpaired electron. In the magnetic field these unpaired electrons are oriented in a unipolar direction for a given amount of time (TE = excitation time). When the field influence is removed, the electrons reorient themselves in random fashion; this period is the relaxation time (TR). The longer the TR, the more random the orientation. Based on the relative TE/TR, a differential image can be produced. T1 images have a shorter TR than T2 images. In the orbit, the highest water content structure outside the globe is fat tissue. This produces a bright image which obscures orbital detail. This effect is most pronounced on T1 images. When T2 imaging is used, the fat compartment is less bright, resulting in greater detail. One disadvantage of the T2-weighted images is that the long imaging time requires a very cooperative patient. To obtain better orbital images with shorter imaging times, a variety of techniques have been used.

Eidelberg et al.[1] performed MRI with short T1 inversion recovery sequence (STIR) on 20 patients with chronic unilateral optic neuropathy. The STIR sequence helped to distinguish the optic nerve from the surrounding orbital fat. In 7 of the patients, no mass was noted on standard MRI but was apparent when the STIR sequence was applied.

The development of paramagnetic contrast material has increased the sensitivity of MRI in the central nervous system. Currently the most widely used contrast material is gadolinium-diethylenetriamine pentaacetic acid (Gd-DTPA). Intracanalicular and chiasmal lesions are imaged best this way. When applied to intraorbital lesions, Gd-DTPA generally decreases the contrast between orbital fat and the suspected lesion. Haik et al.[2] describe a patient with an optic nerve meningioma. While the intraorbital tumor was imaged with both CT and non-contrast MRI, the intracranial extension was only appreciated with Gd-DTPA–enhanced MRI. The authors describe the mechanism by which Gd-DTPA improves the imaging capabilities of MRI. We have also seen a number of cases in which Gd-DTPA–enhanced MRI was superior to either CT or non-enhanced MRI for demonstrating intracranial spread of meningiomas. In one case, a patient was followed up for 12 years with a suspected apical optic nerve meningioma. There was progressive loss of vision, but no evidence of intracranial spread on CT scans or non-enhanced MRI. A Gd-DTPA–enhanced MRI was ultimately obtained and demonstrated extension of the tumor through the optic canal. A fronto-orbitotomy was performed, and pathologic studies revealed a choristoma of the optic nerve. We have found Gd-DTPA enhancement to be of value in all cases in which intracranial spread of orbital disease is suspected. It is also of value when evaluating any intracranial mass, especially those involving the cavernous sinus and chiasm as it combines the improved level of resolution with the multiplanar capabilities of MRI.

In two articles, Simon and Szumowski[3, 4] provide us with another algorithm for increasing the sensitivity of MRI in the orbit. To avoid high fat signal intensity without increasing the TR to prohibitively long intervals, the authors have applied a chemical shift imaging (CSI) fat-suppression algorithm. The authors believe their technique has advantages over the STIR fat-suppression technique. These reports are the first of what will be many attempts by neuroradiologists to maximize intraorbital contrast techniques to improve the resolution of MRI. We enthusiastically anticipate their introduction.

Two fascinating case reports present unusual magnetic resonance images. Applegate and Pribman[5] present the MRI findings of a case of sudden proptosis in a 16-year-old girl with neurofibromatosis and blindness secondary to bilateral optic nerve gliomas. As the patient was blind, decompression was not attempted. The patient was followed up with MRI, which provided a serial study of the paramagnetic properties of a resolving hemorrhage. Brodsky et al.[6] present the first magnetic resonance images of a patient who had a pathologically proven surgical excision of an optic nerve glioma that postoperatively appears intact on MRI and CT.

We think that CT and MRI are complementary imaging techniques when applied to orbital disease. In the intracanalicular and intracranial spaces, MRI is far superior to CT since it is not subject to signal averaging artifact from the surrounding bone. The use of Gd-DTPA in these cases further enhances resolution. One further advantage of MRI is the multiplanar capabilities. In the intraorbital space, CT still holds a small advantage based on the high fat content, familiarity with the images generated, and the relative speed of the examination. However, with the expanding data base of images that is defining MRI in the orbit and the expanding number of algorithms to increase the resolution of MRI in fat compartments, we may ultimately see MRI supplant CT.

Atta[7] provides an excellent review of ultrasound of the optic nerve. A detailed description of the 30 degree test for the detection of fluid within the optic nerve sheath is included. We agree with his conclusions that ultrasound provides a safe, inexpensive screening test that meets with little patient resistance. We think that, as a dynamic test, ultrasound provides information unavailable on the static CT or MRI. An interesting historical review of orbital imaging from the discovery of x-rays by Roentgen in 1895 to MRI is provided by Taveras and Haik.[8]

FINE NEEDLE ASPIRATION BIOPSY

The use of fine needle aspiration biopsy to diagnose tumors of the orbit was introduced in this country in 1979 by Kennerdell et al.[9] Since that time, the technique has gained slow acceptance primarily for the diagnosis of solid intraorbital tumors. There has been one previous report of a diagnostic biopsy of an optic nerve glioma. de Keizer et al.[10] report an optic nerve glioma with intraocular extension and iris tumors in a 3-year-old boy with neurofibromatosis. In addition to noninvasive imaging, fine needle biopsy was performed.

Pennelli et al.[11] report a case of juvenile pilocytic astrocytoma diagnosed with fine needle aspiration biopsy. A CT-guided biopsy was consistent with the histologic diagnosis made on the resected intraorbital nerve. The authors discuss the rationale for the use of the fine needle technique.

We are in full agreement that fine needle biopsy is an essential tool in the management of orbital disease. It is especially useful in those cases in which the diagnosis would obviate extensive surgery or be necessary prior to proceeding with a radical operation. The concerns regarding seeding the needle tract with tumor cells have proven to be justified only with pancreatic cancer. There have been no reports of tumor seeding in all other sites.

OPTIC NERVE GLIOMAS

Unquestionably the most exhaustive review of the collective experience with optic nerve and chiasmal gliomas in the literature was undertaken by Alvord and Lofton.[12] Six hundred twenty-three cases of optic gliomas were reviewed with particular attention to the prognosis of the disease based on the patient's age, tumor site, form of treatment, presence of neurofibromatosis, and intracranial extension. They found each of these parameters was statistically significant. Despite the generally held belief that these tumors are a homogenous group of low-grade astrocytomas, they found them to be very inhomogeneous, with a wide spectrum of growth rates. With a mathematical model they found that some grew rapidly but most behaved as though the growth rate progressively decelerated. The authors think that these results are inconsistent with these tumors being classified as hamartomas. Among the most important conclusions are the following:

1. Optic nerve gliomas have an excellent prognosis following excision and only slightly worse prognosis following radiation therapy.
2. Twenty-five percent of optic nerve gliomas have invaded the optic chiasm at the time of diagnosis, and 5% of optic nerve gliomas recur in the optic chiasm following intraorbital excision. There were no reports of recurrence following complete intracranial excision.
3. Patients with neurofibromatosis have a two times greater recurrence rate following complete excision of intraorbital glioma.
4. Chiasmal gliomas are slightly to moderately responsive to doses of greater than 4,500 rad.
5. There is no difference in prognosis in patients with neurofibromatosis following radiation therapy of chiasmal gliomas.
6. They were unable to comment on the efficacy of chemotherapy as it has been used for too short a time.
7. There is a greater incidence of death due to tumor in patients greater than 20 years of age and especially in those older than 50 years of age.

Wright et al.[13] report on the follow-up of the 31 patients first presented in 1980 with optic nerve gliomas. They divide the patients into two groups. One group was clinically stable over a period of up to 13.5 years. In this group, neurofibromatosis was relatively common (11 of 16). In the remaining 15 patients, the tumor continued to grow as documented by loss of vision or progressive proptosis. Four of these patients had neurofibromatosis, and 11 underwent neurosurgical exploration. None received radiation therapy as either a primary or adjunctive therapy. They propose a decision tree for the treatment of patients with optic nerve tumors. Visual acuity and radiologic evidence of involvement of the optic canal and chiasm are the most critical elements of the decision tree. Readers are referred to the discussion. They refer to the accompanying paper describing the aggressive behavior of optic nerve meningiomas in the pediatric age group, which leads them to be all the more aggressive with tumors in this age group. They excise these tumors when there is poor vision or documented growth.

Flickinger et al.[14] report the results of treating 36 patients who had gliomas of the optic nerve or chiasm. Pathologic confirmation was obtained in 32 patients. Tumor initially confined to the optic nerve recurred in 1 case after complete excision. The surgical procedure was not described. Twenty-five patients with biopsy proven gliomas of the optic chiasm were treated with radiation therapy. All were low-grade astrocytomas. Radiation therapy was administered with a variety of delivery systems. The dose of 4,500 to 5,040 rad to the 95% isodose line with 180-rad fractions was the optimum for tumor control and avoided late complications. Survival at 5, 10, and 15 years was 96%, 90%, and 90%, respectively, and the progression-free survival was 87% at 5, 10, and 15 years. Vision improved or stabilized in 86% of patients after radiation therapy. The authors include an exhaustive review of the often conflicting literature in this area.

Wechsler-Jentzsch[15] present 12 patients, 3 with high-grade astroyctomas and 9 with low-grade astrocytomas in a variety of sites including 1 patient with an optic nerve glioma. The authors measure the tumor volume response to radiation therapy as measured with CT or MRI. In the patient with an optic nerve glioma, a stable 59% reduction in tumor volume over a 4-year period was achieved. The radiation therapy dose was generally 5,000 to 5,580 rad delivered in 10-rad fractions. There is an interesting discussion of tumor growth kinetics in the two groups as it relates to the response to radiation therapy.

Seven cases of optic nerve gliomas in adults have been reported.[16] One patient was 61 years old. Both clinically and histologically these tumors resembled those in the pediatric population. Unlike optic chiasma gliomas, which are clinically aggressive and histologically are malignant astrocytomas,[17] these tumors had a very benign course. The authors advocate excision of the tumor from the globe to the optic chiasm without enucleation. There was a recurrence in only one case after resection; however, in two cases in which there was incomplete excision, there was no recurrence up to 21 years later. The authors conclude that these tumors should be managed conservatively, as they are in the pediatric population.

As part of a report that also contains data on patients with optic nerve meningiomas, Gabivov et al.[18] treated 28 patients with optic nerve gliomas. The surgical approach they use is novel. They begin with a low fronto-craniotomy. The intracranial portion of the nerve is removed from the optic chiasm to the optic canal. The optic canal is not unroofed, rather, the intracanalicular segment of the optic nerve is simply coagulated. The intraorbital nerve is removed medially up to the posterior globe. There was only one recurrence at the stump of infraorbital nerve at the posterior globe.

Bilgic et al.[19] report a series of 24 patients with intraorbital or intracranial optic nerve glioma. Interestingly, they used only plain radiographs of the optic canal to decide if the tumor had extended intracranially. Based on this information, patients with intracranial disease underwent a craniotomy with excision of the optic nerve to the optic chiasm and postoperative radiation therapy. The 16 patients with evidence of intracranial disease did poorly: only 37% survived for an average of 8 years. The authors suggest that the disease in this group of patients was more advanced at the time of diagnosis. We would agree with this conclusion and add that this study confirms the major advantage conferred with CT and especially MRI in defining early spread of tumor into the intracanalicular space before it involves the optic chiasm. We are happy to rid ourselves of the vagaries of diagnosis that plagued the age of plain film radiology.

Liesternick et al.[20] performed CT on 65 children diagnosed with neurofibromatosis type 1 and no previously noted ophthalmic abnormalities. Optic gliomas were detected in ten (15%) of these children. Three had unilateral tumors, three had bilateral tumors, and four had involvement of the optic chiasm. Abnormalities in vision were found in only two children. These results suggest a role for routine CT or MRI examination as part of the evaluation of children with neurofibromatosis.

A 27-year-old man with a documented optic nerve tumor who presented with sudden proptosis and vision loss to no light perception was reported.[21] CT showed a markedly swollen optic nerve. He was treated emergently with corticosteroids, the nerve sheath was surgically decompressed, and the tumor was debulked. Vision returned to 20/25. The authors entertain the possible mechanisms for sudden vision loss in this patient. An optic chiasm mass presumed to be a glioma in an 8-year-old child with poor vision was presented.[22] Review of the case included the evaluation, diagnostic tests to be ordered, salient features of the appropriate neuroimaging, and options of biopsy and treatment as discussed by three noted experts. The reader is directed to this paper for their comments.[22] Gower et al.[23] describe an unusually large cystic pilocytic astrocytoma of the optic chiasm, with extensions into the third ventricle and hypothalamus. The MRI features are discussed as are the surgical procedure and postoperative radiation therapy and chemotherapy.

There were two cases of optic nerve glioma diagnosed with fine needle biopsy. These are described previously.[10, 11]

We currently use CT and MRI in all cases of suspected optic nerve gliomas. Surgical excision via combined fronto-orbitotomy is recommended in all cases with poor vision, documented enlargement, or involvement of the optic canal. In all cases, we attempt to remove the entire optic nerve from optic chiasm to the posterior globe. We often find it possible to remove the intracanalicular segment without unroofing the canal and dividing the annulus of Zinn. If there is gross or microscopic involvement of the optic chiasm, radiation therapy (5,000 rad) is considered. We have not had extensive experience with chemotherapy for the treatment of the most aggressive and invasive tumors and await the results of national collaborative studies currently underway.

OPTIC NERVE MENINGIOMAS

Wright et al.[24] report the largest series of patients with optic nerve sheath meningiomas. A majority of their patients were middle-aged women; however, a large fraction (13/50) were less than 30 years old. With both MRI and CT, they reported a 90% rate of correct diagnosis. They emphasize the significantly more aggressive behavior of these tumors in the pediatric age group and speculate on the cause. They note that once the tumor has invaded the middle cranial fossa, there is no chance of eradicating the disease. Therefore their approach to these tumors is based on the site of the tumor, its growth, and, most importantly, the age of the patient. They no longer advocate local excision of the tumor as it invariably leads to vision loss and may produce aggressive orbital disease that requires exenteration. In all patients under the age of 30 years, they advocate excision of the tumor via frontal craniotomy to remove the full extent of the tumor. In the patients over 30 years old, medical observation is advocated until vision is severely impaired; then the optic nerve is removed. They used radiation therapy in only two patients but were encouraged by the results. In cases in which the tumor invaded the sphenoid ridge, they advocate surgical debulking and adjuvant radiation therapy.

Nine patients with primary optic nerve sheath meningiomas were studied by Clark et al.[25] They studied two patients with MRI and were impressed with the superior resolution of MRI compared to that of CT. All of the patients underwent surgical excision of the tumors: six via lateral orbitotomy, three via fronto-orbitotomy. None of the patients were treated with radiation therapy. All had postoperative loss of vision. They classify the tumors based on location and make some conclusions about the pathogenesis of the tumor. The authors think that growth of the anteriorly placed tumors is not constrained by the dural sheath, which may lead to extradural extension without optic nerve compression or invasion. These tumors can however lead to proptosis. The growth of posterior tumors is restricted by the dural sheath, which leads to optic nerve compression, blood vessel compromise, and invasion of the optic nerve. By any of these three mechanisms there is often a profound loss of vision. These are also the tumors that result in optocilliary shunt vessels resulting from the blood vessel compromise. In their series, 22% of the patients had optocilliary shunt vessels as is reported in other studies. They do not use radiation therapy either primarily or as adjuvant treatment.

The management of seven optic nerve meningiomas and four cases of intraorbital extension of an intracranial meningioma were described.[26] Partial or total excision was attempted in five of the seven optic nerve tumors. There was some improvement in vision in all but one of the patients, although no measure of the preoperative and postoperative vision was reported. In one case, an apical tumor was removed with an ultrasonic aspirator and the patient had no light perception postoperatively. Treatment was limited to 4,000 to 5,000 rad of radiation therapy in two inoperable cases. In one of these cases, the vision stabilized. In the other, there was improvement in both the vision and shrinkage of the tumor volume on CT. The follow-up period was 2 years. They also note the infrequent occurrence of meningiomas in patients less than 20 years of age. The findings on high-resolution CT and MRI help to distinguish these tumors from gliomas, which are more common in this age group. They conclude that optic nerve meningiomas are difficult to remove without sacrificing vision. We agree and are particularly reluctant to approach apical lesions surgically. Instead we prefer radiation therapy (5,000 to 5,500 rad) when there is progressive loss of vision. When there is no useful vision left, the optic nerve is removed via combined fronto-orbitotomy to preclude intracranial spread.

Gabibov et al.[18] reviewed a series of 63 patients, 35 of whom had optic nerve meningiomas and the remainder of whom had gliomas (see previous paragraph). All presented with decreased vision, and 27 had proptosis. Plain X-rays and CT scans were obtained on all patients. Patients were grouped according to the degree of vision loss and CT findings. The indications for surgery are not clearly stated. In all cases in which a subtotal excision was attempted, vision was lost and in one case the patient had no light perception. Radiation therapy was not used. There were six recurrences.

A 12-year study of optic nerve meningiomas was published by Kennerdell et al. Thirty-eight patients (39 eyes) were observed or treated with surgery, radiation therapy, or a combination of the two. Patients in whom the tumor was believed to be confined to the orbit and caused little or no functional deficit were observed. Radiation therapy (5,000 to 5,500 rad) delivered via linear accelerator was used in cases in which the tumor was confined to the orbit and there was functional or progressive visual loss (visual acuity of 20/40 or worse). Excision of the tumor or observation was offered to patients with intracranial tumors and no useful vision. In those patients with severe disease and intracranial spread, surgical excision of both the intracranial and intraorbital nerve followed by radiation therapy was advocated. Early success with excision of nerve sheath meningiomas was not supported by more recent experience. In all of the more recent cases, the final visual outcome was poor and there exists the possibility of permitting a recurrence within the orbit that would require exenteration. As a result, we no longer advocate this form of treatment. Tissue diagnosis was not required for treatment with radiation therapy: only one of the cases in this group was diagnosed with fine needle aspiration biopsy prior to therapy. We depended instead on characteristic neuroradiologic features. With one exception, these patients were older than 30 years, and as a group the lesions did not progress rapidly, although none of the patients in the series maintained vision of 20/50 or better without treatment with radiation therapy or surgery. All six patients treated primarily with radiation therapy demonstrated improved visual acuity or visual fields for 3 to 7 years.

There were two reports of meningiomas with atypical presentations. McNab and Wright[28] report three cases of optic nerve sheath cysts. All the patients underwent surgical decompression of the optic nerve sheath. Biopsy specimens obtained at surgery revealed a meningioma in each case. There was improvement in vision in only one case. The authors review other reports of optic nerve cysts and the associated pathologic states and speculate on the pathogenesis of these tumors. Since optic nerve cysts that occur without related pathologic conditions are rare, the authors caution that this group of patients be followed up for extended periods with repeated CT and MRI as the size of the tumors at the time of initial presentation may be below the level of resolution of these imaging techniques. Castillo et al.[29] report a case of a massive meningioma involving the optic nerves, optic chiasm, and optic tracts in an 11-year-old girl. They describe the CT and MRI features helpful in distinguishing the lesion from a glioma, a much more common lesion in this age group. A review of the literature is included as well as a discussion of the particularly aggressive behavior of these lesions in the pediatric age group. These reports encourage us to be vigilant for the unsuspected diagnosis in the otherwise typical case.

OTHER OPTIC NERVE TUMORS

While the vast majority of optic nerve tumors are gliomas and meningiomas, a number of interesting tumors were described. Shuey and Blacharski[30] represent a case of acute vision loss in a 22-year-old man with a melanocytoma of the optic nerve head. A discussion of the differential diagnosis and the mechanism of the vision loss is included. The authors thought that the most likely causes were central retinal artery occlusion and ischemic necrosis of the optic nerve head.

Nerad et al.[31] describe a patient with von Hippel-Lindau disease and an optic nerve hemangioblastoma diagnosed with incisional biopsy. The tumor continued to enlarge after the biopsy, producing blindness and disfiguring proptosis. It was ultimately excised via lateral orbitotomy. It is impossible to remove the tumors and preserve vision since its growth is inseparable from the surrounding neural tissue. They note that these tumors must be distinguished from optic gliomas and meningiomas. They caution that these patients should be fully evaluated for other evidence of angiomatosis and followed up for an extended period since some will ultimately develop other signs of the disease. Whether such a tumor arising in the optic nerve can extend intracranially is unknown.

The first case of an isolated metastasis to the optic nerve from a cerebellar medulloblastoma (a rare, poorly differentiated embyronal tumor) was reported 28 months after the primary tumor was treated by resection and radiation therapy.[32] The authors discuss the embryologic origin and biologic behavior of the tumor as well as treatment.

The third case of optic nerve ganglioglioma was reported by Bergin et al.[33] The tumor most often occurs on the floor of the third ventricle and in the hypothalamus where it is generally slow-growing. The authors describe the pathologic findings and discuss the theories of pathogenesis. On CT scans, the tumor was indistinguishable from an optic nerve glioma and did not extend intracranially. The tumor was excised via combined medial and lateral orbitotomy. One year later, there was no evidence of recurrence.

The treatment of a 24-year-old woman with a cavernous angioma of the optic nerve was discussed.[34, 35] CT features are presented as are the first magnetic resonance images of an optic nerve angioma. The T2-weighted images show the tumor as being clearly separate from the surrounding hemosiderin. The authors advocate the surgical excision of these tumors to avoid complications from spontaneous hemorrhage.

REFERENCES

1. Eidelberg D, Newton MR, Johnson G, et al: Chronic unilateral optic neuropathy: A magnetic resonance study. *Ann Neurol* 1988; 24:3–11.

2. Haik BG, Zimmerman R, Louis LS: Gadolinium-DTPA enhancement of an optic nerve and chiasml meningioma. *J Clin Neuro-ophthalmol* 1989; 9:122–125.

3. Simon JH, Szumowski J: Chemical shift imaging with paramagnetic enhancement for improved lesion depiction. *Radiology* 1989; 171:539–543.

4. Simon JH, Szumowski J, Totterman S: Fat suppression magnetic resonance imaging of the orbit. *AJNR* 1988; 9:961–968.

5. Applegate LJ, Pribram HFW: Hematoma of optic nerve glioma-A cause of sudden proptosis. *J Clin Neuro-ophthalmol* 1989; 9:15–19.

6. Brodsky MC, Hoyt WF, Newton DR: The "phantom" optic nerve. *J Clin Neuro-ophthalmol* 1988; 8:67–86.

7. Atta HR: Imaging of the optic nerve with standardised echography. *Eye* 1988; 2:358–366.

8. Taveras JL, Haik BG: Radiography of the eye and orbit: A historical overview. *Surv Ophthalmol* 1988; 32:361–368.

9. Kennerdell JS, Dekker A, Johnson BL, et al: Fine-needle aspiration biopsy. Its use in orbital tumors. *Arch Ophthalmol* 1979; 97:1315–1317.

10. de Keizer RJW, de Wolff-Rouendaal D, Bots GTAM, et al: Optic glioma with intraocular tumor and seeding in a child with neurofibromatosis. *Am J Ophthalmol* 1989; 108:717–725.

11. Pennelli N, Monntaguti A, Carteri A, et al: Juvenile pilocytic astrocytoma of the optic nerve diagnosed by fine needle aspiration biopsy. *Acta Cytologica* 1988; 32:395–398.

12. Alvord EC, Lofton S: Gliomas of optic nerve or chiasm. *J Neurosurg* 1988; 68:85–98.

13. Wright JE, McNab AA, McDonald WI: Optic nerve glioma and the management of optic nerve tumors in the young. *Br J Ophthalmol* 1989; 73:967–974.

14. Flickinger JC, Torres C, Deutsch M: Management of low-grade gliomas of the optic nerve and chiasm. *Cancer* 1988; 61:635–642.

15. Wechsler-Jentzsch K, Witt JH, Fitz CR, et al: Unresectable gliomas in children: Tumor-volume response to radiation therapy. *Radiology* 1988; 169:237–242.

16. Wulc AE, Bergin DJ, Barnes D, et al: Orbital optic nerve glioma in adult life. *Arch Ophthalmol* 1989; 107:1013–1016.

17. Hoyt WF, Meshal LG, Lessel S, et al: Malignant optic glioma of adulthood. *Brain* 1973; 96:121–132.

18. Gabibov GA, Blinkov SM, Tcherekayev VA: The management of optic nerve meningiomas and gliomas. *J Neurosurg* 1988; 68:889–893.

19. Bilgic S, Erbengi A, Tinaztepe B, et al: Optic glioma of childhood: Clinical, histopathological, and histochemical observations. *Br J Ophthalmol* 1989; 73:832–837.

20. Listernick R, Charrow J, Greenwald MJ, et al: Optic gliomas in children with neurofibromatosis type 1. *J Pediatr* 1989; 114:788–792.

21. Jordan DR, Anderson RL, White GL, et al: Acute vision loss due to a calcified optic nerve glioma. *Can J Ophthalmol* 1989; 24:335–339.

22. Gittinger JW: To image or not to image. *Surv Ophthalmol* 1988; 32:350–356.

23. Gower DJ, Pollay M, Shuman RM, et al: Cystic optic glioma. *Neurosurgery* 1990; 26:133–137.

24. Wright JE, McNab AA, McDonald WI: Primary optic nerve sheath meningioma. *Br J Ophthalmol* 1989; 73:960–966.

25. Clark WC, Theofilos CS, Fleming JC: Primary optic nerve sheath meningiomas. *J Neurosurg* 1989; 70:37–40.

26. Ito M, Ishizawa A, Miyaoka M, et al: Intraorbital meningiomas. *Surg Neurol* 1988; 29:448–453.

27. Kennerdell JS, Maroon JC, Malton M, et al: The management of optic nerve sheath meningiomas. *Am J Ophthalmol* 1988; 106:450–457.

28. McNab AA, Wright JE: Cysts of the optic nerve: Three cases associated with meningioma. *Eye* 1989; 3:355–359.

29. Castillo M, Davis PC, Ross WK, et al: Meningioma of the chiasm and optic nerves: CT and MR findings. *J Comput Assist Tomogr* 1989; 13:679–681.

30. Shuey TF, Blacharski PA: Pigmented tumor and acute vision loss. *Surv Ophthalmol* 1988; 33:121–126.

31. Nerad JA, Kersten RC, Anderson RL: Hemangioblastoma of the optic nerve. *Ophthalmology* 1988; 95:398–402.

32. Garrity JA, Herman DC, Dinapoli RP, et al: Isolated metastisis to the optic nerve from medulloblastoma. *Ophthalmology* 1989; 96:207–210.

33. Bergin DJ, Johnson TE, Spencer WH, et al: Ganglioglioma of the optic nerve. *Am J Ophthalmol* 1988; 105:146–149.

34. Hassler W, Zentner J, Peterson D: Cavernous angioma of the optic nerve. *Surg Neurol* 1989; 31:444–447.

35. Hassler W, Zentner J, Wilhelm H: Cavernous angiomas of the anterior visual pathways. *J Clin Neuro-ophthalmol* 1989; 9:160–164.

CHAPTER 3

Other Optic Nerve Disorders

Myles M. Behrens, M.D.

Professor of Clinical Ophthalmology, Columbia-Presbyterian Medical Center, New York, New York

Jeffrey G. Odel, M.D.

Assistant Professor of Clinical Ophthalmology, Columbia-Presbyterian Medical Center, New York, New York

The past 2 years have yielded advances in the study of optic nerve diseases including, in particular, major advances in the understanding of the pathogenesis, and the diagnosis of, Leber's hereditary optic neuropathy; increasing literature on the use of optic nerve sheath decompression in papilledema with progressive visual loss and its newly suggested use in progressive anterior ischemic optic neuropathy, and increasing attention to clarification of the management of traumatic optic neuropathy.

HEREDITARY

Nikoskelainen et al.[1] reemphasized the value of fundus examination of family members (maternal relatives) for the telltale angiopathy of Leber's hereditary optic neuropathy in determining the etiology of otherwise cryptogenic cases of optic neuropathy. In reviewing their few presumably sporadic cases, they found them to actually be familial. They doubt the existence of sporadic cases. In Finnish families, half of the sons of a carrier woman develop optic atrophy, and 27% of asymptomatic men have peripapillary microangiopathy. Nearly all daughters of carrier women become carriers; 18% of them develop optic atrophy. Thirty-two percent are asymptomatic but have peripapillary microangiopathy.

In Leber's hereditary optic neuropathy, a point mutation has been found at position 11778 in the mitochondrial genome, the mitochondrial DNA responsible for the production of one of the enzymes in the respiratory chain. It is present in some but not all mitochondria. Adenosine triphosphate (ATP) is manufactured but at a lower level, leading to variable involvement of different systems. Wallace et al.[2] found the mutation in all maternal-related members, whether or not affected, in 9 of 11 families with Leber's hereditary optic neuropathy, but in none of the control subjects. As pointed out by Singh et al.,[3] restriction fragment analysis in three independent families has indicated at least two independent occurrences. Parker et al.[4] found corroboratory levels of the affected enzyme in blood platelets of patients with Leber's hereditary optic neuropathy. This important discovery provides a definitive diagnostic blood test when positive.

It would seem likely that the development of a clinical optic neuropathy in close sequence in the two eyes reflects some added, possibly environmental, precipitating factor. In view of the premonitory and coinciding dilatation of peripapillary vessels (and perhaps attendant ischemic axonal swelling and dysfunction) in the setting of an underlying defect in the respiratory enzyme chain, it would seem reasonable that such a factor might be cyanide.[3, 4] Further circumstantial evidence for a role of cyanide was provided in a recent study in which elevated blood cyanide levels were found in patients with the acute, but not the chronic, stage of Leber's hereditary optic neuropathy.[5] However, leukocyte rhodanese levels were normal in all. This would lend support to the use of hydroxocabalamine after the first eye is affected and perhaps the use of medication for long-term prophylaxis in those predisposed by the fundus findings, family history, or positive blood test. The avoidance of tobacco, alcohol, and foods containing cyanide might also be a helpful measure.

Further studies by Wallace's group[6] of the mixture of mutant and normal mitochondrial DNA molecules (heteroplasmy) within families and the tissues of individuals with Leber's hereditary optic neuropathy have shown that the proportion of mutant mitochondrial DNA varies in both circumstances. Cases appearing sporadic may represent the first clinical manifestation of a mutation, closer to its origin and more likely heteroplasmic.[7] In one such isolated case with homoplasmy, heteroplasmy was found in the patient's mother and in some of his siblings.[6] The variability in the proportion of mutant mitochondrial DNA in family members and within their various tissues is likely a factor in determining whether or when optic neuropathy occurs.[7]

PAPILLEDEMA

The 30 degree test with standardized A-scan echography, which has been used to demonstrate fluid within the optic nerve sheaths, was carried out immediately before and after lumbar puncture in a patient with asymptomatic papilledema from pseudotumor cerebri.[8] Opening pressure was 320 mm of cerebrospinal fluid. Anterior optic nerve thickness was initially 4.6 mm in the right eye and 4.1 mm in the left eye in the primary position with the presence of compressible fluid. Thickness was 3.1 mm in eccentric gaze (normal values, 2.22 to 3.3 mm). After lumbar puncture, the thickness was 2.6 mm in the right eye and 2.8 mm in the left eye without change on eccentric gaze in the absence of compressible fluid. Gittinger and Asdourian[9] remind us of the occurrence of macular changes that may be symptomatic in patients with papilledema from pseudotumor cerebri as has previously been reported.[10] These changes may be consequent to macular edema or traction on the macula.

Verplanck et al.[11] found that contrast grating sensitivity was a valuable adjunct to conventional perimetry in detecting visual loss in 15 women with the acute onset of pseudotumor cerebri. Visual evoked potentials rarely proved helpful. Contrast sensitivity was abnormal in 18 eyes and was the only abnormality in 9. Perimetry was abnormal in 13 and was the only abnormality in 5. The visual evoked response was abnormal in 5 and was the only abnormality in 1. Tytla and Buncic[12] also studied contrast sensitivity in obstructive hydrocephalus and pseudotumor cerebri before and after shunting. In the first 3 days after shunting, contrast sensitivity was unchanged but rapidly became normal by day 4 to 6 and remained normal for up to a year. They used these data in considering four possible mechanisms for the reversible impairment. Simple conduction block could have been expected to have resolved when the pressure had become normal (within 24 hours). Remyelination takes too long for demyelination to be the basis. Accumulation of intraaxonal material takes too long to resolve as indicated by the delay in recovery of the papilledema. The fourth mechanism, which they favored, was ischemia from compression of fine vessels by swollen axons. They pointed out that endoneural pressure "gradually subsides, slowly decompressing the vasculature until perfusion becomes adequate and then functional responsiveness can be expected abruptly to return." Another report of unilateral papilledema in pseudotumor cerebri[13] focused on asymmetry in sheath transmission. This is certainly a factor in some cases, but they did not consider the alternative explanation proposed by Muci-Mendoza et al.[14] in a prior volume. Muci-Mendoza et al. thought that some local disk factor was important in at least some cases.

Pasquale et al.[15] reported a patient with pseudotumor cerebri from dural sinus thrombosis. A search for coagulation abnormalities discovered a possible protein S deficiency and dysfibrinogenemia. Two patients were reported with pseudotumor cerebri attributed to danazol.[16] One of them had venous sinus thrombosis and the other had no apparent mechanism. Two patients with severe visual loss from chronic papilledema were found to have large intracranial arteriovenous malformations.[17] The POEMS (polyneuropathy, organomegaly, endocrinopathy, M protein, skin changes) syndrome was reviewed in a study from the Mayo Clinic.[18] Of the 148 patients in their study with monoclonal gammopathy and peripheral neuropathy, 11 were found to have POEMS syndrome. Eight of the 11 patients and two thirds of patients in other series have had disk swelling. In some, but not all, it is the result of increased intracranial pressure.

The October 1988 issue of the Archives of Ophthalmology contains reports of three substantial series of patients[19, 20, 21] treated effectively for chronic papilledema and progressive visual loss consequent to pseudotumor cerebri with optic nerve sheath fenestration. There was an accompanying editorial in the same issue by Keltner.[22] The first series[19, 20] used a medial orbital approach as originally described by Galbraith and Sullivan.[23] Sergott et al.[20] modified the procedure by adding multiple slits in an attempt to avoid plugging with orbital fat and also the use of lysis of arachnoidal adhesions to attempt to prevent loculation.

The third series[21] used a lateral orbitotomy. They preferred this because they thought it allowed more direct visualization of the optic nerve and because it is a procedure that is more familiar to orbital surgeons. The procedure was described in detail in a separate article.[24] Lateral orbitotomy of course requires general anesthesia and a skin incision, and there is a greater potential for damage to the ciliary ganglion. The medial approach provides quicker access to the nerve, but there is a greater chance of damaging the medial rectus muscle and producing transient diplopia. In some cases approached medially, a lateral orbitotomy must be added for better exposure. It would appear that both procedures are satisfactory. The mechanism of action of fenestration is controversial and summarized by Keltner.[22] It may be continued filtration or it may be that scarring develops in the subarachnoid space of the nerve which prevents accumulation of fluid. There is evidence supporting both mechanisms, but we also think that ongoing filtration is most likely to be the mechanism.

Brourman et al.[19] reported that 4 of 6 patients enjoyed relief of headache after optic nerve sheath decompression. They also noted that in 4 patients, iopamidol injected intrathecally completely filled the subarachnoid space of the nerve 1 day to 4 months after surgery. In the series of Sergott et al.,[20] 12 of 17 cases of unilateral sheath decompression showed bilateral resolution of papilledema and in 13 of these cases, headache improved or resolved. In the series of Corbett et al.,[21] 9 of 16 patients showed bilateral resolution of papilledema after unilateral sheath decompression. In 10, headache improved. Keltner[22] suggested that the variable pattern of communication between the orbital and intracranial subarachnoid spaces is the explanation for the variability in the degree of resolution of contralateral papilledema and relief of headache. He concurs with the recommendation of Sergott et al.[20] of multiple openings in the optic nerve sheath and lysis of subarachnoid trabeculae to maximize the potential for filtration. Keltner further suggested that ongoing filtration may not be of sufficient magnitude to produce a measurable decrease in intracranial pressure.

In the three series reported in the Archives of Ophthalmology, the visual response was generally excellent after optic nerve sheath decompression. Vision improved in all 10 operated eyes of 6 patients in one series,[19] in 21 of 23 patients in the second series (the other 2 improved after re-operation that was necessitated by fat plugging the window),[20] and in 12 of 40 eyes of 28 patients in the third series.[21] In that series, 22 eyes were unchanged.

The reason for the less favorable results in the series of Corbett et al. are not completely clear, but probably the difference cannot be solely the result of differenes in surgical technique. Complications also were more prevalent in their series. Keltner[22] mentioned the deaths of two patients with secondary pseudotumor cerebri (vasculitic or thrombotic) after sheath decompression. This would indicate the advisability of careful preoperative study of patients for possible predisposition to complications.

Overall, these three series indicate that optic nerve sheath decompression is safe and effective in preventing, and perhaps even reversing, progressive visual loss. It also may lessen headache. Sergott et al.[20] point out that subsequent shunt or corticosteroid therapy was not required in any of their patients for headache. Keltner concludes that optic nerve sheath fenestration has become the favored alternative to lumboperitoneal shunt when surgery is indicated for progressive visual loss in pseudotumor cerebri. However, we agree with Keltner that lumboperitoneal shunts in our experience have been better than the authors of the three series would suggest. Unilateral sheath decompression is recommended unless severe bilateral visual loss or anesthesia risk justify a bilateral procedure. Multiple openings and lysis of trabeculae are warranted. The other eye should be operated on if there is continuing papilledema with progressive visual loss in the fellow eye before irreversible optic atrophy supervenes.[22] Unfortunately, the patency of the fenestration cannot be determined in instances of progressive postoperative visual loss except with repeat surgery. Readers are also advised to read the excellent review by Corbett and Thompson[25] on the management of pseudotumor cerebri. They reemphasize the importance of frequent visual evaluations in pseudotumor cerebri. Quantitative perimetry should be performed monthly. They discount the value of the visual evoked response or measurement of the intracranial pressure with frequent lumbar punctures.

There was an additional report of optic nerve fenestration by Herzau[26] in 15 of 50 patients with pseudotumor cerebri. There was resolution of papilledema in nearly all cases but there was less improvement in vision than that reported in the other series. Three patients had progression. Herzau noted that the operation was ineffective in patients with severe chronic atrophic papilledema. Guy et al.[27] reported the association of pseudotumor cerebri with renal insufficiency. Again, optic nerve sheath decompression appeared to be of benefit. Some of the aggravating factors that might have been important included hypertension and elevation of the vitamin A level (from impaired excretion). The possibility of hypotension with renal dialysis was mentioned as an indication for sheath decompression in such patients.

ISCHEMIC OPTIC NEUROPATHY

A fifth study[29] confirmed that crowding of the optic disk appears to predispose patients to non-arteritic anterior ischemic optic neuropathy (AION). This has been found repeatedly in prior studies of cup-disk diameter. In the present study, horizontal disk diameter and area (but not vertical disk diameter) were smaller in the fellow eyes of patients with AION than they were in control subjects.

Tomsak and Remler[30] reported elevated intraocular pressure in 5 of 56 consecutive patients with AION who had been referred for neuro-ophthalmologic consultation. All of them had very small optic cups. This suggests an increased incidence of elevated intraocular pressure. As they indicated, Hayreh had found this association in patients with early AION after cataract[31, 32] and presumed that the pressure changes had decreased the arteriovenous perfusion gradient. Katz[33] had reported higher peaks of intraocular pressure in patients with AION. It was over 21 mm Hg in 7 of 16 of his patients but in none of the age- and race-matched control subjects. It is as yet uncertain as to whether intraocular pressure elevation plays a role in the pathogenesis of AION. In patients with elevated intraocular pressure who have AION, it is widespread neuro-ophthalmologic practice to bring down the intraocular pressure to avoid any possible contribution to the progression of the disease. Tomsak and Remler[30] emphasized the possible importance of prophylaxis for the fellow eye.

Borchert and Lessell[34] emphasized the occurrence of stepwise, gradual or even prolonged progression of visual impairment in AION. They also reported late recurrences (after resolution of disk swelling), which probably occurred in two of their patients. They reminded us of the hypothesis originally suggested by Lavin and Ellenberger,[35] with which we are in agreement, that decreased disk crowding from atrophy explains the rarity of late recurrence by preventing the cascading effect of disk swelling leading to further small vessel compromise as well summarized by Beck et al.[36] Borchert and Lessell[34] further suggested that relative sparing of axons initially might also render patients susceptible to progression during the period of swelling. As they suggested, their cases (except perhaps for case 10) buttressed this predisposition to progression or recurrence, a term that we reserve for late recurrence. It has been our experience as well that late recurrence tends to reflect milder initial involvement, which we suspect likely to also be the case when there is progression. We should also mention that we have occasionally observed late progression of the visual deficit even in the absence of disk edema.

The possible importance of preserved axons as a factor predisposing to progression and recurrence might justify the suggestion made by one of us (J. G. O.) that panretinal laser photocoagulation of the fellow eye might be of value in preventing involvement. In collaboration with Dr. L. Yannuzzi, we are considering a trial. However, we note that the cup-disk ratios were not affected in a series of 100 patients with diabetic retinopathy in which one eye was treated with argon laser or xenon arc and compared after 1 year with the fellow eye.[37] That study was prompted by the observation of visual field defects and disk pallor after panretinal photocoagulation. The atrophy clearly is a consequence of heavy photocoagulation at least in experimental circumstances.[38]

The progressive course of some patients with AION as in Borchert and Lessell's report[34] (two with progression over several months) lends potential value to the expedited publication of preliminary favorable results by Sergott et al.[39] in a study of optic nerve sheath decompression in the progressive form of AION. They found that visual function improved in 12 (clearly so according to our interpretation in 8) of 14 cases but in only 1 of 3 with the nonprogressive variety and in 2 of 15 with nonprogressive AION who were not subjected to surgery. While four examiners were involved, this was not a conclusive rigorous study. As the authors themselves point out, the study was not done in masked fashion. The rationale underlying the initiation of the surgical trial was the capacity of vision to be reversed in chronic papilledema following optic nerve sheath decompression. This was buttressed by their finding at surgery that "the optic nerve sheaths were distended, similar in appearance to the nerve sheaths we have observed in pseudotumor cerebri," with which the authors have extensive experience. They thought that the nerve itself appeared grossly normal and "incision of the retrobulbar meningeal sheath resulted in the release of considerable amount of clear cerebrospinal fluid (CSF)." It seems surprising to us that "the quantity of CSF was insufficient for chemical analysis." Certainly if the optic nerve sheaths are distended (the reason for which is unclear in any case), there would be rationale for decompression in the face of ongoing progression of visual loss in AION over a period of weeks. The authors suggest that there was reversibility in cases performed between 4 and 30 (mean 20) days. Even though the results are preliminary, this procedure would seem reasonable in some cases, hopefully some in a well-organized study.

Improvement of an involved fellow eye in two of the cases is astounding, but one of us (M.B.) has seen this occur in a patient without surgery. The authors suggest that it may reflect decompression of the perineural subarachnoid space of the fellow eye as in pseudotumor cerebri surgery. It also could be that effort on the part of the patient and/or the examiner could explain some of the improvement. The findings of Sergott et al. would suggest that distal optic nerve appearance should be studied with ultrasound (possibly with the 30 degree test by A scan) and with thin section computed tomography and/or magnetic resonance imaging in AION. If the authors' finding of sheath distension in progressive cases is substantiated by these tests, it would further justify use of the procedure and also help to determine in which cases it is apt to be useful. In the meantime, their cautious advocacy of surgery in special cases seems reasonable. Those cases would be of AION with continuing progression over weeks.

Sergott et al.[40] also found that optic nerve sheath decompression was useful in treating the optic neuropathy associated with acute retinal necrosis syndrome. An enlarged optic nerve silhouette had been demonstrated in all six patients who underwent decompression.

Portnoy et al.[41] reported a case of embolic AION. That patient had apoplectic onset and multiple retinal cholesterol emboli of carotid atherosclerotic origin. There was also choroidal hypoperfusion adjacent to a mildly swollen disk. Temporal field loss was present.

There was another report of recurrent but otherwise characteristic AION in young adults.[42] Again, the relatively mild involvement in youth with persistent crowding may favor recurrence. Drusen were ruled out with computed tomography. The possibility of migraine was raised, although there was no evidence for it in the history. They also discussed the possible connection to the big blind spot syndrome and optic disk vasculitis.

Another study[43] pertinent to amiodarone-related papillopathy (see the previous volume) also suggested a toxic basis. A patient on amiodarone without papillopathy had evidence on post-mortem examination of "selective accumulation of intracytoplasmic lamellar inclusions in the large axons" of the optic nerve on electron microscopy.

There was an additional report[44] of a case of bilateral uremic optic neuropathy. It had not responded to corticosteroid therapy but did improve with dialysis. As pointed out in the accompanying editorial,[45] this resembled some of the cases reported by Knox et al.,[46] which were reviewed in the last volume. There was an additional report[47] of three patients with bilateral optic neuropathy occurring while they were receiving hemodialysis that was attributed to other specific etiologies. This study pointed up the heterogeneity of the optic neuropathy in patients with uremia. One case was reversible and attributed to deferoxamine chelation therapy. Another was from chronically increased intracranial pressure. Finally, there was one with typical but severe consecutive AION.

TRAUMA AND DECOMPRESSION

The optimal management of posttraumatic optic neuropathy has not yet been determined. Lessell[48] summarized his experience with 33 cases in the era of computed tomography over 11 years. Thirty of the cases were unilateral. The optic canal was affected by a fracture in only 7, although 10 others had skull fractures elsewhere. The fracture and the optic neuropathy are both consequences of mechanical trauma but not interrelated in most cases as to cause and effect. Twenty-seven of the patients had loss of consciousness, which correlated poorly with final visual acuity.

Of particular importance was the follow-up data on outcome in relation to therapy. Vision improved in 5 of 25 untreated patients, 1 of 4 treated with corticosteroids, and 3 of 4 treated with corticosteroids and transethmoidal optical canal decompression. In neither group was megadose corticosteroids used initially as suggested by Anderson et al.[49] in delayed visual loss. This is the only situation in which we, in the tradition of Walsh, have been therapeutically aggressive. Lessell pointed out that in none of his patients was vision lost after the first examination.

This may explain the relatively high number of untreated patients. Fractures, two of the canal and one adjacent, were present in 3 of the 4 cases that were surgically decompressed. He pointed out that improvement occurred in a higher percentage of those treated with corticosteroids and surgery and that the numbers were too small for meaningful conclusions. In addition, since 2 patients with immediate loss of light perception had some recovery without treatment, he made the valid point that the interdiction of surgery in all such cases is illogical. This is certainly true for the use of corticosteroid therapy, which is increasingly offered in high doses to such patients.

Further support for this mode of therapy comes from a recent study on the early treatment of acute spinal cord injury.[50] Lessell concluded that a randomized prospective study would be desirable to clarify the optimal management but was impractical and suggested that the approach to this might be with a central data bank. This suggestion was echoed by Wolin and Lavin,[51] who reported four patients with traumatic optic neuropathy, although not pure indirect trauma in view of associated ocular and orbital injury in which there was immediate loss of light perception but substantial recovery of vision without surgical intervention. In one patient, recovery began after 6 days without corticosteroids and in two others, the recovery began before corticosteroid therapy was initiated. Their experience led them to question the need for surgical decompression in the absence of a compressive lesion not only in cases of immediate visual loss but also with delayed visual loss not responding to high-dose corticosteroid therapy.

Three of Lessell's cases were bilateral with a presumed optic nerve basis. In the era of magnetic resonance imaging, one case has been reported[52] with delayed progressive bilateral visual loss due to hemorrhage and swelling within the optic nerves and chiasm following frontal trauma. These abnormalities were not appreciated on computed tomography. There was moderate recovery, apparently without corticosteroid therapy.

Orbital complications of sinus surgery were reviewed in nine patients,[53] including one case in which both optic nerves were transected during bilateral intranasal endoscopic ethmoidectomy. In three, there was intraoperative orbital hemorrhage during external or intranasal ethmoidectomy. To assist in early recognition of orbital involvement during sinus surgery, it was suggested that the eye remain uncovered intraoperatively and that tarsorrhaphy be avoided. Intraoperative recognition of subtle eye movement abnormalities, lid retraction, or subconjunctival hemorrhage should suggest orbital penetration. A strategy for treating an expanding orbital hematoma to prevent loss of vision was presented.

Guy et al.[54] reported the successful treatment of severe optic neuropathy in five patients with thyroid ophthalmopathy. They used 1 g of methylprednisolone each day for 3 days and maintained the remission with oral prednisone and radiation therapy. This seems an appropriate means of treatment in patients who fail to respond to oral prednisone, as pointed out in the discussion by Feldon. It is a logical conclusion to the early recognition by Day and Carroll[55] of the beneficial effect of systemic corticosteroid therapy in such patients when administered in sufficient dosage. They drew attention to the risks of complications with prolonged therapy, but this may be obviated by the addition of radiation therapy as in the current report.

Surgical decompression of the orbit for thyroid ophthalmopathy was reviewed in 60 consecutive patients by Mourits et al.[56] Twenty-five patients were treated with surgery alone for optic neuropathy (bilateral in all but 1). The authors compared three approaches and found that each approach worked in two thirds of the cases. For cosmetic reasons, they favored a coronal approach. Leone et al.[57] advocated medial and lateral (two-wall) decompression. They thought that this minimized the complications associated with removal of the orbital floor. They found that this procedure was adequate in the 8 patients in their study, 2 of whom had an optic neuropathy.

A case of pseudo-Schnabel's cavernous degeneration of the optic nerve was reported.[58] Coalescent globules of silicone oil had infiltrated the optic nerve following enucleation for painful glaucoma several years after vitrectomy and silicone oil implantation. This supports the hypothesis that fluid from the vitreous cavity fills the cystic spaces in cavernous degeneration of the optic nerve.[59]

Delayed radiation necrosis of the anterior visual pathway is a serious complication that is difficult to treat. A follow-up report on the value of hyperbaric oxygen concluded that there was no benefit.[60] This is in contrast to the initial suggestion from the same group[61] that it was of value! Thirteen patients were treated (11 also with corticosteroids), and there was no improvement in any of them during or after treatment. The follow-up period was 1 to 4 years. However, hyperbaric oxygen therapy has been valuable in radiation necrosis of bone[62] and possibly earlier treatment might be of value. There were other reports of delayed radiation necrosis of the anterior visual pathway,[63, 64] including the not-surprising occurrence of necrosis after radiation therapy for an optico-hypothalamic glioma.[63] These authors emphasized (and we agree) that the onset occasionally is somewhat sooner than generally believed, about 5 months. The authors also reminded us about the detrimental effects of radiation on the developing brain.

TOXICITY

A case of methanol-induced optic neuropathy was reported[65] in which early recognition was achieved, before the availability of blood levels, by elevation of the anion and osmolal gaps. This also occurs with ethylene glycol ingestion and allowed proper correction of the metabolic acidosis as well as the administration of ethanol and removal of methanol with hemodialysis.

A case of remitting optic neuropathy was reported[66] in a patient receiving therapeutic doses of phenobarbital to which it was attributed. This must be an exceedingly rare occurrence. Although an alternative etiology was not found, it cannot be ruled out. The asymmetry of involvement with a relative afferent pupillary defect is somewhat against a toxic origin. Similar considerations led Miller to caution against accepting a case report of a single small dose of vincristine as a cause of optic atrophy.[67] Vrabec et al.[68] reported a patient with bilateral centrocecal scotomas following large and prolonged oral doses of ciprofloxacin hydrochloride (Cipro). It improved at the cessation of this broad-spectrum antibiotic, which is structurally similar to other quinolone compounds that have been associated with an optic neuropathy. The patient's remote alcoholism was convincingly discounted as a factor. The authors advised monitoring optic nerve function in patients receiving high doses of ciprofloxacin hydrochloride.

ANOMALIES

The definitive clinical diagnosis of optic nerve hypoplasia in a young child has been made easier by Romano,[69] who reported horizontal optic nerve diameter in 35-mm transparencies taken with one of the standard fundus cameras. The range was 3.44 to 4.70 mm (mean, 3.88 mm) in 55 healthy children, all of whom were under the age of 18 years and had no significant refractive error. In 16 eyes with clinically confirmed optic nerve hypoplasia, the range was 1.80 to 3.27 mm (mean, 2.64 mm). There was no overlap, leading him to conclude that a 3.4-mm horizontal optic disk diameter in a standardized 35-mm photograph can be used as a dividing line; smaller nerves are considered hypoplastic. This is certainly helpful with regard to frank hypoplasia of clinical significance; however, minor forms may remain in the indeterminant zone, and segmental hypoplasia would not be detected by this means.[70] The author is continuing to collect data for further clarification of the extent of the gap between hypoplastic and normal disk.

Septo-optic dysplasia received attention in several reports. Roessmann[71] reviewed its historical evolution (the DeMorsier syndrome) since the important reports of Hoyt et al.[72] and Kaplan et al.[73] in 1970. With increased recognition and the new noninvasive neuroimaging techniques, there has been a mushrooming of reported cases with varied presence and prominence or absence of components of the syndrome as appreciated ophthalmologically, endocrinologically, or neuroradiologically. In two patients with optic nerve hypoplasia and endocrine defects but normal computed tomography scans of midline brain anatomy, Kaufman et al.[74] found hypoplasia of the pituitary stalk on magnetic resonance imaging. A recent report[75] described a full-blown syndrome of septo-optic dysplasia in two siblings, raising the possibility of autosomal-recessive inheritance. The presence of neurologic abnormalities in both patients prompted the authors to review published reports, which they found to include 48 cases in which the neurologic status was described. Forty-two percent of these cases showed such defects. Among them, half had seizures, 40% were retarded, and 15% had hemiparesis.

An infant with deletion of chromosome 17 was reported with unilateral symptomatic optic nerve hypoplasia in association with congenital optic disk pigmentation. This gave the appearance of gray optic disks, the differential diagnosis of which was discussed.[76]

Bass and Sherman[77] recorded delays in the visual evoked response to pattern stimuli in a series of patients with the tilted disk syndrome. In some of their cases, however, other factors such as amblyopia might contribute.

Nearly half of a family of 35 were affected by a spectrum of cavitary optic disk abnormalities (optic nerve pit or coloboma and large anomalous disk) with some evidence of prior macula elevation in some instances.[78] An autosomal-dominant inheritance with variable expressivity was presumed to be the basis for this spectrum of anomalies that they did not attribute to simple failure of closure of the embryonic fissure of the globe, since none had typical colobomas. The authors postulated failure of formation of the fissure posteriorly with a secondary anomalous course of the primitive hyaloid artery.

An infant was reported[79] with bilateral optic nerve hypoplasia with deep central excavation, suggesting colobomas. These were in continuity with retrobulbar cystic masses which on magnetic resonance imaging appeared to contain vitreous. These resemble the lesion illustrated in the last volume. The electroretinogram was normal but the visual evoked response was not elicited.

Another instance of progressive visual loss in the presence of an optic disk anomaly, in this instance coloboma, appropriately prompted computed tomography. This demonstrated a middle fossa arachnoid cyst compressing the optic nerve.[80] A patient with optic nerve head disk drusen was reported with apparently related peripapillary central serous choroidopathy with a typical focal leak[81] without evidence of subretinal neovascularization, which is known to occur with disk drusen. A 25-year-old woman with disk drusen was reported,[82] who also had migraine and developed central retinal artery occlusion in both eyes without any other evident basis. The occlusion in the second eye followed the first by 8 years during which time she had episodic fleeting amaurosis. She had been given one 20 mg propranolol tablet the day before the central retinal artery occlusion. Katz[83] had pointed out a possible relationship of this medication with vascular occlusion. It was suggested, as seems reasonable, that the combination of disk drusen and migraine diathesis may have been responsible since retinal vascular occlusion may occur with either disease in a young patient.

REFERENCES

1. Nikoskelainen E, Nummelin K, Savontaus M-L: Does sporadic Leber's disease exist? *J Clin Neuro Ophthalmol* 1988; 8:225–229.
2. Wallace DC, Singh G, Lott MT, et al: Mitochondrial DNA mutation associated with Leber's hereditary optic neuropathy. *Science* 1988; 242:1427.
3. Singh G, Lott MT, Wallace DC: A mitochondrial DNA mutation as a cause of Leber's hereditary optic neuropathy. *N Engl J Med* 1989; 320:1300–1305.
4. Parker WD Jr, Oley CA, Karks JK: A defect in mitochondrial electron-transport activity (NADH-coenzyme Q oxidoreductase) in Leber's hereditary optic neuropathy. *N Engl J Med* 1989; 320:1331–1333.

5. Berninger TA, Meyer LV, Siess E, et al: Leber's hereditary optic atrophy: Further evidence for a defect of cyanide metabolism. *Br J Ophthalmol* 1989; 73:314–316.

6. Lott MT, Voljavec AS, Wallace DC: Variable genotype of Leber's hereditary optic neuropathy patients. *Am J Ophthalmol* 1990; 109:625–631.

7. Newman NJ, Wallace DC: Mitochondria and Leber's hereditary optic neuropathy. *Am J Ophthalmol* 1990; 109:726–727.

8. Galetta S, Byrne SF, Smith JL: Echographic correlation of optic nerve sheath size and cerebrospinal fluid pressure. *J Clin Neuro Ophthalmol* 1989; 9:79–82.

9. Gittinger JW Jr, Asdourian GK: Macular abnormalities in papilledema from pseudotumor cerebri. *Ophthalmology* 1989; 96:192–194.

10. Morris AT, Sanders MD: Macular changes resulting from papilledema. *Br J Ophthalmol* 1980; 64:211–216.

11. Verplanck M, Kaufman DI, Parson T, et al: Electrophysiology versus psychophysics in the detection of visual loss in pseudotumor cerebri. *Neurology* 1988; 38:1789–1792.

12. Tytla ME, Buncic JR: Recovery of spatial vision following shunting for hydrocephalus. *Arch Ophthalmol* 1990; 108:701–704.

13. To KW, Warren FA: Unilateral papilledema in pseudotumor cerebri. *Arch Ophthalmol* 1990; 108:644–645.

14. Muci-Mendoza R, Arruga J, Hoyt WF: Distension bilateral del Espacio Subaracnoideo Perioptico en el Pseudotumor Cerebri con Papiledema Unilateral: Su demonstracion a traves de la tomografia computarizada de la orbita. *Rev Neurol (Barc)* 1981; 39:11.

15. Pasquale LR, Moster ML, Schmaier A: Dural sinus thrombosis with abnormalities of protein S and fibrinogen. *Arch Ophthalmol* 1990; 108:644.

16. Hamed LM, Glaser JS, Schatz NJ, et al: Pseudotumor cerebri induced by danazol. *Am J Ophthalmol* 1989; 107:105–110.

17. Kashii S, Solomon SK, Moser FG, et al: Progressive visual field defects in patients with intracranial arteriovenous malformations. *Am J Ophthalmol* 1990; 109:556–562.

18. Bolling JP, Brazis PW: Optic disk swelling with peripheral neuropathy, organomegaly, endocrinopathy, monoclonal gammopathy, and skin changes (POEMS syndrome). *Am J Ophthalmol* 1990; 109:503–510.

19. Brourman ND, Spoor TC, Ramocki JM: Optic nerve sheath decompression for pseudotumor cerebri. *Arch Ophthalmol* 1988; 106:1378.

20. Sergott RC, Savino PJ, Bosley TM: Modified optic nerve sheath decompression provides long-term visual improvement for pseudotumor cerebri. *Arch Ophthalmol* 1988; 106:1384–1390.

21. Corbett JJ, Nerad JA, Tse DT, et al: Results of optic nerve sheath fenestration for pseudotumor cerebri. *Arch Ophthalmol* 1988; 106:1391–1397.

22. Keltner JL: Optic nerve sheath decompression. How does it work? Has its time come? *Arch Ophthalmol* 1988; 106:1365–1369.

23. Galbraith JEK, Sullivan JH: Decompression of the perioptic meninges for relief of papilledema. *Am J Ophthalmol* 1973; 76:687–692.

24. Tse DT, Nerad JA, Anderson RL, et al: Optic nerve sheath fenestration in pseudotumor cerebri. *Arch Ophthalmol* 1988; 106:1458–1462.

25. Corbett JJ, Thompson HS: The rational management of idiopathic intracranial hypertension. *Arch Neurol* 1989; 46:1049–1051.

26. Herzau V: Fenestration of optic nerve sheaths in pseudotumor cerebri. *Neuro Ophthalmol* 1989; 9:65–72.

27. Guy J, Johnston PK, Corbett JJ, et al: Treatment of visual loss in pseudotumor cerebri associated with uremia. *Neurology* 1990; 40:28–32.

29. Mansour AH, Shoch D, Logani S: Optic disk size in ischemic optic neuropathy. *Am J Ophthalmol* 1988; 106:587–589.

30. Tomsak RL, Remler BF: Anterior ischemic optic neuropathy and increased intraocular pressure. *J Clin Neuro Ophthalmol* 1989; 9:116–118.

31. Hayreh SS: Anterior ischemic optic neuropathy IV. Occurrence after cataract extraction. *Arch Ophthalmol* 1980; 98:1410–1416.

32. Serrano LA, Behrens MM, Carroll FD: Postcataract extraction ischemic optic neuropathy. *Arch Ophthalmol* 1982; 100:1177.

33. Katz B, Weinreb RN, Wheeler D: Ischemic optic neuropathy and intraocular pressure (abstract). *Ophthalmology* 1987; 94:92.

34. Borchert M, Lessell S: Progressive and recurrent nonarteritic anterior ischemic optic neuropathy. *Am J Ophthalmol* 1988; 106:443–449.

35. Lavin PJM, Ellenberger C Jr: Recurrent ischemic optic neuropathy. *Neuro Ophthalmology* 1983; 3:193–198.

36. Beck RW, Servais GE, Hayreh SS: Anterior ischemic optic neuropathy IX. Cup-to-disc ratio and its role in pathogenesis. *Ophthalmology* 1987; 94:1503–1508.

37. Johns KJ, Leonard-Martin T, Feman SS: The effect of panretinal photocoagulation on optic nerve cupping. *Ophthalmology* 1989; 96:211–216.

38. Radius RL, Anderson DR: The mechanism of disc pallor in experimental optic atrophy: A fluorescein angiographic study. *Arch Ophthalmol* 1979; 97:532–537.

39. Sergott RC, Cohen MS, Bosley TM, et al: Optic nerve decompression may improve the progressive form of nonarteritic ischemic optic neuropathy. *Arch Ophthalmol* 1989; 107:1743–1754.

40. Sergott RC, Anand R, Belmont JB, et al: Acute retinal necrosis neuropathy. Clinical profile and surgical therapy. *Arch Ophthalmol* 1989; 107:692–696.

41. Portnoy SL, Beer PM, Packer AJ, et al: Embolic anterior ischemic optic neuropathy. *J Clin Neuro Ophthalmol* 1989; 9:21–25.

42. Hamed LM, Purvin L, Rosenberg M: Recurrent anterior ischemic optic neuropathy in young adults. *J Clin Neuro Ophthalmol* 1988; 8:239–246.

43. Mansour AM, Puklin JE, O'Grady R: Optic nerve ultra-structure following amiodarone therapy. *J Clin Neuro Ophthalmol* 1988; 8:231–237.

44. Saini JS, Jain JS, Dhar S, et al: Uremic optic neuropathy. *J Clin Neuro Ophthalmol* 1989; 9:131–133.

45. Editorial Comment. Optic neuropathy in uremia. *J Clin Neuro Ophthalmol* 1989; 9:134–135.

46. Knox DL, Hanneken AM, Hollows C, et al: Uremic optic neuropathy. *Arch Ophthalmol* 1988; 106:50–54.

47. Hamed LM, Winward KE, Glaser JS, et al: Optic neuropathy in uremia. *Am J Ophthalmol* 1989; 108:30–35.

48. Lessell S: Indirect optic nerve trauma. *Arch Ophthalmol* 1989; 107:382–386.

49. Anderson RL, Panje WR, Gross CE: Optic nerve blindness following blunt forehead trauma. *Ophthalmology* 1982; 89:445–455.

50. Bracken MB, Shepard MJ, Collins WF, et al: A randomized, controlled trial of methylprednisolone or naloxone in the treatment of acute spinal-cord injury: Results of the second National acute spinal cord injury study. *N Engl J Med* 1990; 322:1405–1411.

51. Wolin MJ, Lavin PJM: Spontaneous visual recovery from traumatic optic neuropathy after blunt head injury. *Ophthalmology* 1990; 109:430–435.

52. Crowe NW, Nickles TP, Troost BT, et al: Intrachiasmal hemorrhage: A cause of delayed post-tramatic blindness. *Neurology* 1989; 39:863–865.

53. Buus DR, Tse DT, Farris BK: Ophthalmic complications of sinus surgery. *Ophthalmology* 1990; 97:612–619.

54. Guy JR, Fagien S, Donovan JP, et al: Methylprednisolone pulse therapy in severe dysthroid optic neuropathy. *Ophthalmology* 1989; 96:1048–1053.

55. Day RM, Carroll FD: Corticosteroids in the treatment of optic nerve involvement. *Arch Ophthalmol* 1968; 79:279–282.

56. Mourits M, Koornneef L, Wiersinga WM, et al: Orbital decompression for Grave's ophthalmopathy by inferomedial, by inferomedial plus lateral, and by coronal approach. *Ophthalmology* 1990; 97:636–641.

57. Leone CR Jr, Piest KL, Newman RJ: Medial and lateral wall decompression for thyroid ophthalmopathy. *Am J Ophthalmol* 1989; 108:160–166.

58. Shields CL, Eagle RC Jr: Pseudo-Schnabel's cavernous degeneration of the optic nerve secondary to intraocular silicone oil. *Arch Ophthalmol* 1989; 107:714–717.

59. Zimmerman LE, deVenicia G, Hamasaki DI: Pathology of the optic nerve in experimental acute glaucoma. *Invest Ophthalmol Vis Sci* 1967; 6:109–125.

60. Roden D, Bosley TM, Fowble B, et al: Delayed radiation injury to the retrobulbar optic nerves and chiasm. Clinical syndrome and treatment with hyperbaric oxygen and corticosteroids. *Ophthalmology* 1990; 97:346–351.

61. Guy J, Schatz NJ: Hyperbaric oxygen in the treatment of radiation induced optic neuropathy. *Ophthalmology* 1986; 93:1083–1088.

62. Grim PS, Gottlieb LJ, Boddie A, et al: Hyperbaric oxygen therapy. *JAMA* 1990; 263:2216–2220.

63. Warman R, Glaser JS, Quencer RM: Radionecrosis of optico-hypothalamic glioma. *Neuro Ophthalmol* 1989; 9:219–226.

64. Pasquier F, Leys D, Dubois F, et al: Chiasm and optic nerve necrosis following radiation therapy. Report of two cases. *Neuro Ophthalmol* 1989; 9:331–336.

65. Greiner JV, Pillai S, Limaye SR, et al: Sterno-induced methanol toxicity and visual recovery after prompt hemodialysis. *Arch Ophthalmol* 1989; 107:643.

66. Homma K, Wakakura M, Ishikawa S: A case of phenobarbital-induced optic neuropathy. *Neuro Ophthalmol* 1989; 9:357.

67. Teichman KD, Dabbagh N: Severe visual loss after a single dose of vincristine in a patient with spinal cord astrocytoma. *Surv Ophthalmol* 1989; 34:149.

68. Vrabec TR, Sergott RC, Jaeger EA, et al: Reversible visual loss in a patient receiving high-dose ciprofloxacin hydrochloride (Cipro). *Ophthalmology* 1990; 97:707–710.

69. Romano PE: Simple photogrammetric diagnosis of optic nerve hypoplasia. *Arch Ophthalmol* 1989; 107:824–826.

70. Kim RY, Hoyt WF, Lessell S, et al: Superior segmental optic hypoplasia. A sign of maternal diabetes. *Arch Ophthalmol* 1989; 107:1312–1315.

71. Roessmann U: Septo-optic dysplasia (SOD) or DeMorsier syndrome. *J Clin Neuro Ophthalmol* 1989; 9:156–159.

72. Hoyt WF, Kaplan SL, Grumbach MM, et al: Septo-optic dysplasia and pituitary dwarfism. *Lancet* 1970; 1:893–894.

73. Kaplan SL, Grumbach MM, Hoyt WF: A syndrome of hypopituitary dwarfism, hypoplasia of optic nerves and malformation of porencephalon. *Pediatr Res* 1970; 4:480–481.

74. Kaufman LM, Miller MT, Mafee MF: Magnetic resonance imaging of pituitary stalk hypoplasia. A discrete midline anomaly associated with endocrine abnormalities in septo-optic dysplasia. *Arch Ophthalmol* 1989; 107:1485–1489.

75. Benner JD, Preslan MW, Gratz E, et al: Septo-optic dysplasia in two siblings. *Am J Ophthalmol* 1990; 109:632–637.
76. Brodsky MC, Buckley EG, McConkie-Rosell A: The case of the gray optic disc! *Surv Ophthalmol* 1989; 33:367–372.
77. Bass SJ, Sherman J: Visual evoked potential (VEP) delays in tilted and/or oblique entrance of the optic nerve head. *Neuro Ophthalmol* 1988; 8:109–122.
78. Slusher MM, Weaver RG Jr, Greven CM, et al: The spectrum of cavitary optic disc anomalies in a family. *Ophthalmol* 1989; 96:342–347.
79. Slamovits TL, Kimball GP, Friberg TR, et al: Bilateral optic disc colobomas with orbital cysts and hypoplastic optic nerves and chiasm. *J Clin Neuro Ophthalmol* 1989; 9:172–177.
80. Rosenberg LF, Burde RM: Progressive visual loss caused by an arachnoidal brain cyst in a patient with an optic nerve coloboma. *Am J Ophthalmol* 1988; 106:322–325.
81. Moisseiev J, Cahane M, Treister G: Optic nerve head drusen and peripapillary central serous chorioretinopathy. *Am J Ophthalmol* 1989; 108:202.
82. Newman NJ, Lessell S, Brandt EM: Bilateral central retinal artery occlusions, disk drusen, and migraine. *Am J Ophthalmol* 1989; 107:236–240.
83. Katz B: Migrainous central retinal artery occlusion. *J Clin Neuro Ophthalmol* 1986; 6:69.

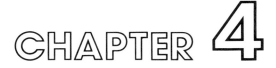

CHAPTER 4

The Optic Chiasm

Joel S. Glaser, M.D.

Professor, Ophthalmology, Neurology, and Neurologic Surgery, Bascom Palmer Eye Institute, Department of Ophthalmology, University of Miami School of Medicine, Miami, Florida

ANATOMY

The position of the optic chiasm in the suprasellar cistern has been subjected to analysis with magnetic resonance imaging (MRI).[1] The author determined an average optic chiasm-to-tuberculum distance of 3.8 mm (2.6 mm for women, 4.3 mm for men). The anatomic material was from 131 healthy individuals without sellar or optic chiasm disease and was studied in the sagittal plane. Because of difficulty in identifying the dorsum or diaphragma sellae, the distance of the optic chiasm to these important structures was not measured. All optic chiasma lay on a line roughly 45 degrees posterosuperior to the tuberculum, and none was observed wholly anterior to the tuberculum, although 15% of optic chiasma were positioned "very close" to the tuberculum. A comparison is made with the previous pneumographic studies of Bull (1956),[2] the autopsy cases of Bergland et al. (1968),[3] and the fine anatomic dissections of Rhoton et al. (1985).[4]

CONGENITAL ANOMALIES

Six autopsy cases of alobar holoprosencephaly[5] disclosed glioneuronal heterotopia most prominent and extensive in the prosencephalic base around the optic chiasm; the adjacent floor of the third ventricle was intermingled with excessive mesenchymal elements. These cases variably are associated with congenital hypopituitarism and eye anomalies. A rare familial occurrence of septo-optic dysplasia (SOD; deMorsier syndrome) is recorded in a sister and brother[6]; these cases are also associated with a hypoplastic corpus callosum and a diffusely dilated ventricular system. MRI in two cases of SOD with optic disk hypoplasia and multiple hormone insufficiencies disclosed absent pituitary stalks.[7] The association of *astigmatism* and optic nerve hypoplasia (ONH), with and without SOD, is reported,[8] which highlights the importance of careful retinoscopy to identify and correct refractive errors in children with ONH/SOD.

Brodsky et al.[9] provide high resolution MR images of 15 cases of optic nerve hypoplasia. On coronal and sagittal views, thin nerves with attenuated signals were demonstrable; all patients with severe bilateral hypoplasia showed diffuse optic chiasm hypoplasia. Orbital coronal sections were considered not useful because of chemical-shift artifacts and eye movements. Optic disk colobomas in association with orbital cysts and MRI evidence of hypoplastic optic nerves and chiasm is the subject of a case report.[10]

NEOPLASMS

Pituitary Adenomas

The pituitary gland in pregnancy was the subject of a histologic and immunocytochemical study of 69 autopsy specimens from women who died during pregnancy, after abortion, or in the postpartum period.[11] There was an accumulation of large mitosing chromophobic "pregnancy cells" immunoreactive for prolactin only. Hyperplasia of such prolactin cells was evident at 1 month gestation and, in some cases, accumulation resembled microadenomas. Among the 69 pituitary glands studied, there were eight noninvasive microadenomas (seven contained prolactin only). Prolactinomas were no more numerous or larger than those encountered in nonpregnant women or in men, suggesting that pregnancy neither initiates nor accelerates the growth of prolactin-secreting tumors.

What do you do with an incidentally discovered pituitary adenoma? First, consider that Kernohan and Sayre[12] reported that asymptomatic adenomas occur in more than 20% of pituitary glands examined at autopsy, and that some degree of adenomatous hyperplasia can be found in almost every pituitary gland. Another postmortem study[13] comprised pituitary glands removed from 120 individuals without clinical evidence of pituitary tumors, revealed a 27% incidence of microadenomas, of which 41% stained for prolactin without a gender difference.

To generalize, more than 1 in 10 people in the general population dies harboring a prolactinoma! The incessant parade of this clinical problem is, then, no surprise. Reincke et al.[14] now describe 18 patients with "incidentaloma" discovered with computed tomography (CT) or MRI performed for unrelated disease. Average mass size was estimated at 13 mm (range, 5 to 25 mm), and there were 2 instances of bitemporal hemianopia, partial hypopituitarism in 5 patients, and growth hormone secretion without acromegaly in one case. Fourteen patients were treated conservatively with repeat imaging and 4 underwent surgical procedures. The authors conclude that "it is rational to observe the clinical course carefully in patients with normal visual acuity and normal pituitary function." Serial neuroimaging, pituitary function tests, and ophthalmologic reexamination [quantitative perimetry, ideally] are, of course, indicated in chronically observed cases.

Bynke and Hillman[15] provide a summary of a Swedish experience with transsphenoidal management of 59 consecutive cases of pituitary adenomas with suprasellar extension (Hardy-Wilson grades A,B,C). "Radical surgical removal" of suprasellar portions was possible in all but 6 cases, and 4 underwent secondary intracranial surgery for large tumor remnants.

A series of eight patients with field defects due to prolactinomas enjoyed improved visual function with bromocriptine treatment only.[16] The authors advocate bromocriptine as a primary treatment for these tumors, but caution that neuro-ophthalmologic, endocrinologic, and imaging studies must be continued indefinitely.

The long-acting somatostatin analog SMS 201–995 has been shown to be effective in the treatment of somatotropic and thyrotropic adenomas. In some cases, it suppresses hormone secretion and reduces tumor size. This agent was administered subcutaneously to eight patients[17] with adenomas of several types and with advanced field defects: six patients recovered acuity and field, two during the first 4 to 6 hours of treatment! Maximal improvement occurred within 6 to 45 days. This effect seemed independent of adenoma type, including growth-hormone secreting, thyroid stimulating hormone and silent corticotropic secreting, and nonsecreting adenomas. In all cases but one, no tumor shrinkage could be demonstrated, suggesting that visual improvement is independent of reduction in tumor volume.

Pituitary enlargement occurs in primary hypothyroidism as a result of pituitary thyrotroph hyperplasia, but sellar changes are rare. Three children with growth failure presented with primary hypothyroidism and pituitary masses with suprasellar extension.[18] Levothyroxine therapy reversed the pituitary masses, but no information is provided regarding visual function before or after treatment.

Silent pituitary "apoplexy" implies nonsymptomatic hemorrhage within pituitary adenomas. In a series of 12 patients with neuroimages (CT and/or MRI) consistent with hemorrhages in adenomas, only 3 had clinical courses of "pituitary apoplexy."[19] MRI signals suggestive of pituitary hemorrhage were mimicked by a primary intrasellar melanoma in a 35-year-old woman.[20] Bright signal on

T1-weighted images and dark signal on T2-weighted images simulated blood, but the paramagnetic effect of stable free radicals of melanin is thought to account for these MRI signal characteristics.

Optic Gliomas

Optic pathway gliomas in neurofibromatosis-type 1 (NFB-1) are reviewed by Hoyt and Imes,[21] topics including: incidence, ophthalmic findings, CT and MRI characteristics, neuropathologic findings, and long-term behavior. This is a handy 6-page summary that concludes: "It is agreed that the main bulk of an optic pathway glioma is a low-grade neoplasm with unpredictable growth potential. . . . It is not possible to demonstrate clear histological differences between tumors with limited growth rate and tumors that will grow."

A Turkish series from 1968 to 1982 is reported,[22] consisting of 8 intraorbital and 16 intracranial optic gliomas, all histologically confirmed. The authors state that the 16 cases of intracranial gliomas ". . . underwent biopsy, subtotal or total (!!) tumour resection" and postoperative administration of 5,500 rad radiation and carmustine (BCNU) therapy. Seven of the patients died within 1 month to 7 years. Extraordinarily, during a mean follow-up of 8 years, the survival rate was only 37.5%! The causes of deaths are not disclosed, and certainly this is not a typical experience.

Another study was undertaken to determine the frequency of optic gliomas in patients with NFB-1.[23] CT scans were obtained from 65 children with NFB-1 and no visual or ocular abnormalities, and ten (15%) optic gliomas were detected: three unilateral nerve, three bilateral, and four optic chiasm plus one or both optic nerves. Interestingly, Lewis et al.[24] previously reported a 15% incidence of optic gliomas in 217 patients with NFB-1 aged 4 to 69 years.

The efficacy of radiation therapy is assessed by Pierce et al.,[25] who reviewed the results of 24 irradiated gliomas of optic nerve and chiasm. Acuity and/or visual fields were said to improve or stabilize in 91%, with a 6-year progression-free interval in 88%, and 6-year survival in 100%; 15 of 18 patients developed a deficiency of growth hormone.

A case of *multicentric gliomas* is reported[26] with pilocytic astrocytomas of the optic chiasm, brain stem, and spinal cord; there were no stigmata of NFB. Spinal metastases are documented[27] in a child with otherwise typical pilocytic optic chiasm glioma, without signs of anaplasia. A 3-year-old boy with NFB and pilocytic optic nerve glioma showed intraocular extension and iris seeding[28]; in the optic canal three foci of malignant astrocytoma grade 3 were found, leading the authors to conclude that optic gliomas are true astrocytomas and not hamartomas, and that there is a continuum from benign to malignant transformation. Wilson et al.[29] also report giant cyst formation said to be arising from an optic chiasm and optic tract glioma, 4 years following conventional radiation therapy. The authors concluded that the cyst was "an unusual feature of the tumor growth, degeneration, or both. . . ."

The confusion between benign *spasmus nutans* and nystagmus associated with optic chiasm gliomas is further clarified in an important paper by Gottlob et al.,[30] who analyzed clinical findings and eye/head movement recordings. Ten cases had spasmus nutans-like disease associated with intracranial anomalies (including two optic chiasm gliomas), but head or eye movement recordings do not allow distinction between spasmus nutans and nystagmus accompanying such intracranial lesions, neuroimaging being required.

Lymphomas

A detailed review of visual system disease, including anterior pathways, with non-Hodgkin's lymphoma has been published in *Clinical Neurology and Neurosurgery*[31]; the bibliography is ample. Single cases of primary optic chiasm lymphoma[32] and of Hodgkin's disease of the optic chiasm[33] are also reported. A 58-year-old woman presenting with visual loss, decreased hearing, and headaches was found to have steroid-responsive primary central nervous system (CNS) lymphoma, including massive enlargement of the optic chiasm.[34] An MRI-guided stereotactic biopsy was performed, but unfortunately, was neither illustrated nor further described (!). In this case, radiologic regression is said to be a phenomenon that is characteristic of (or defines?) ghost-cell tumors.

Miscellaneous Tumors

Meningiomas.—The use of gadolinium diethylenetriamine pentaacetic acid (Gd-DTPA)–enhanced MRI in demonstrating and defining basal meningiomas is discussed by Haik et al.[35] and Zimmerman et al.[36] The latter is a series of six patients with unilateral optic nerve sheath meningiomas with variable intracranial extension. In nonenhanced MRI, meningioma tends to be isointense to brain tissue and difficult to delineate, but with Gd-DTPA, tumor tissue is made distinct. Three cases of meningioma that became rapidly visually symptomatic during pregnancy are documented[37]; the authors speculate that accelerated tumor growth is related to stimulation of predominantly progesterone receptors, but the authors do not specify if a receptor assay was performed on material from the two cases subjected to surgery during and just after pregnancy. An instance of optic nerve sheath meningioma accompanied by contralateral internal carotid artery aneurysm is recorded.[38]

Craniopharyngioma.—Thirty patients with craniopharyngiomas were assessed preoperatively and postoperatively to determine the extent of visual recovery.[39] Visual acuity was reduced in 42% of eyes before surgery, and 1 week postoperatively, acuity was reduced in 23% of eyes. Importantly, there was no long-term improvement in acuity or visual fields in patients with defects present after the first postoperative month. Optic atrophy was present in 12 of 24 eyes of patients younger than 18 years, and in 11 of 36 eyes in the patients older than 18 years. Many visual fields did not show typical bitemporal depression of peripheral isopters.

Gerinomas.—A case report and literature review of germinomas in the suprasellar area is provided by Bowman and Farris.[40] Of 64 reviewed cases, 87.5% had diabetes insipidus, 83% had visual loss, and 56% had hypopituitarism. These lesions are more frequent in women, with a peak incidence in the 10- to 20-year-old age group.

RADIATION DAMAGE

Delayed radiation damage to the anterior visual pathways is recognized with apparently increasing frequency. In a paper reporting radiation necrosis of an optico-hypothalamic glioma, Warman et al.[41] provide a literature review and analysis of cumulative data, which indicate that the time interval from treatment to onset of visual collapse is shorter than previously thought. In fact, the 8 to 13 month post-irradiation interval encompasses two thirds of all cases, as opposed to former estimates of peak incidence at 1 to 1½ years. In a more technical review, the visual outcome following proton irradiation of 20 upper clivus tumors was analyzed[42]; a complication rate of 1 in 5 is observed when the optic nerve is exposed to a dosage of 65 cobalt Gray equivalent (CGE), and complication rates of 2 in 16 and 1 in 13 at a dose of 55 CGE for optic nerve and chiasm, respectively.

The good news is that gadolinium-enhanced MRI shows a characteristic picture of optic nerve and/or optic chiasm thickening and excludes other mechanisms of visual loss (e.g., tumor recurrence, prolapsed optic chiasm).[43, 44] The bad news is that there is very little evidence that radiation injury to the optic nerves or chiasm is alleviated with hyperbaric oxygenation and/or massive corticosteroid regimens.[45] In this report, 13 patients were treated for visual loss that evolved 4 to 35 months after radiation therapy, but no patient enjoyed improved vision. In a rebuttal letter, Guy and Schatz[46] emphasize that this series included only patients treated from 2 to 12 weeks after loss of vision.

INFLAMMATIONS AND SARCOID

The application of MRI in the diagnosis of multiple sclerosis (MS) and other demyelinating diseases provokes a paradox: the correlation (or lack thereof) of radiologically definable lesions with clinical signs and symptoms. In a Japanese study[47] of 30 patients with optic neuritis, including 21 with MS, optic chiasm signal abnormalities were found in 5 cases, but MRI signal abnormalities did not correlate well with Goldmann visual field defects.

Sarcoidosis of the CNS has a well-known predilection for the leptomeninges at the base of the brain. A retrospective study[48] strongly supports the efficacy of MRI in detecting gadolinium-enhanced abnormalities in 17 of 20 patients with CNS sarcoidosis; lesions were detected with nonenhanced MRI in only 3 cases, but all 17 demonstrated gadolinium-enhancing lesions in leptomeninges, dura, brain parenchyma, hypothalamus, periventricular white matter, optic chiasm, and pituitary gland. A single case of optic chiasm sarcoidosis was documented,[49] presenting with visual loss, papilledema, and diabetes insipidus.

ANEURYSMS AND VASCULAR LESIONS

Aneurysms of the ophthalmic artery are either rare or previously imprecisely defined lesions, but A. L. Day of the University of Florida has provided an excellent anatomic description and pertinent clinical-surgical analysis.[50] Day distinguishes two sites for aneurysm formation of the ophthalmic segment (paraclinoidal) of the internal carotid artery (ICA): (1) just distal to the origin of the ophthalmic artery (41 cases), usually pointing superomedially; and (2) at the superior hypophyseal artery (39 cases) above the dural ring at the medial bend of the ICA, with a tendency to burrow beneath the anterior clinoid. There was a marked preponderance of affected women (7:1), and 45% disclosed multiple aneurysms. The author describes his surgical approaches and reports an experience in clipping 52/54 lesions with low operative and visual morbidity.

A feature photo of bitemporal hemianopia with CT evidence of internal carotid artery dolicho-ectasia is available.[51]

Cavernous Angiomas/Malformations

These processes that affect the optic chiasm and tracts are seemingly not so rare, presenting typically with new headache and visual loss—a syndrome of "optic chiasm apoplexy"—and with some hope of visual recovery with surgical excision or hematoma evacuation.[52–54] An arteriovenous malformation of the optic chiasm was associated with a second vascular anomaly of the maxillary antrum, thought to represent the Bonnet-Dechaume-Blanc (Wyburn-Mason) syndrome, but without retinal or orbital lesions.[55]

Corboy and Galetta[56] have documented an instance of optic chiasm apoplexy secondary to cavernous angioma, with several family members also found to have various CNS vascular malformations. MRI can disclose symptomatic and asymptomatic carriers of cavernous angiomas. Asymptomatic lesions should be followed.

EMPTY SELLA AND CYSTS

Kaufman et al.[57] from Case Western Reserve have documented the morphologic and clinical characteristics of herniation of the anterior visual pathways and third ventricle structures into primary and secondary empty sellae. High-resolution MRI is superior to CT in accurately demonstrating anatomic relationships. Progression of visual symptoms is not inevitable, and there was little correlation between the degree of herniation and relative severity of visual defects. Nagata et al.[58] document a similar case, which the authors term a new variety of primary empty sella syndrome.

A case of symptomatic Rathke's cleft cyst is described.[59] MRI afforded optimal visualization of the intrasellar and suprasellar disposition of the pituitary gland, optic chiasm, infundibulum, and carotid vessels.

MISCELLANEOUS CONDITIONS AND OBSERVATIONS

Indirect trauma to the optic chiasm is rarely documented with specific neuroimaging abnormalities, but Crowe et al.[60] report a 49-year-old man with progressively blurred vision presenting 9 days following head trauma. MRI showed hemorrhage and swelling within the optic nerves and chiasm. A more typical case of reduced vision and bitemporal hemianopia, with neither CT nor MRI optic chiasm abnormalities but with fractures of the sella turcica is documented.[61]

"Selected Neurologic Complications of Pregnancy" is the topic recently reviewed by Fox et al.,[62] including a brief discussion of the management of pituitary tumors during pregnancy. (See also JS Sunness: The pregnant woman's eye.[63]) Also, during the 30th week of pregnancy, a 26-year-old woman developed decreased vision, left temporal hemianopia, and a symmetric homogeneous sellar mass on CT and MRI. The mass regressed spontaneously after delivery and was diagnosed as lymphocytic adenohypophysitis, although no evidence was arrayed that this was not simply an instance of major pituitary hypertrophy during pregnancy.[64]

Pattern-reversal visual-evoked potentials (VEPs) were recorded in 38 patients with optic chiasm lesions, comparing full-field to half-field stimulation.[65] Temporal half-field (crossed fibers) stimulation showed a 80% abnormality rate (vs. 66% full-field), and the nasal field (uncrossed fibers) showed a 32% abnormality rate.

An 18-year-old girl with recurrent tunnel vision demonstrated an hysterical bitemporal hemianopia on automated perimetry,[66] and myelinated retinal nerve fibers in a man with one eye regressed after a pituitary adenoma was resected.[67]

REFERENCES

1. Doyle AJ: Optic chiasm position on MR images. *AJNR* 1990; 11:553–555.
2. Bull J: The normal variations in the position of the optic recess of the third ventricle. *Acta Radiol* 1956; 46:72–80.
3. Bergland RM, Ray BS, Torack RM: Anatomical variations in the pituitary gland and adjacent structures in 225 autopsy cases. *J Neurosurg* 1968; 28:93–99.
4. Rhoton AL, Renn WH, Harris FS: Microsurgical anatomy of the sellar region and cavernous sinus, in Rand RW (ed): *Microneurosurgery*. St Louis, Mosby, 1985, p 113.
5. Mizuguchi M, Morimatsu Y: Histopathological study of alobar holoprosencephaly, marginal glioneural heterotopia and other gliomesenchymal abnormalities. *Acta Neuropathol* 1989; 78:183–188.
6. Benner JD, Preslan MW, Gratz E, et al: Septo-optic dysplasia in two siblings. *Am J Ophthalmol* 1990; 109:632–637.
7. Kaufman LM, Miller MT, Mafee MF: Magnetic resonant imaging of pituitary stalk hypoplasia: A discreet midline anomaly associated with endocrine abnormalities in septo-optic dysplasia. *Arch Ophthalmol* 1989; 107:1485–1489.
8. Zeki SM: Optic nerve hypoplasia and astigmatism: A new association. *Br J Ophthalmol* 1990; 74:297–299.
9. Brodsky MC, Glasier CM, Pollock SC, et al: Optic nerve hypoplasia. Identification by magnetic resonance imaging. *Arch Ophthalmol* 1990; 108:1562–1567.
10. Slamovits TL, Kimball GP, Friberg TR, et al: Bilateral optic disc colobomas with orbital cysts and hypoplastic optic nerves and chiasm. *J Clin Neuro Ophthalmol* 1989; 9:172–177.
11. Scheithauer BW, Sano T, Kovacs KT, et al: The pituitary gland in pregnancy: A clinicopathologic and immunohistochemical study of 69 cases. *Mayo Clin Proc* 1990; 65:461–474.
12. Kernohan JW, Sayre GP: Tumors of the pituitary gland and infundibulum, in *Atlas of Tumor Pathology, Series 1, Fascicle 36*. Washington DC, Armed Forces Institute of Pathology, 1956.
13. Burrow GN, Wortzman G, Rewcastle NB, et al: Microadenomas of the pituitary and abnormal sellar tomograms in an unselected autopsy service. *N Engl J Med* 1981; 304:156–161.
14. Reincke M, Allolio B, Saeger W, et al: The 'incidentaloma' of the pituitary gland. Is neurosurgery required? *JAMA* 1990; 263:2772–2776.
15. Bynke O, Hillman J: Role of transsphenoidal operation in the management of pituitary adenomas with suprasellar extension. *Arch Neurochir* 1989; 100:50–55.
16. Lesser RL, Zheutlin JD, Boghen D, et al: Visual function improvement in patients with macroprolactinomas treated with bromocriptine. *Am J Ophthalmol* 1990; 109:535–543.
17. Warnet A, Timsit J, Chanson P, et al: The effect of somatostatin analogue on chiasmal dysfunction from pituitary adenomas. *J Neurosurg* 1989; 75:687–690.
18. Atchison JA, Lee PA, Albright AL: Reversible suprasellar pituitary mass secondary to hypothyroidism. *JAMA* 1989; 262:3175–3177.
19. Ostrov SG, Quencer RM, Hoffman JC, et al: Hemorrhage within pituitary adenomas: How often associated with pituitary apoplexy syndrome? *AJNR* 1989; 10:503–510.
20. Chappell PM, Kelly WM, Ercius M: Primary sellar melanoma simulating hemorrhagic pituitary adenoma: MR and pathologic findings. *AJNR* 1990; 11:1054–1056.
21. Hoyt WF, Imes RK: Optic gliomas of neurofibromatosis-1 (NF-1): Contemporary perspectives, in Ishibashi Y, Hori Y (eds): *Tuberous Sclerosis and Neurofibromatosis: Epidemiology, Pathophysiology, Biology and Management*. Amsterdam, Excerpta Medica, 1990, pp 239–246.
22. Bilgec S, Erbengi A, Tinaztepe B, et al: Optic gliomas of childhood: Clinical, histopathological, and histochemical observations. *Br J Ophthalmol* 1990; 73:832–837.

23. Listernick R, Charrow J, Greenwald MJ, et al: Optic gliomas in children with neurofibromatosis type 1. *J Pediatr* 1989; 114:788–792.

24. Lewis RA, Gerson JP, Axelson KA, et al: von Recklinghausen's neurofibromatosis. II. Incidence of optic gliomas. *Ophthalmology* 1984; 91:929–935.

25. Pierce SM, Barnes PD, Loeffler JS, et al: Definitive radiation therapy in the management of symptomatic patients with optic gliomas: Survival and long-term effects. *Cancer* 1990; 65:45–52.

26. Matsumoto T, Uekusa T, Abe H, et al: Multicentric astrocytomas of the optic chiasm, brain stem and spinal cord. *Acta Pathol Jpn* 1989; 39:664–669.

27. Kocks W, Kalff R, Reinhardt V, et al: Spinal metastasis of pilocytic astrocytoma of the chiasma opticum. *Childs Nerv Syst* 1989; 5:118–120.

28. De Keizer RJW, De Wolff-Rouendaal D, Bots GTAM, et al: Optic glioma with intraocular tumor and seeding in a child with neurofibromatosis. *Am J Ophthalmol* 1989; 108:717–725.

29. Wilson WB, Finkel RS, McCleary L, et al: Large cystic optic glioma. *Neurology* 1990; 40:1898–1900.

30. Gottlob I, Zubcov A, Catalano RA et al: Signs distinguishing spasmus nutans (with and without central nervous system lesions) from infantile nystagmus. *Ophthalmology* 1990; 97:1166–1175.

31. Maiuri F: Visual involvement in primary non-Hodgkin's lymphoma. *Clin Neurol Neurosurg* 1990; 92:119–124.

32. Cantore GP, Raco A, Artico M, et al: Primary chiasmatic lymphoma. *Clin Neurol Neurosurg* 1989; 91:71–74.

33. McFadzean RM, McIlwaine GG, McLellan D: Hodgkin's disease at the optic chiasm. *J Clin Neuro Ophthalmol* 1990; 10:248–254.

34. Gray RS, Abrahams JJ, Hufnagel TJ, et al: Ghost-cell tumor of the optic chiasm. Primary CNS lymphoma. *J Clin Neuro Ophthalmol* 1989; 9:98–104.

35. Haik BG, Zimmerman R, Saint Louis L: Gadolinium-DTPA enhancement of an optic nerve and chiasmal meningioma. *J Clin Neuro Ophthalmol* 1989; 9:122–125.

36. Zimmerman CF, Schatz NJ, Glaser JS: Magnetic resonance imaging of optic nerve meningiomas. Enhancement with gadolinium-DPTA. *Ophthalmology* 1990; 97:585–591.

37. Wan WL, Geller JL, Feldon SE, et al: Visual loss caused by rapidly progressive intracranial meningiomas during pregnancy. *Ophthalmology* 1990; 97:18–21.

38. Landau K, Horton JC, Hoyt WF, et al: Aneurysm mimicking intracranial growth of optic nerve sheath meningioma. *J Clin Neuro Ophthalmol* 1990; 10:185–187.

39. Repka MX, Miller NR, Miller M: Visual outcome after surgical removal of craniopharyngiomas. *Ophthalmology* 1989; 96:195–199.

40. Bowman CB, Farris BK: Primary chiasmal germinoma. A case report and review of the literature. *J Clin Neuro Ophthalmol* 1990; 10:9–17.

41. Warman R, Glaser JS, Quencer RM: Radionecrosis of optico-hypothalamic glioma. *Neuro Ophthalmol* 1989; 9:219–226.

42. Habrand IL, Austin-Seymour M, Birnbaum S, et al: Neurovisual outcome following proton radiation therapy. *Int J Radiat Oncol Biol Phys* 1989; 16:1601–1606.

43. Croisile B, Piperno D, Bascoulergue Y, et al: Radionécrose chiasmatique après irradiation de la selle turcique à doses conventionnelles. *Rev Neurol (Paris)* 1990; 146:57–60.

44. Zimmerman CF, Schatz NJ, Glaser JS: Magnetic resonance imaging of radiation optic neuropathy. *Am J Ophthalmol* 1990; 110:389–394.

45. Roden D, Bosley TM, Fowble B, et al: Delayed radiation injury to the retrobulbar optic nerves and chiasm. Clinical syndrome and treatment with hyperbaric oxygen and corticosteroids. *Ophthalmology* 1990; 97:346–351.

46. Guy J, Schatz NJ: Effectiveness of hyperbaric oxygen in treating radiation injury to the optic nerves and chiasm (letter). *Ophthalmology* 1990; 10:1246–1247.

47. Kakisu Y, Adachi-Usami E, Kojima S, et al: Magnetic resonance imaging in the diagnosis of optic neuritis and neuropathy. *Nippon Ganka Gakkai Zasshi* 1989; 93:281–286.

48. Sherman JL, Stern BJ: Sarcoidosis of the CNS: Comparison of unenhanced and enhanced MR images. *AJR* 1990; 155:1293–1301.

49. Walker FO, McLean WT, Elster A, et al: Chiasmal sarcoidosis. *AJNR* 1990; 11:1205–1207.

50. Day AL: Aneurysms of the ophthalmic segment. A clinical and anatomical analysis. *J Neurosurg* 1990; 72:677–691.

51. Slavin ML: Bitemporal hemianopia associated with dolichoectasia of intracranial carotid arteries. *J Clin Neuro Ophthalmol* 1990; 10:80–81.

52. Regli L, de Tribolet N, Regli F, et al: Chiasmal apoplexy: Hemorrhage from a cavernous malformation in the optic chiasm. *J Neurol Neurosurg Psychiatry* 1989; 52:1095–1099.

53. Castel JP, Delorge-Kerdiles C, Rivel J: Angiome caverneux du chiasma optique. *Neurochirurgie* 1989; 35:252–256.

54. Zentner J, Grodd W, Hassler W: Cavernous angioma of the optic tract. *J Neurol* 1989; 236:117–119.

55. Gibo H, Watanabe N, Kobayashi S, et al: Removal of an arteriovenous malformation in the optic chiasm. A case of the Bonnet-Dechaume-Blanc syndrome without retinal involvement. *Surg Neurol* 1989; 31:142–148.

56. Corboy JR, Galetta SL: Familial cavernous angiomas manifesting with an acute chiasmal syndrome. *Am J Ophthalmol* 1989; 108:245–250.

57. Kaufman B, Tomsak RL, Kaufman BA, et al: Herniation of the suprasellar visual system and third ventricle into empty sellae: Morphologic and clinical considerations. *AJR* 1989; 152:597–608.

58. Nagata K, Joshita H, Matsui T, et al: Primary empty sella syndrome caused by abnormal dilation of the optic recess. *Surg Neurol* 1989; 31:323–329.

59. Wagle VG, Nelson D, Rossi A, et al: Magnetic resonance imaging of symptomatic Rathke's cleft cyst: Report of a case. *Neurosurgery* 1989; 24:276–278.

60. Crowe NW, Nickles TP, Troost BT, et al: Intrachiasmal hemorrhage: A cause of delayed post-traumatic blindness. *Neurology* 1989; 39:863–865.

61. Dette TM, Ohrloff C, Solimosy L, et al: Chiasmalasion nach schwerem Schadel-Hirn-Trauma. Klinische, funktionelle und neuroradiologische Charakteristik am Bespiel eines seltenen Falles. *Fortschr Ophthalmol* 1989; 86:676–678.

62. Fox MW, Harms, Davis DH: Selected neurologic complications of pregnancy. *Mayo Clin Proc* 1990; 65:1595–1618.

63. Sunness JS: The pregnant woman's eye. *Surv Ophthalmol* 1988; 32:219–238.

64. Mikami T, Uozumi T, Yamanaka M, et al: Lymphocytic adenohypophysitis: MRI findings of a suspected case. *No Shinkei Geka* 1989; 17:871–876.

65. Brecelj J, Denislic M, Skrbec M: Visual evoked potential abnormalities in chiasmal lesions. *Doc Ophthalmol* 1989; 73:139–148.

66. Fish RH, Kline LB, Hanumanthu VK et al: Hysterical bitemporal hemianopia "cured" with contact lenses (letter). *J Clin Neuro Ophthalmol* 1990; 10:76–78.

67. Gupta A, Khandalavala B, Bansal RK, et al: Atrophy of myelinated nerve fibers in pituitary adenoma. *J Clin Neuro Ophthalmol* 1990; 10:100–102.

CHAPTER 5

The Retrochiasmal Visual Pathways

Carl Ellenberger, Jr., M.D.

Medical Director, Lebanon Magnetic Imaging, Lebanon, Pennsylvania

The pursuit of new information on the retrochiasmal visual pathways allows one to range widely. In a restrictive sense, that title means the geniculocalcarine pathway, but visual signals also travel through the complex prestriate or association networks and beyond, all of which are retrochiasmal and vulnerable to the same diseases. I attempted to stop at the threshold of higher cortical functions, but couldn't resist glancing occasionally in that direction. I still wandered into territory covered by other chapters on migraine, stroke, neuroimaging, etc., hoping to see from a different perspective. I don't presume to be authoritative on the understanding of the visual process, but still find this work fascinating and include a small number of reports to guide an interested reader into some of the active areas within that very comprehensive network.

THE VISUAL PROCESS

A new volume covers recent investigations of the visual process by authorities in a wide variety of disciplines, from biochemistry to artificial intelligence.[1] It progresses from the functional and pharmacologic organization of the retina to the effects of Alzheimer's disease and Parkinson's disease as explained with current visual theory.

The diverse approaches to understanding vision are linked by several common themes, particularly the theory of parallel pathways in visual processing.[1] This is admirably discussed by Margaret Livingstone: "Segregation of Form, Color, Movement and Depth Processing in the Visual System: Anatomy, Physiology, Art and Illusion." She explains several well-known illusions, such as Leonardo da Vinci's observation that depth seems greater when we view a two-dimensional illustration with one eye, and equiluminance of colors, a phenomenon modern advertising artists use to their advantage.

Evoked potentials can demonstrate parallel visual pathways in humans. Berninger et al. selectively excited each of two parallel visual pathways (each named for a lamina of the lateral geniculate body: the magnocellular and the parvocellular) by choosing the appropriate wavelength of visual stimulus to generate evoked potentials.[2] The polarity of the evoked potentials both in retina and in cortex depended on which of these pathways was stimulated. The findings of Rimmer et al. are also consistent with the theory of parallel processing.[3] They found that latency of the pattern electroretinogram, pattern visually evoked potential, and retinocortical time all varied with the spatial frequency of the stimulus, i.e., exhibited spatial selectivity.

Another common theme in recent investigations is the concept of functional anatomy. Raichle briefly reviews work begun by Roy and Sherrington, the first to postulate an automatic mechanism that provides for a local variation of the blood supply in response to activity in regions of the brain.[4] Their experiments gave them the first in vivo look at the human visual system. Raichle has found that local increases in functional activity (as when we view an image) are best reflected in parallel increases in blood flow—not in glucose or oxygen consumption, a premise that underlies much of our current understanding. Current physiologic-anatomic data could be inaccurate if based on standard cranial tomographic reference planes (e.g., the orbitomeatal line). Raichle has developed a new strategy for anatomic localization with neurosurgical sterotaxy and image averaging.[5]

As confirmation of the accuracy of his method, Raichle finds a retinotopic organization of the living human visual cortex very similar to that already precisely mapped in animals—with an impressive accuracy of as little as 3 mm. He also studied the anatomy of the processing of passively presented words. These stimuli activated striate cortex bilaterally, but also three inferior, lateral-prestrite areas, one on the left and two on the right, extending as far anteriorly as the temporooccipital boundary, areas that may comprise a network that codes for visual word form and may be damaged in patients with pure alexia.

Also using stereotactic methods, Lueck et al. compared the results of positron emission tomography (PET) scans of subjects viewing multicolored and black-and-white displays and identified a region of normal human cerebral cortex specialized for color vision.[6] This region, the lingual and fusiform gyri in the inferior occipital lobes, is probably homologous to area V4 in prestriate cortex, shown by physiologic studies to be a color center in macaque monkeys. Clinical observations of patients with acquired dyschromatopsia (see previous editions) have suggested that this approximate region is important for color processing.

When a large black dog chases a small calico cat in the same part of our visual field, how does the brain associate the various properties of each so that we don't attribute the color, size, speed, and other features of the dog to the cat? Stryker considers the question beginning with the oldest theory of the grandmother cell, a hypothetical cell at the top of the hierarchy of the visual network that responds only to the image of one's grandmother.[7] According to this fanciful concept, other cells exist with equally specific requirements for excitation, as many cells as required to respond to all possible visual images in the world. This idea has shortcomings, not the least of which is the astronomical number of cells required.

A second theory to explain how the brain puts together the various representations of the visual features of an object was offered years ago by Crick, who thinks that these representations are combined only transiently, rather than in fixed receptive fields. This temporary association might be effected by neurons of the thalamic reticular nucleus unifying the perceptual qualities represented in different cortical areas, a sort of neural searchlight simultaneously illuminating all the neurons that are activated by the same object in the world.

Recent studies of Gray, Singer, and Eckhorn suggest another mechanism for this temporary association: neurons in the visual cortex activated by the same object in the world may discharge rhythmically and in unison. Gray and Singer have found that visual stimuli can cause many neurons in visual cortex to discharge rhythmically at 40 to 50 Hz.[8] They hypothesize that the synchronization of oscillatory responses of spatially distributed, feature-selective cells might be a way to establish relations between features in different parts of the visual field. In support of this hypothesis, they demonstrate that neurons in spatially separate columns can synchronize their oscillatory responses.[9] Eckhorn found oscillatory field potentials evoked by some stimuli are in phase even between the two primary areas of visual cortex (areas 17 and 18).[10] Visually related activities can thus be transiently labeled by a temporal code that signals their momentary association. Will this newly demonstrated importance of brain rhythms bring new life to the electroencephalogram (EEG)?

A third theme emerging from recent studies is the similarity between the human and monkey visual systems, a reassuring confirmation of the validity of decades of work in animals. Tolhurst and Ling review the evidence relating to the similarity between the human and monkey striate cortex.[11] Limited available data suggest that the human linear magnification factor is about 1.6 times greater than that in the macaque. This is consistent with observations that the human striate cortex, compared with that of the macaque, has over two times the area, and has neurons with longer dendrites, wider ocular dominance columns, and more widely separated cytochrome oxidase blobs. Surprisingly perhaps, the striate cortices in both species have the same total number of neurons. The foveal magnification factor in the macaque is believed to be about 15 mm/degree, so Tolhurst and Ling estimate the human foveal value to be about 20 to 25 mm/degree rather than the currently accepted value of 8 to 11 mm/degree. The magnification factor falls more rapidly with eccentricity than current estimates suggest.

Hockfield et al. compare human and macaque visual cortices in another way.[12] With the monoclonal antibody Cat-301 that recognizes an antigen in human cortex that is closely related, if not identical, to the antigen in laboratory animals, they show that the organization of human area V1 (striate cortex) correlates with the organization of ocular dominance columns demonstrated by cytochrome oxidase histochemistry. The organization demonstrated with Cat-301 in human area V2 (extrastriate cortex) correlates with the thick stripes of the cytochrome oxidase pattern. These observations provide evidence for a visual pathway in human cortex homologous to the magnocellular pathway in the macaque, a pathway involved in processing the low-contrast, achromatic, and moving components of visual stimuli.

Burkhalter and Bernardo studied visual cortical circuitry in humans with a fluorescent perchlorate dye as an axonal marker.[13] They traced projections of V1 and V2 visual cortex in the postmortem, fixed human brain. V1 projects forward to layers 3 and 4 of V2, and V2 projects back to layers 1, 2, 3, 5, and 6 of V1. V2 projections, probably from cytochrome oxidase (CO)-reactive stripes, also reach layer 4B of V1. Differential connections between CO-rich (blobs) and CO-poor regions (interblobs) also exist within V1; blobs are connected to blobs and interblobs are connected to interblobs. Again, these results show that the connections in human visual cortex resemble those of nonhuman primates and that their organization is consistent with the concept of multiple processing streams in the visual system.

Retinal ganglion cells represent the visual image with a spatial code in which each cell conveys information about a small region in the image. In contrast, cells of primary visual cortex use a hybrid space-frequency code in which each cell conveys information about a region that is local in space, spatial frequency, and orientation. For the mathematically sophisticated, Watson and Ahumada describe a mathematical model for this transformation: a multilevel hexagonal orthogonal-oriented quadrature pyramid transform.[14] In the biological model, the input lattice is the retinal ganglion cell array. The resultant scheme generates receptive fields that resemble those of the primary visual cortex.

Rizzo and Robin call attention a metaphor for a group of operations that gate the processing of information in the brain.[15] Every educator knows that attention can critically alter learning and performance. (Pay attention!) The operations of attention selectively allocate our limited processing capacity to the barrage of simultaneous incoming signals. Psychologically defined functions such as concentration, search, readiness, and vigilance are components of attention, but their neural substrate is uncertain. On the premise that the actions of attention can be understood from an information-processing perspective, Rizzo and Robin studied a patient with simultanagnosia from bilateral superior occipital strokes to: (1) learn how disordered attention may affect cognitive abilities that are vision-based; and to (2) inquire how such defects may relate to current insights on visual processing. Their findings and discussion, too complex to summarize here in a few sentences, are a fascinating bridge between the theoretical and often obscure hypotheses of the computationists and the everyday world of patients with strokes. Rizzo and Robin conclude that simultanagnosia in their patient related to an inability to sustain visuospatial attention across an array, corresponding to processing failure at a level of long-range (global) spatiotemporal interactions among converging inputs from early vision. The operations for orienting and sustaining attention may be dissociable at visual association cortex levels.

Illustrating the interdependence of the several components of the visual system, Rizzo and Hurtwig found in a man with extensive bilateral occipital lesions acquired at birth that smooth pursuit of suprathreshold targets was mostly saccadic and did not improve with added nonvisual cues.[16] The results suggest that the visual cortex is crucial to the development of eye movements. The foveal representation in the occipital lobes, missing in this subject, is needed for development of normal smooth pursuit.

STROKE

A curmudgeon chides us to abandon a neurologic household word, lacune.[17] According to Landau, that is a "noun of historical interest . . . [which] never did provide statistically justified information regarding the nature of clinical symptoms, pathologic process, anatomic location, dynamic pathogenesis, prognosis, or rational treatment." He advocates the soft-drink classification: small, medium, and large. The argument has merit, but just for our purposes here, I'll use a different scheme.

Large Artery Disease

Mayo authors describe four patients with episodic binocular visual impairment related exclusively to light exposure.[18] Each had bilateral high-grade stenosis or occlusion of the internal carotid arteries. They propose that this phenomenon relates to bilateral simultaneous retinal ischemia that delays regeneration of visual pigments in the pigment epithelial layer. This symptom, perhaps akin to transient visual obscuration, should be distinguished from bilateral occipital lobe ischemia caused by disease in the vertebrobasilar system.

Although a variant posterior cerebral artery may arise directly from the internal carotid artery, carotid artery disease rarely causes occipital infarction. But we can no longer rest assured that sudden isolated hemianopia indicates vertebrobasilar disease. Pessin et al. describe a patient with hemianopia from occipital infarction as an initial manifestation of occlusive carotid disease.[19] A fetal posterior cerebral artery branched from the internal carotid artery. Cohen contributed an almost identical example.[20]

Branch Artery Disease

Computed tomography (CT) and magnetic resonance imaging (MRI) have called to our attention small infarctions deep in the brain. Caplan and his group have described several syndromes caused by small branch arterial occlusion in the territory of both anterior and posterior cerebral arteries.[21, 22]

When a patient with atherosclerotic risk factors presents with sudden hemianopia, we may not think of lacunar (or small) stroke, an observation that supports Caplan's contention that branch athermatous disease is a neglected concept. However, the anterior choroidal artery is one such branch artery, and hemianopia may result from its occlusion because of infarction of the optic tract. Paradoxically, with branch arterial disease, hemianopia indicates disease in middle cerebral arterial territory, while occlusion of a small proximal branch of the posterior cerebral artery, the thalamogeniculate branch, does not cause hemianopia unless the main trunk of the posterior cerebral artery is also occluded to cause occipital infarction. Disease in other small branches may cause small deep infarcts too: thalamostriate, Huebner's, thalamoperforating, paramedian, and short circumferential basilar branches. Hypertension is not a prerequisite for these small strokes, and treatment with platelet inhibitors may be indicated.

Bruno and colleagues also elucidate the mechanisms of anterior choroidal artery territorial infarctions.[23] Their findings also suggest that these infarctions usually result from small-vessel disease as described by Caplan. Associated carotid artery stenosis and potential sources of cardiac emboli are rare and may even be coincidental. Risk factors among the 31 patients in their study were hypertension in 20, smoking in 17, diabetes mellitus in 10, age greater than 69 years in 8, and elevated serum cholesterol concentration in 3. Ghika et al. also found a high incidence (42%) of small artery disease among 100 patients with infarcts in the territory of the deep perforators of the carotid system, including the anterior choroidal arteries (23%).[24] Hypertension and diabetes mellitus were the "most common etiologic factors. . . . However, large-artery disease and cardioembolism may be more important than previously assumed."

From the Oops! department comes a report of three patients who had complete homonymous hemianopia with clinical and neuroimaging characteristics of ipsilateral optic tract infarction after anterior temporal lobectomy for seizure control.[25] The authors attribute this injury to irritative vasospasm of the anterior choroidal artery. This "pure" optic tract syndrome is different from the more common naturally caused one where a compressive lesion causes an incongruous defect because it also squeezes the ipsilateral optic nerve.

In contrast to the deep distribution of branch arterial infarcts, Ringelstein et al. found that 92% of proven embolic brain infarctions were distributed in the territory of the pial arteries.[26]

TUMORS

Vascular Malformations

Cavernous Angiomas.—Often cryptic (40% are invisible on angiogram), the shy cavernous angioma has come into its own during the age of MRI. It has now been exposed as the cause of some idiopathic seizures, headaches, and other symptoms, the causes of which were formerly elusive. Lee and Spetzler correctly distinguish these as examples of vascular malformations rather than arteriovenous malformations (AVM) because they lack AV communication.[27] They are masses of abnormally dilated vascular spaces with no intervening brain parenchyma, not thrombosed arteriovenous malformations as formerly suspected. Often discovered incidentally, they have a characteristic appearance on MRI: larger lesions appear as areas of mixed signal intensity surrounded by a rim (hemosiderin) of low signal intensity on T2-weighted images, while smaller lesions appear as dots of decreased signal intensity on T2-weighted images.

Lance described a 26-year-old man with frequent transient episodes of left homonymous hemianopia and hallucinations that proved to be partial seizures caused by a small cavernous angioma in the occipital lobe.[28] Resistant to anticonvulsants, the angioma was treated with fine-beam radiation therapy (gamma knife), and the seizures subsided.

Rigamonti et al. studied 24 patients with histologically verified cerebral cavernous malformations.[29] Thirteen were members of 6 unrelated Mexican-American families. Eleven percent of relatives of these families had seizures, and cavernous malformations were found in 14 of the 16 who underwent MRI. Eleven images demonstrated multiple lesions. The authors concluded: (1) cavernous malformations are more prevalent than previously reported; (2) a familial form of the disorder exists; (3) patients with the familial form tend to have multiple angiomas; and (4) Mexican-American families have a higher prevalence of angiomas. MRI is the radiographic technique of choice for the identification and follow-up of these lesions.

Mason et al. also found cavernous angiomas among 18 members of three generations of an Hispanic family.[30] The inheritance was autosomal dominant, some had multiple lesions, and some patients with lesions lacked symptoms. Others have noted the tendency for hereditary cavernous angiomas to be multiple, but mistakenly call them AVMs.[31] Perhaps the high sensitivity of MRI for small vascular malformations will outmode the term "cryptic" (i.e., invisible by arteriography). Rigamonti et al. call attention to the possibility that a cavernous angioma may be a silent unexpected neighbor of a symptomatic venous malformation.[32]

What to do, if anything, with a cavernous angioma after its discovery remains to be determined in each case. Gamma knife radiation surgery as well as conventional surgery seem promising, especially for stopping seizures, and even for angiomas in the brain stem, if you are quick about it.[33-37]

Arteriovenous Malformations.—By coincidence, two groups report the unusual association of intracranial hypertension and arteriovenous malformations.[38, 39] Kashii et al. maintain that their two patients had visual field defects because of chronic papilledema, ignoring what appears to be a left hemianopic defect in one patient with a large right occipito-temporal AVM, which they describe as hyperdense on MRI. (It is hypointense.) Six patients of Chimowitz had intracranial hypertension associated with an AVM. Although most of these had transient visual obscurations related to papilledema, the visual field defects in three patients related directly to the location of the AVM. Four AVMs would have escaped detection with routine unenhanced CT, and the erroneous diagnosis would have been made of benign intracranial hypertension. The raised pressure seems to be due to high flow draining into the superior sagittal sinus.

Other Tumors.—Two authorities conclude that available evidence does not justify aggressive therapy of all low-grade gliomas of the cerebral hemispheres.[40] They cite several trials in progress to gather more information. A 24-year-old man with recent-onset seizures was found to have an occipital lobe ganglioglioma with homonymous quadrantanopia and transsynaptic atrophy of retinal nerve fibers.[41] This association indicates that gangliogliomas may arise during neural development and exist for many years before the onset of symptoms.

Castillo and colleagues studied MRI, CT, and clinical features of 18 cases of pathologically proven intracranial gangliogliomas.[42] These are relatively benign tumors that are diagnosed after long-standing symptoms. About half are solid and affect the temporal lobe; the others are cystic and found most often in cerebellum. They may contain calcium, and the tendency of both the cystic and solid forms to enhance is variable.

HEMIANOPIA

I have preferred the term "hemianopia" for the visual deficit caused by chiasmal or retrochiasmal lesions because the adjectival form is an efficient shorthand way to localize the cause of visual loss; saying "hemianopic" throws the ball to the neuro-ophthalmologist. Alas, the Medical Subject Headings from the National Library of Medicine chose "hemianopsia," so perhaps we should talk about "hemianopsic" field defects. Then there are those who use "hemianoptic."[43] These authors were taken to task for using entopic instead of the more accurate entoptic to indicate images that arise from within (ent) the optic globe.

The infallibility of the new-fangled computerized gadgets was further eroded when a patient learned to produce a factitial quadrantanop(s)ia on a field analyzer.[44] If the subject fails to respond to the light stimulus in the chosen quadrant at the beginning of the test—when light stimuli are directed in four points, one per quadrant, the field analyzer directs only bright stimuli to that quadrant, providing clues to the confabulator.

Vision may be abnormal in the homonymous hemifield opposite a hemianopic field. Hess and Pointer measured spatial and temporal contrast sensitivity in three healthy subjects with hemianopia in whom stable visual loss was caused by striate cortical lesions and exhibited foveal sparing.[45] In comparison with the normal control sensitivities, spatial and temporal sensitivities in the sighted hemifield were both reduced. None of the patients had blindsight in the hemianopic field.

Hemianopia may cause spurious results on the FM-100 hue test for color vision.[46] Those with left homonymous hemianopia performed worse when they performed the FM-100 test in the conventional left-right direction than when they did it in the reverse direction. The same difference occurred in the reverse with patients who had right homonymous hemianopia.

What first seems to be hemianopia may instead be hemispatial visual inattention.[47] A patient with right thalamic and temporo-occipital lesions had a left visual field defect when her eyes were directed either straight ahead (midsagittal plane) or toward left hemispace. But the defect disappeared when her eyes were directed to right hemispace, suggesting that the patient had hemispatial visual inattention rather than hemianopia. One suspects that this deficit had a better prognosis for recovery.

In the age of modern neuroimaging, the clinical localizing value of optokinetic nystagmus (OKN) may be obsolescent. Just as well, because Kolmel tested 15 patients with unilateral strictly occipital lesions and complete homonymous hemianopia and compared the findings with those of healthy control subjects.[48] Quantitative analysis of the results in the patients revealed a bilateral disorder of OKN, but there was greater decrease in gain and amplitude when the stimulus moved toward the side of the lesion.

Rehabilitation of Hemianopia

Prognosis for recovery of hemianopia caused by ischemic cerebral lesions is generally poor. Complete recovery of visual fields occurred in only 14 (17%) of the 81 patients with a complete homonymous hemianopia admitted with stroke and in 13 (72%) of the 18 patients with a partial hemianopia.[49] Cumulative fatality at 28 days was greater in patients with a complete hemianopia (49%) compared with patients with partial defects (11%).

Patients with hemianopia read slowly. Recordings of ocular movements during reading showed that the increase in global reading time related mainly to the increase in number of movements of progression and regression in right hemianopia and to the time to return to the next line in left hemianopia.[50] Comparing these recordings with those of the same patients during elementary ocular movements and simulated reading suggested to the authors that the reading difficulties are not only linguistic and/or cognitive but also may relate to basic sensory factors, such as size of words or spaces between words.

Several workers continue to try to restore the vision of patients with ischemic hemianopia. Zihl maintains that the majority of patients with hemianopic defects suffer from reading disabilities (which he calls hemianopic dyslexia) because the residual visual field is too small for complete comprehension of words and sentences.[51] They also typically show a reduction of searching movements in the affected hemifield. He maintains that adequate adaptation of reading and searching strategies to the field disorder does not take place spontaneously, and so systematic treatment with an electronic device is helpful. I remain skeptical because of the impossibility of controls. (No two lesions are identical.) But one can't argue with good intentions.

Schweitzer employs a practical and comprehensive approach to visual rehabilitation, recognizing the wide variety of associated deficits in patients with hemianopia.[52] His ergotherapy tries to improve "difficulty dressing, . . . poor spatial orientation, . . . difficulty construing spatial relations or reading." Ergotherapy seems a very practical approach, giving help with activities of everyday life, such as household training, functional games, craft skills, etc. In a well-protected environment, the patient learns to judge his or her capabilities and to make the best of his or her strengths and weaknesses in daily life. Such therapy is not likely to be reimbursed in the United States or to turn much of a profit for investors!

The simpler technique of using press-on Fresnel prisms would seem more suited to the health care system in the United States.[53] The authors claim that it helped 26% of 41 patients with homonymous hemianopia over a 10-year period, usually those patients with good acuity and an otherwise normal neurological status and proper motivation.

Functional Hemianopia

Gittinger reviews the controversial history of functional hemianopia from Briquet's 1859 monograph on 430 cases of hysteria, through the 19th century works of Charcot, Freud, and Janet, and the observations of Fox and Wilbrand and Saenger in the early 20th century.[54] Neetens and Smet allow that the causes for functional visual loss are variable: conversion symptoms, malingering, easy suggestibility, and the like.[55] Generally, the task falling to the ophthalmologist is indeed to prove the absence of serious organic pathologic conditions, but it is a task that many of us focus on to the neglect of the more complex underlying problems that cause the visual symptoms. Demonstrating the functional nature of these visual symptoms is usually easy and made easier with modern neuroimaging. Many of these patients have broader problems related to difficulty in coping with life. We should avoid labeling all patients with functional visual loss as "hysteric." Bell et al. found hemifield pattern-onset more helpful than pattern-reversal visually evoked potentials in reaching the correct diagnosis in a patient with functional overlay and negative imaging.[56]

Sectoral Hemianopia

Glickstein links the cortical map of the visual field to the Russo-Japanese war.[57] The precise occipital lesions caused by the higher velocity and smaller caliber of bullets from a new Russian rifle enabled Tatsuji Inouye to correct earlier conclusions of Henschen and show that the macular region is represented at the occipital poles and is magnified in relation to the peripheral parts of the field. Inouye's work was overshadowed by the similar conclusion of Gordon Holmes and William Lister, studying soldiers injured in World War I, because the drawings of Holmes and Lister were easier to interpret. Inouye argued in favor of bilateral representation of the macula, Holmes against it.

How can an extrastriate lesion with irregular borders cause an homonymous altitudinal field defect with a linear horizontal edge? Areas V2, V3, and V3A each contain a second order transformation of the visual hemifield, splitting along the representation of the horizontal meridian to form thin belts wrapped around striate cortex. In this manner, the multiple extrastriate representations of the upper visual quadrant are physically separated form those of the lower visual quadrant. An irregular lesion placed within areas V2, V3, V3A may be sufficient to create a visual field defect. Horton and Hoyt argue that, although the lesion may straddle these areas without regard to isoazimuth and isoelevation lines, it will produce a quadrantic field defect with a clean horizontal border because of the inherent arrangement of the upper and lower visual hemifield representations in extrastriate cortex.[58] Thus, they maintain that a horizontal border of a hemianopic visual field defect is a clue to the extrastriate location of the lesion.

Lakhanpal and Selhorst describe two patients who suffered strokes and had absolute, complete, binocular inferior altitudinal hemianopic defects (AVFDs) that involved both nasal and adjacent temporal quadrants and respected the horizontal meridian.[59] They remind us that only AVFDs due to occipital infarcts spare fixation because of the anastomotic blood supply of the occipital pole. The infarcts appeared to be in the posterior aspect of the occipital lobe, superior to the calcarine fissure, but not localized well enough on CT scans to test Horton and Hoyt's theory. Another patient with congruous homonymous superior quadrantanopia had infarction of the striate cortex at autopsy.[60] Despite pathologic examination, the infarcts, described as patchy, were again not localized well enough to test Horton and Hoyt's theory.

Gunderson and Hoyt's report of horizontal homonymous sectoral defects as an indication of geniculate hemianopia,[61] and then Frisén's association of a similar defect with the distal anterior choroidal artery,[62] created opportunities for later authors to report exceptions. Grossman et al. describe a patient with such a defect caused by infarction of the territory of a penetrating branch of the calcarine artery in the area of the calcarine fissure.[63]

Macular Sparing

Coincidentally, sector retinitis pigmentosa caused monocular hemianopia that respected the vertical meridian and spared macular vision.[64] Manor used the entoptic phenomenon called Haidinger's Brushes to study macular sparing.[43] Most patients with postgeniculate lesions had it and most with pregeniculate lesions did not. This subjective test may not have been sensitive enough to detect the foveal sparing related to nasotemporal overlap demonstrated in anatomic studies.

ALZHEIMER'S DISEASE

Evidence is growing to support the idea that Alzheimer's disease (AD) affects parts of the brain. It follows that the visual deficits may be specific. Developing a correspondence between anatomy and pathology will take some time, however, at least partly because of the difficulty in making reliable quantitative observations among these patients.

Examining toluidine blue-stained and also paraphenylene diamine flat-mount preparations, Sadun and Bassi found that early AD has a predilection for retinal ganglion cells with the largest axons.[65] Thus, they postulate that selective involvement of the M-cell system (ganglion cells that project to magnocellular layer in lateral geniculate body, to cortex, to middle temporal (MT) area) might explain deficits in contrast sensitivity, spatial orientation, and eye movement control with only minimal effects on visual acuity.

Beach and associates discovered selective involvement of neuronal populations within area 17 of the visual cortex.[66] Staining with the monoclonal antibody, Alz-50, which identifies pathologically involved neuronal systems in patients with AD, revealed strong positive staining only in AD cases (not in healthy subjects). The pattern of staining was highly lamina-selective: laminae I-IVa and V were intensely stained, lamina VI was moderately intense, and laminae IVb and IVc were relatively unstained. The results support the growing consensus that cortical pathology in AD is not generalized, but affects specific neuronal populations.

Mendez et al. begin to sort out the visual deficits that may prove specific to AD.[67] Despite preserved visual acuity and color recognition, patients with AD were impaired in the visual evaluation of common objects, famous faces, spatial locations, and complex figures. All had disturbances in figure-ground analysis; 57% had difficulty visually recognizing actual objects. A subgroup of younger patients had Balint's syndrome; they may present to the ophthalmologist with visuo-spatial difficulties, particularly in locating objects in space. They have constriction of their effective visual fields, difficulty exploring space, poor hand-eye coordination, and abnormal control of eye movements. In trying to explain these deficits, the authors remind us that neurofibrillary tangles, associated with severity of dementia, are rare in area 17, increase 20-fold in area 18, and nearly double again in area 20.

Consistent with these selective pathologic findings, single photon emission computed tomography (SPECT) and PET also show hypoperfusion and hypometabolism in the posterior parietotemporal regions and relative sparing of the visual cortex that correlate with the severity of the disease.[68]

The involvement of the anterior visual pathway in AD is perhaps surprising, but is confirmed with electrical studies. Two other groups have also found that mean amplitude of the pattern-reversal electroretinogram in patients with AD is significantly less than that of a control group, probably because of axon depletion in the optic nerve and degeneration of retinal ganglion cells.[69, 70] Patients with AD had normal pattern-reversal evoked cortical potentials but a delayed second component of the flash evoked potential, the latter a confirmation of an established finding.

CORTICAL BLINDNESS

Several new causes of cortical blindness have been described since the last edition. A patient suffered 90 minutes of cortical blindness during a hypotensive episode caused by postpartum pulmonary embolism. Recovery of vision and cardiopulmonary function were good.[71] A young patient with a blood cyclosporine level almost six times the usual therapeutic value experienced transient cortical blindness associated with continuous focal occipital EEG discharge. Seizures are a well-recognized complication of cyclosporine toxicity. Phenytoin is useful for two reasons: (1) to act as an anticonvulsant; and (2) to accelerate the hepatic oxidative metabolism of cyclosporine.[72]

Four patients experienced transient cortical blindness after intraarterial injection of an iodinated contrast agent.[73] Immediate CT showed abnormal contrast enhancement in the occipital lobes in all four cases, and one of two patients had high signal intensity on T2-weighted MRI images in the occipital lobes. Follow-up CT scans were obtained in two cases and had returned to normal. Duncan et al. describe three patients with cortical blindness during eclampsia.[74] Hyperintensity on T2-weighted MRI and hypointensity on T1-weighted MRI indicated that the lesions were ischemic rather than hemorrhagic. Vision improved in all three patients.

HALLUCINATIONS

Lance has postulated that visual hallucinations arise from the visual association cortex when it is deprived of inflow from striate cortex and are not unusual when a patient has a visual field defect.[28] Benson described a patient who experienced formed hallucinations as the sole presenting feature of hemianopia caused by an occipital infarct.[75] Lepore reviews the characteristics of visual hallucinations among 104 patients with lesions affecting vision.[76] The visual images were elementary in 51% and complex in 21% (people, faces, animals, etc); no reasons can be found to account for the difference. Unlike the irritative kind, these hallucinations do not aid in localization. They are more frequent when visual acuity is less than 20/50, whether caused by pre- or post-geniculate lesions. Lepore reaffirms previous observations that purely visual hallucinations are not characteristic isolated symptoms of a psychiatric disorder; rather, they occur in patients with eye and neurologic diseases.

INFECTIOUS/INFLAMMATORY DISEASE

Acquired Immunodeficiency Syndrome

A major discussion of the visual complications of the acquired immunodeficiency syndrome (AIDS) belongs in another chapter, because visual symptoms in patients with AIDS usually relate to involvement of the eyeball. Nevertheless, visual symptoms occasionally arise from focal cerebral lesions, which occur in 10% of patients with AIDS. Half of the mass lesions are toxoplasmosis; lymphoma is next most common. Encephalopathy and cryptococcosis rarely cause focal symptoms.

In apparent contrast to that general rule, in a pathologic study, Mizusawa et al. found a surprisingly high incidence (34%) of cerebrovascular lesions in 83 patients with AIDS.[77] Cerebral hemorrhage had occurred in 4 cases, cerebral infarct in 23 cases, and both in 1 case. Most of the 24 infarctions were asymptomatic, multiple, and small and involved the striatum, cerebral cortex, and brain stem. Mural thickening small blood vessels, seen in 50% of cases with infarcts, may have been pathogenetic. Other causes of the infarcts included vasculitis, perivascular lymphocytic infiltration, thromboembolism, and systemic ischemia/anoxia.

Central nervous system (CNS) manifestations herald the onset of AIDS in about 10% of cases. Slavin et al. describe a patient with isolated homonymous hemianopia as a first manifestation.[78] Eventually, additional cerebral lesions developed that suggested progressive multifocal leukoencephalopathy. The patient died 4 months after the initial symptoms, but postmortem studies were not done. Toxoplasmosis caused a partial hemianopic defect in another patient.[79]

Other Infectious and Inflammatory Diseases

Stressing that isolated angiitis of the nervous system is a diagnosis made only after specific causes of granulomatous angiitis are excluded, Moore advocates aggressive therapy with prednisone and cyclophosphamide.[80] She reports five patients with this often fatal illness who responded well to this therapy.

The diagnosis of isolated angiitis must rest on more than segmental arterial narrowing on an arteriogram, which can be caused by a variety of other conditions, including postpartum hypertension.[81] Cocaine abuse can cause cerebral vasculitis with symptoms including cortical blindness.[82] The symptoms in two cocaine abusers were prolonged but eventually improved. Among other specific causes for cerebral vasculitis recently was acute infection with a non-spotted fever group *Rickettsia,* most likely either *Rickettsia typhi* or *R. canada.*[83] Serum samples from a mouse trapped at the patient's home contained antibody only to *R. canada.*

Another 16-year-old patient with progressive encephalopathy caused by cerebral vasculitis proved to have borreliosis.[84] During and after antibiotic treatment, all clinical symptoms and pathologic changes in the cerebrospinal fluid almost completely disappeared. Two other patients had arteriographic signs suggesting vasculitis of the basilar artery that were caused by *Borrelia burgdorferi* basilar meningitis.[85] The authors prefer the term neuroborreliosis. One of six patients with CNS manifestations of infection with *B. burgdorferi* had a brain biopsy specimen that showed microgliosis without an inflammatory infiltrate or vasculitis.[86] Weeks to years after initial infection, these patients presented with behavioral changes, ataxia, and/or weakness in bulbar or peripheral muscles. Only four responded well to penicillin therapy. MRI abnormalities in the brains in two patients resembled those of demyelination.

Sotelo et al. had good success in treating neurocysticercosis with albendazole, even when they shortened the usual period of therapy from 1 month to 1 week.[87]

NEUROIMAGING

Srebro and Purdy used evoked scalp potentials, CT, and MRI to localize cortical activity evoked by visual stimuli in humans.[88] Veraart et al. studied glucose utilization in the visual cortex of blind human subjects with PET.[89] In six subjects who became blind early in life, metabolism in the visual cortex was elevated compared with that in healthy subjects with the eyes open. By contrast, glucose utilization in the visual areas of six human subjects who became blind after completion of visual development was decreased, slightly lower than in healthy volunteers studied with the eyes closed. The authors postulate that the difference between early and late blind subjects might reflect the persistence, in early blindness, of supranumerary synapses that would escape the normal developmental decrease in synaptic density during infancy.

Kiyosawa et al. studied the effects of optic radiation infarctions on the metabolism of the visual cortex.[90] Previous reports had shown that ischemia in the calcarine cortex reduces glucose metabolism in those areas of cortex corresponding to the visual field loss, and that lesions in the optic radiations cause less of a reduction.[91] The authors studied eight patients using ^{18}F-fluorodeoxyglucose PET after an isolated stroke had damaged the optic radiations. They found diffuse hypometabolism throughout the damaged cerebral hemisphere, even in cortical areas not infarcted. Glucose metabolism in primary and association visual cortex of the damaged hemisphere was decreased by more than 47%, almost as great a reduction as that found in the infarcted region. Metabolism in the undamaged hemisphere was less affected, but significant decrements were found in calcarine and lateral occipital cortex. The authors postulate that the contralateral effects were the result of transcallosal diaschisis due to damaged callosal connections between homologous regions of hemisphere.

Focal lesions cannot account for many of the neuropsychiatric manifestations of lupus erythematosus (SLE). Although MRI is sensitive in the demonstration of focal lesions, Stoppe et al. suggest that PET may be the best means of studying the changes that underlie the attention and orientation difficulties, memory impairment, etc., caused by SLE, which may relate to widespread antibody mediated neuronal deactivation.[92]

Two of three patients with hypertensive encephalopathy (HTE) were unable to see.[93] MRI demonstrated focal, symmetric increased signal intensity in white matter and cortex, with occipital lobe involvement in each case. These results support the concept that HTE is caused by the extravasation of fluid and proteins across the blood-brain barrier during a breakdown of cerebral autoregulation. The lesions, which have proved to be highly nonspecific MRI findings, resolved in several weeks during treatment.

BLINDSIGHT

Blindsight refers to residual visual capability within visual field defects caused by destruction of part of the striate cortex even though visual stimuli presented in the field defect are not consciously perceived. Some patients can detect and localize unseen stimuli, movement, and orientation when they are required to guess. Although still to some degree controversial, this phenomenon has raised interesting questions regarding the nature of consciousness and the role of the extrastriate pathways in visual processing.

By measuring sensitivity to light of different wavelengths in patients with blindsight, Stoerig and Cowey show that spectral sensitivity in the blind fields is surprisingly high, with a reduction of only 1 log unit or less across the visible spectrum.[94] The sensitivity curve is also essentially normal in form, whether the patients are adapted to light or dark. A shift in peak sensitivity from medium to shorter wavelengths in adaptation to the dark (the Purkinje shift) and the presence of discontinuities in the light-adapted curve together show that blindsight involves both rod and cone contributions, and that some color opponency remains. Marshall and Halligan report an analogous dissociation between overt and covert perception in a patient with visuo-spatial neglect.[95] The patient had left homonymous hemianopia and neglect, the latter not a direct consequence of the former. Examiners presented simultaneously two line drawings of a house; in one, the left side was on fire. She judged that the drawings were identical; yet when asked to select where she would prefer to live, she reliably chose the house that was not burning. A 30-year-old woman after occipital lobectomy could detect moving luminance gratings in her blind hemifield in 68% of trials, but saw stationary gratings only at a chance level.[96]

MIGRAINE

Hupp et al. review the visual symptoms associated with migraine and current theories of pathophysiology.[97] They offer a diagnostic algorithm to help differentiate migraine from more serious conditions. In another report, two adults experienced new-onset migrainous-type visual disturbances and had filling defects near the torcular Herophili on angiography, indicating venous sinus thrombosis.[98] Neither patient had a visual field deficit nor CT evidence of an occipital infarction. Another patient with migraine had a 14-year history of diplopia, using either eye alone or both.[99] One MRI showed the ubiquitous and nonspecific multifocal white-matter lucencies, but a follow-up MRI did not. Patients with migraine are far more likely to experience discomfort when viewing black-and-white striped patterns.[100]

Welch and Levine ask three questions regarding the relationship of migraine and stroke, review the evidence, and answer yes to each: (1) Does stroke occur in the course of a migraine attack, causing true migraine-related cerebral infarction? (2) Does migraine cause stroke because other risk factors for stroke are present to interact with the migraine-induced pathogenesis? (3) Can stroke present as a migraine syndrome, i.e., symptomatic migraine?[101] The authors view migraine-related stroke as a result of interaction of coagulation, hemodynamic, and neuronal factors.

Careful perimetry disclosed some form of visual field abnormality in a surprising 35% of 60 patients with migraine (defined by the Ad Hoc Committee on Headache).[102] The prevalence of field loss increased with increasing age and duration of the migraine problem. Three patients had hemianopic defects. The abnormalities were significant when compared with the age-matched normal values of the Humphrey Field Analyzer. The authors didn't determine how many defects were permanent and found some initially abnormal fields to be normal on retesting. Still, the possibility of lasting visual loss strengthens indications for treating a relatively benign problem.

REFERENCES

1. Cohen B, Bodis-Wollner I (eds): Vision and the Brain, vol 67. New York, Raven Press, 1990.

2. Berninger TA, Arden GB, Hogg CR, et al: Separable evoked retinal and cortical potentials from each major visual pathway: Preliminary results. *Br J Ophthalmol* 1989; 73:502–511.

3. Rimmer S, Iragui V, Klauber MR, et al: Retinocortical time exhibits spatial selectivity. *Invest Ophthalmol Vis Sci* 1989; 30:2045–2049.

4. Raichle ME: Developing a functional anatomy of the human visual system with positron emission tomography, in Cohen B, Bodis-Wallner I (eds): *Vision and the Brain*. New York, Raven Press, 199.

5. Mintun MA, Fox PT, Raichle ME: A highly accurate method of localizing regions of neuronal activation in the human brain with positron emission tomography. *J Cereb Blood Flow Metab* 1989; 9:96–103.

6. Lueck CJ, Zeki S, Friston KJ, et al: The color centre in the cerebral cortex of man. *Nature* 1989; 340:386–389.

7. Stryker MP: Cortical physiology. Is grandmother an oscillation? *Nature* 1989; 338:297–298.

8. Gray CM, Singer W: Stimulus-specific neuronal oscillations in orientation columns of cat visual cortex. *Proc Natl Acad Sci USA* 1989; 86:1698–1702.

9. Gray CM, Konig P, Engel AK, et al: Oscillatory responses in cat visual cortex exhibit intercolumnar synchronization which reflects global stimulus properties. *Nature* 1989; 338:334–337.

10. Eckhorn R, Bauer R, Jordan W, et al: Coherent oscillations: A mechanism of feature linking in the visual cortex? Multiple electrode and correlation analyses in the cat. *Biol Cybern* 1988; 60:121–130.

11. Tolhurst DJ, Ling L: Magnification factors and the organization of the human striate cortex. *Hum Neurobiol* 1988; 6:247–254.

12. Hockfield S, Tootell RB, Zaremba S: Molecular differences among neurons reveal an organization of human visual cortex. *Proc Natl Acad Sci USA* 1990; 87:3027–3031.

13. Burkhalter A, Bernardo KL: Organization of corticocortical connections in human visual cortex. *Proc Natl Acad Sci USA* 1989; 86:1071–1075.

14. Watson AB, Ahumada AJ Jr: A hexagonal orthogonal-oriented pyramid as a model of image representation in visual cortex. *IEEE Trans Biomed Eng* 1989; 36:97–106.

15. Rizzo M, Robin DA: Simultanagnosia: A defect of sustained attention yields insights on visual information processing. *Neurology* 1990; 40:447–455.

16. Rizzo M, Hurtig R: The effect of bilateral visual cortex lesions on the development of eye movements and perception. *Neurology* 1989; 39:406–413.

17. Landau WM: Au clair de lacune: Holy, wholly, holey logic. *Neurology* 1989; 39:725–730.

18. Wiebers DO, Swanson JW, Cascino TL, et al: Bilateral loss of vision in bright light. *Stroke* 1989; 20:554–558.

19. Pessin MS, Kwan ES, Scott RM, et al: Occipital infarction with hemianopsia from carotid occlusive disease. *Stroke* 1989; 20:409–411.

20. Cohen SN: Occipital infarction with hemianopsia from carotid occlusive disease. *Stroke* 1989; 20:1433–1434.

21. Caplan LR: Intracranial branch atheromatous disease: A neglected, understudied, and underused concept. *Neurology* 1989; 39:1246–1250.

22. Caplan LR, DeWitt LD, Pessin MS, et al: Lateral thalamic infarcts. *Arch Neurol* 1988; 45:959–964.

23. Bruno A, Graff-Radford NR, Biller J, et al: Anterior choroidal artery territory infarction: A small vessel disease. *Stroke* 1989; 20:616–619.

24. Ghika J, Bogousslavsky J, Regli F: Infarcts in the territory of the deep perforators of the carotid system. *Neurology* 1989; 39:507–512.

25. Anderson DR, Trobe JD, Hood TW, et al: Optic tract injury after anterior temporal lobectomy. *Ophthalmology* 1989; 96:1065–1070.

26. Ringelstein EB, Koschorke S, Holling A, et al: Computed tomographic patterns of proven embolic brain infarctions. *Ann Neurol* 1990; 26:759–765.

27. Lee KS, Spetzler RF: Cerebral cavernous malformations. *Arch Neurol* 1989; 46:1273.

28. Lance JW, Smee RI: Partial seizures with visual disturbance treated by radiotherapy of cavernous hemangioma. *Ann Neurol* 1989; 26:782–785.

29. Rigamonti D, Hadley MN, Drayer BP, et al: Cerebral cavernous malformations. Incidence and familial occurrence. *N Engl J Med* 1988; 319:343–347.

30. Mason I, Aase JM, Orrison WW, et al: Familial cavernous angiomas of the brain in an Hispanic family. *Neurology* 1988; 38:324–326.

31. Allard JC, Hochberg FH, Franklin PD: Magnetic resonance imaging in a family with hereditary cerebral arteriovenous malformations. *Arch Neurol* 1989; 46:184–187.

32. Rigamonti D, Spetzler RF: The association of venous and cavernous malformations. Report of four cases and discussion of the pathophysiological, diagnostic, and therapeutic implications. *Acta Neurochir (Wien)* 1988; 92:100–105.

33. Farmer J-P, Cosgrove GR, Villemure J-G, et al: Intracerebral cavernous hemangiomas. *Neurology* 1988; 38:1699–1704.

34. Altschuler EM, Lunsford LD, Coffey RJ, et al: Gamma knife radiosurgery for intracranial arteriovenous malformations in childhood and adolescence. *Pediatr Neurosci* 1989; 15:53–61.

35. Seifert V, Trost HA, Dietz H: Cavernous angiomas of the supratentorial compartment. *Zentralbl Neurochir* 1989; 50:89–92.

36. Fahlbusch R, Strauss C, Huk W, et al: Surgical removal of pontomesencephalic cavernous hemangiomas. *Neurosurgery* 1990; 26:449–456.

37. Kashiwagi S, van Loveren HR, Tew JM Jr, et al: Diagnosis and treatment of vascular brain-stem malformations. *J Neurosurg* 1990; 72:27–34.

38. Kashii S, Solomon SK, Moser, et al: Progressive visual field defects in patients with intracranial arteriovenous malformations. *Am J Ophthalmol* 1990; 109:556–562.

39. Chimowitz MI, Little JR, Awad IA, et al: Intracranial hypertension associated with unruptured cerebral arteriovenous malformations. *Ann Neurol* 1990; 27:474–479.

40. Cairncross JG, Laperriere NJ: Low-grade glioma: To treat or not to treat? *Arch Neurol* 1989; 46:1238–1239.

41. Fletcher WA, Hoyt WF, Narahara MH: Congenital quadrantanopia with occipital lobe ganglioglioma. *Neurology* 1988; 38:1892–1894.

42. Castillo M, Davis PC, Takei Y, et al: Intracranial ganglioglioma: MR, CT, and clinical findings in 18 patients. *AJNR* 1990; 11:109–114.

43. Manor RS: Entoptic [corrected] phenomena in pregeniculate and postgeniculate hemianopsia with splitting of macula by perimetry *Am J Ophthalmol* 1989; 108:585–591.

44. Glovinsky Y, Quigley HA, Bissett RA, et al: Artificially produced quadrantanopsia in computed visual field testing. *Am J Ophthalmol* 1990; 110:90–91.

45. Hess RF, Pointer JS: Spatial and temporal contrast sensitivity in hemianopia. A comparative study of the sighted and blind hemifields. *Brain* 1989; 112:871–894.

46. Zihl J, Roth W, Kerkhoff G, et al: The influence of homonymous visual field disorders on color sorting performance in the FM 100-hue test. *Neuropsychologia* 1988; 26:869–876.

47. Kooistra CA, Heilman KM: Hemispatial visual inattention masquerading as hemianopia. *Neurology* 1989; 39:1125–1127.

48. Kolmel HW, Nabel HJ: Optokinetic nystagmus in homonymous hemianopia due to a strictly occipital lesion. *Eur Arch Psychiatry Neurol Sci* 1989; 238:199–202.

49. Gray CS, French JM, Bates D, et al: Recovery of visual fields in acute stroke: Homonymous hemianopia associated with adverse prognosis. *Age Ageing* 1989; 18:419–421.

50. Eber AM, Metz-Lutz MN, Strubel D, et al: Electro-oculographic study of reading in hemianopic patients. *Rev Neurol (Paris)* 1988; 144:515–518.

51. Zihl J: Homonymous hemianopsia and its rehabilitation. *Klin Monatsbl Augenheilkd* 1988; 192:555–558.

52. Schweizer V: Rehabilitation of the hemianopsia patient from the viewpoint of the ergotherapist. *Klin Monatsbl Augenheilkd* 1988; 192:559–564.

53. Hedges TR Jr, Stunkard J, Twer A: Fresnel prisms—their value in the rehabilitation of homonymous hemianopsias. *Klin Monatsbl Augenheilkd* 1988; 192:568–571.

54. Gittinger JW Jr: Functional hemianopsia: A historical perspective. *Surv Ophthalmol* 1988; 32:427–432.

55. Neetens A, Smet H: Functional monocular hemianopsia. *Klin Monatsbl Augenheilkd* 1988; 192:551–554.

56. Bell RA, Biersdorf WR, Beck RW: Homonymous hemianopia and pattern onset hemifield visual evoked potentials. *Arch Ophthalmol* 1989; 107:1429–1430.

57. Glickstein M: The discovery of the visual cortex. *Sci Am* 1988; 259:118–127.

58. Horton JC, Hoyt WF: Occipital visual field defects respecting the horizontal meridian: A hallmark of extrastriate cortical lesions. Presented at the 16th Annual North American Neuro-ophthalmological Society Meeting, Steamboat Springs, Colo, Feb 1990.

59. Lakhanpal A, Selhorst JB: Bilateral altitudinal visual fields. *Ann Ophthalmol* 1990; 22:112–117.

60. Gomez CR, Bhat MH, Chung HD: Homonymous quadrantic visual field defect resulting from vertebrobasilar insufficiency: Report of a case. *Angiology* 1990; 41:151–155.

61. Gunderson CH, Hoyt WF: Geniculate hemianopia: Incongruous homonymous field defects in two patients with partial lesions of the lateral geniculate nucleus. *J Neurol Neurosurg Psychiatry* 1971; 34:1–6.

62. Frisén L: Quadruple sectoranopia and sectoral optic atrophy. A syndrome of the distal anterior choroidal artery. *J Neurol Neurosurg Psychiatry* 1979; 42:590–594.

63. Grossman M, Galetta SL, Nichols CW, et al: Horizontal homonymous sectoral field defect after ischemic infarction of the occipital cortex. *Am J Ophthalmol* 1990; 109:234–236.

64. Johnson LN, Rabinowitz YS, Hepler RS: Hemianopia resecting the vertical meridian and with foveal sparing from retinal degeneration. *Neurology* 1989; 39:872–873.

65. Sadun AA, Bassi CJ: The visual system in Alzheimer's disease, in Cohen B, Bodis-Wollner (eds): *Vision and the Brain,* vol 67. New York, Raven Press, 1990, pp 331–347.

66. Beach TG, Walker R, McGeer EG: Lamina-selective A68 immunoreactivity in primary visual cortex of Alzheimer's disease patients. *Brain Res* 1989; 501:171–174.

67. Mendez MF, Mendez MA, Martin R, et al: Complex visual disturbances in Alzheimer's disease. *Neurology* 1990; 40:439–443.

68. DeKosky ST, Shih WJ, Schmitt FA, et al: Assessing utility of single photon emission computed tomography (SPECT) scan in Alzheimer disease: Correlation with cognitive severity. *Alzheimer Dis Assoc Disord* 1990; 4:14–23.

69. Katz B, Rimmer S, Iragui V, et al: Abnormal pattern electroretinogram in Alzheimer's disease: Evidence for retinal ganglion cell degeneration? *Ann Neurol* 1989; 26:221–225.

70. Trick GL, Barris MC, Bickler-Bluth M: Abnormal pattern electroretinogram in patients with senile dementia of the Alzheimer type. *Ann Neurol* 1990; 26:226–231.

71. Beck L, Stiller RJ, Leone-Tomaschoff S, et al: Postpartum pulmonary embolus as an unusual cause of cortical blindness. *Am J Obstet Gynecol* 1990; 162:696–697.

72. Rubin AM: Transient cortical blindness and occipital seizures with cyclosporine toxicity. *Transplantation* 1989; 47:572–573.

73. Lantos G: Cortical blindness due to osmotic disruption of the blood-brain barrier by angiographic contrast material: CT and MRI studies. *Neurology* 1989; 39:567–571.

74. Duncan R, Hadley D, Bone I, et al: Blindness in eclampsia: CT and MR imaging. *J Neurol Neurosurg Psychiatry* 1989; 52:899–902.

75. Benson MT, Rennie IG: Formed hallucination in the hemianopic field. *Postgrad Med J* 1989; 65:756–757.

76. Lepore FE: Spontaneous visual phenomena with visual loss: 104 patients with lesions of retinal and neural afferent pathways. *Neurology* 1990; 40:444–447.

77. Mizusawa H, Hirano A, Llena JF, et al: Cerebrovascular lesions in acquired immune deficiency syndrome (AIDS). *Acta Neuropathol (Berl)* 1988; 76:451–457.

78. Slavin ML, Mallin JE, Jacob HS: Isolated homonymous hemianopsia in the acquired immunodeficiency syndrome. *Am J Ophthalmol* 1989; 108:198–200.

79. Girard B, Thenot JC, Topouzis F, et al: Homonymous lateral quadranopsia disclosing cerebral toxoplasmosis in a patient with AIDS. *Bull Soc Ophtalmol Fr* 1989; 89:1373–1378.

80. Moore PM: Diagnosis and management of isolated angiitis of the central nervous system. *Neurology* 1989; 39:167–173.

81. Garner BF, Burns P, Bunning RD, et al: Acute blood pressure elevation can mimic arteriographic appearance of cerebral vasculitis—(a postpartum case with relative hypertension). *J Rheumatol* 1990; 17:93–97.

82. Krendel DA, Ditter SM, Frankel MR, et al: Biopsy-proven cerebral vasculitis associated with cocaine abuse. *Neurology* 1990; 40:1092–1094.

83. Linnemann CC Jr, Pretzman CI, Peterson ED: Acute febrile cerebrovasculitis. A non-spotted fever group rickettsial disease. *Arch Intern Med* 1989; 149:1682–1684.

84. Lock G, Berger G, Grobe H: Neuroborreliosis: progressive encephalomyelitis with cerebral vasculitis. *Monatsschr Kinderheilkd* 1989; 137:101–104.

85. Veenendaal-Hilbers JA, Perquin WV, Hoogland PH, et al: Basal meningovasculitis and occlusion of the basilar artery in two cases of *Borrelia burgdorferi* infection. *Neurology* 1988; 38:1317–1319.

86. Pachner AR, Duray P, Steere AC: Central nervous system manifestations of Lyme disease. *Arch Neurol* 1989; 46:790–797.

87. Sotelo J, Penagos P, Escobedo F, et al: Short course of albendazole therapy for neurocysticercosis. *Arch Neurol* 1988; 45:1130–1133.

88. Srebro R, Purdy PD: Localization of visually evoked cortical activity using magnetic resonance imaging and computerized tomography. *Vision Res* 1990; 30:351–358.

89. Veraart C, De Volder AG, Wanet-Defalque MC, et al: Glucose utilization in human visual cortex is abnormally elevated in blindness of early onset but decreased in blindness of late onset. *Brain Res* 1990; 510:115–121.

90. Kiyosawa M, Bosley TM, Kushner M, et al: Middle cerebral artery strokes causing homonymous hemianopia: Positron emission tomography. *Ann Neurol* 1990; 28:180–183.

91. Mora BN, Carman GJ, Allman JM: In vivo functional localization of the human visual cortex using positron emission tomography and magnetic resonance imaging. *Trends Neurosci* 1989; 12:282–284.

92. Stoppe G, Wildhagen K, Seidel JW, et al: Positron emission tomography in neuropsychiatric lupus erythematosus. *Neurology* 1990; 40:304–308.

93. Hauser RA, Lacey DM, Knight MR: Hypertensive encephalopathy. Magnetic resonance imaging demonstration of reversible cortical white matter lesions. *Arch Neurol* 1988; 45:1078–1083.

94. Stoerig P, Cowey A: Wavelength sensitivity in blindsight. *Nature* 1989; 342:916–918.

95. Marshall JC, Halligan PW: Blindsight and insight in visuo-spatial neglect. *Nature* 1988; 336:766–767.

96. Magnussen S, Mathiesen T: Detection of moving and stationary gratings in the absence of striate cortex. *Neuropsychologia* 1989; 27:725–728.

97. Hupp SL, Kline LB, Corbett JJ: Visual disturbances of migraine. *Surv Ophthalmol* 1989; 33:221–236.

98. Newman DS, Levine SR, Curtis VL, et al: Migraine-like visual phenomena associated with cerebral venous thrombosis. *Headache* 1989; 29:82–85.

99. Sinoff SE, Rosenberg M: Permanent cerebral diplopia in a migraineur. *Neurology* 1990; 40:1138–1139.

100. Marcus DA, Soso MJ: Migraine and stripe-induced visual discomfort. *Arch Neurol* 1989; 46:1129–1132.

101. Welch KMA, Levine SR: Migraine-related stroke in the context of the international headache society classification of head pain. *Arch Neurol* 1990; 47:458–462.

102. Lewis RA, Vijayan N, Watson C, et al: Visual field loss in migraine. *Ophthalmology* 1989; 96:321–326.

CHAPTER 6

Higher Visual Functions

Michael S. Mega, M.D.

Teaching Fellow in Neurology, Department of Neurology, Boston University School of Medicine; Resident in Neurology, Boston Veterans Administration Medical Center, Boston, Massachusetts

Jon Erik Ween, M.D.

Teaching Fellow in Neurology, Department of Neurology, Boston University School of Medicine; Resident in Neurology, Boston Veterans Administration Medical Center, Boston, Massachusetts

Martin L. Albert, M.D., Ph.D.

Professor of Neurology, Boston University School of Medicine; Director, Behavioral Neuroscience, Department of Neurology, Boston University School of Medicine and Boston Veterans Administration Medical Center, Boston, Massachusetts

Two trends emerge as dominant in the current literature on higher visual functions. First is the introduction of a multidisciplinary approach to the study of vision coupled with the application of experimental methods from the field of cognitive neuroscience. Second is the effort to move beyond descriptive phenomena toward the development of neural theories of higher visual functions that are experimentally testable. We shall emphasize these two trends as we review current research in the following categories: disorders of visual attention (neglect syndromes); disorders of perception and visual synthesis (apperceptive agnosia, associative agnosia, prosopagnosia); and disorders of mental imagery.

One popular theoretical and experimental framework for understanding higher visual functions derives from cognitive neuroscience. According to this view, the brain is a computational device that transforms sensory data (input) into behavior (output). The brain accomplishes this computational process by executing many calculations simultaneously (in parallel) rather than one after another (in series) as in a standard computer. Hence for the visual system, rather than functioning as a single processor, many subsystems, or modules, operate in parallel. These subsystems are dependent on widely distributed neural networks that overlap with or share elements of other related networks. However, each operates according to its own set of parameters and constraints.

By the end of this chapter, we will have drawn a picture of higher visual functions as dependent on interlocking sets of functional modules (attention, perception, comprehension, etc.), supported by a neurobiologic substrate of multiple, overlapping neural networks distributed throughout the brain and acting simultaneously in series and in parallel. Higher visual processing begins with attentional mechanisms which, relative to input on body posture, specify the location of a target in space; encoding occurs in the right parietal cortex via tectopulvinar juxtastriate pathways known as the dorsal visual system. This component of the visual system operates in a highly redundant, parallel fashion coordinating the spatial representations of each subsystem. Once attention is focused, invariant features regarding contour and shading of a target are extracted and encoded in the left inferior temporal lobe via geniculostriate pathways known as the ventral visual system. This system is thought to operate in a predominantly serial way.

DISORDERS OF ATTENTION (NEGLECT SYNDROMES)

Kinsbourne[1] developed the (by now well-known) theory of cerebral hemispheric attentional bias that has been further elaborated by Heilman and his collaborators[2] as reduced capacity for activation. The right hemisphere (RH) is thought to activate spatial representational mechanisms in both hemispheres, while the left hemisphere (LH) can activate only its own. Right hemispheric damage (RHD) would then provoke bihemispheric hypoarousal and prevent LH systems from compensating for the deficit, thus resulting in left-sided neglect; whereas LH damage still would allow intact RH mechanisms to function and overcome right-sided neglect. Halligan and Marshall[3] described a patient with a right temporoparietal infarct in whom severe left field neglect resulted when the subject used the right hand, but was much less severe when the mildly paretic left hand was used. Presumably activating the RH by using the left hand stimulated both hemispheres, thereby allowing RH function to overcome the neglect somewhat, whereas stimulating the LH by using the right hand failed to activate the RH representational systems properly. Nichelli and Rinaldi[4] provided further evidence in favor of the attentional bias theory with normal dextrals who showed systematic errors to the left of the true midline during line bisection with their right hand but not when using their left, revealing a surprising lack of hemispheric crosstalk.

If Heilman's theory is correct, then one would expect activation of hemispheric representational systems by other modalities that involve spatial representations to influence the neglect syndrome. This was found by Cappa et al.[5] when vestibular stimulation was shown to decrease the severity of neglect and in some cases abolish it altogether. Passive nonverbal auditory stimulation has also been shown to decrease neglect, presumably due to RH activation, while verbal auditory stimulation failed to modify neglect, since it is thought to stimulate the language-dominant LH only.[6]

A further implication of the attentional bias hypothesis is that the bilateral hypoarousal in RHD should also result in some degree of visual inattention in the ipsilateral field as well; this prediction has been verified by Weintraub and Mesulam.[7] However, the mechanism responsible for the ipsilateral disorder may not be the same as that causing contralateral neglect in RHD. Gainotti et al.[8] have found that patients with ipsilateral inattention have a widespread decrease in attention that also affects verbal memory, while patients with RHD with only contralateral neglect show normal verbal memory.

An alternative interpretation of the attentional bias hypothesis was proposed by Coslett et al.,[2] who suggested that the reduced capacity for activation may translate into a reduced capacity for distributing processes in parallel. Patients with RHD and left field neglect showed greater difficulty with double simultaneous tasks than patients with RHD and no neglect, although each task was performed adequately alone, thus indicating that parallel distribution is particularly affected in left neglect states. Rapcsak et al.[9] applied this theory to visual attention. They found that patients with left field neglect showed significantly worse performance when required to distinguish between targets than when asked to cross out any target in the visual field. They concluded that a serial, low-capacity feature detector was engaged in the former situation, while a parallel, high-capacity preattentive mechanism was used to process large scale representations in the latter situation.

In the work by Nichelli and Rinaldi[8] previously cited, the presence of a cue stimulus preceding the target stimulus caused normal subjects to overestimate the space surrounding the cue. This cue response cannot be accounted for by Heilman's hemispheric activation model. The influence of such preattentive cuing in directing attentive mechanisms has been most intensively studied by Posner and collaborators[10] who describe an active, covert attentional mechanism functioning in three steps: disengaging attention; moving it; and re-engaging it in another location. Normal subjects will display decreased response times when cued to the location at which a target will appear, and increased response times when presented with a cue in a different location, termed valid and invalid cues, respectively. Right parietal lobe lesions that cause neglect are shown to increase the delay associated with invalid cuing, implying a deficiency in disengaging attention. Moreover, response time also increases when the subject is required to move attention in a contralesional direction, even in the nonneglected hemispace, suggesting defects in the movement of attention from one location to another.

The brain stem seems to be implicated in this movement of attention. This is demonstrated by studies of patients with Parkinson's disease who are generally slower in responses than normal subjects but who nevertheless show a benefit from valid cuing similar to that in normal subjects and display a marked decrease in the cost of invalid cuing,[11] thus indicating a facilitated disengagement function. This result isolates the "movement of attention" function as a primary contributor to the overall slowing of covert orientation. Indeed, normal subjects, when given dopamine blocking agents, show a similar reduction in cost of invalid cuing. Anatomically this brain stem influence may be mediated by ascending inhibitory projections from the locus ceruleus that focus cortical activity predominantly in the inferior parietal lobe, but not the geniculostriate inferotemporal system.[12]

Studies of patients with progressive supranuclear palsy, on the other hand, demonstrate a smaller benefit to valid, vertical cuing than patients with Parkinson's disease, linking the attentional movement mechanism to premotor programming.[13, 14] Reuter-Lorenz and Posner[15] found neglect in a visual line bisection task only with scanning from right to left, not left to right. The presence of lateral cues biased a normal control group to err on the side of the cue, and in patients with left field neglect reduced or exacerbated the neglect when cues were presented to the left or right of the true midline, respectively. Robertson[16] studied neglect in a free gaze setting and found similar results.

Thus, studies discussed to this point demonstrate: (1) support for the attentional bias hypothesis as it relates to visual processing; and (2) a strong interaction between attentional and effector mechanisms for orientation in space.

Additional studies have shown alterations in scanning strategies and a predilection for exploring the right hemispace in patients with neglect. Interestingly, the patient reported by Halligan and Marshall in the paper previously cited[3] also demonstrated *right* field neglect when bisecting small lines.[17, 18] Finding that their patient had grossly exaggerated variability in his estimate of line midpoint regardless of line length, they resurrected a theory by E. H. Weber regarding the inherent variability of size estimation. The concept of a "just noticeable difference," in conjunction with an altered scanning strategy of starting on the right rather than the left as in normal subjects, could account for the observed behavior. They hypothesized that neglect may be simply an artifact of altered scanning strategies when the subject becomes less able to discriminate differences in size.

A study by Weintraub and Mesulam[19] showed that arranging stimuli in an orderly array greatly reduces the severity of neglect. By adapting a task to minimize extraocular motion, they found a less pronounced deficit. Using an eye camera to track scanning patterns, Ishiai and Furukawa et al.[20] demonstrated a rightward gaze predilection in normal subjects in a line bisection task. They further observed that patients with left field hemianopia without neglect would search to the left endpoint and bisect the line correctly. Patients with left field hemianopia with neglect, however, would not scan to the left but would fixate on the right end and bisect the line to the right of the true midline. These patients would, however, appreciate their error when forced to fixate on the leftmost aspect of the incorrectly bisected lines. This abnormal scanning pattern was thought to be due either to an attentional bias or to hemispheric hypokinesis from decreased arousal, associated with a completion response where the damaged RH automatically uses available input from the LH via callosal connections to form a complete but inaccurate representation.

Work by Rizzolatti et al.[21] on response times to lateralized cues showed a significant response time barrier at horizontal and vertical meridians, suggesting that representational systems also significantly interact with attentional mechanisms. According to Bisiach (Cappa et al.[5]), the brain represents space in three domains: personal space, peripersonal space, and extrapersonal space. More recent work by Pizzamiglio and Cappa et al.[22] found that in patients with unilateral neglect, handling of peripersonal and extrapersonal space collapsed into a single mode that was clearly dissociated from how they handled personal space, suggesting either that they had lost the ability to distinguish between peripersonal and extrapersonal space or that there are only two principal modes of spatial representation, personal and extrapersonal. The representation of objects in space must proceed relative to some frame of reference. There are three possible alternatives: an object centered frame, an environment centered frame, and a viewer centered frame. How reference frames relate to the representational modes previously described is not yet clear, but assuming that an extrapersonal representation utilizes an environment centered frame of reference and the personal space representation uses a viewer centered frame seems reasonable.

Calvanio et al.[23] studied body and environment centered frames of reference in patients with left neglect and found that the neglect represented both body and environment midlines. Farah et al.[24] found that neglect extended to both environment and viewer centered frames, but found no neglect in an object centered frame. Of course, environmental neglect may occur not only in the horizontal axis but also in the vertical and radial axes.[25]

As Calvanio[23] and Farah[24] both point out, results summarized above imply the existence of a system-specific spatial representation: Spatial orientation requires environment and viewer centered frames of reference and can be altered by damage to the dorsal, right hemisphere predominant system; whereas feature detection requires an object-centered frame which, in left neglect states, is preserved in the intact ventral and left hemispheric predominant system. Animal studies cited by Calvanio[23] indicate that body centered frames are more impaired with anterior lesions, where efferent commands originate. In contrast, environment-centered frames are more affected by posterior lesions where afferent, environment input is received. Thus posterior afferent visual systems use extrapersonal spatial representations relative to an environmental coordinate system, while anterior efferent systems use personal space representations based on a viewer centered frame. It is thought by some[26] that each operating system in the brain has its own representational map, and that the major function of association areas is to provide a transformation from one map to another.

In summary, the distribution and focusing of attention, relative to descriptions of body posture, specify the location of a target in space and are coordinated by the right parietal cortex, receiving stimuli via tectopulvinar juxtastriate pathways known as the dorsal visual system. This system is supported by sets of neural networks that operate in a highly redundant, parallel fashion and organize the spatial representations that are characteristic of each subsystem. Once attention is focused, invariant (or categorical) information regarding the target is extracted and encoded in the left inferior temporal lobe via geniculostriate pathways known as the ventral visual system. This system is thought to operate in a predominantly serial way.

DISORDERS OF PERCEPT FORMATION AND VISUAL SYNTHESIS (AGNOSIAS)

Apperceptive Agnosia

Apperceptive visual agnosia was proposed as a theoretical entity by Lissauer[27] when he divided the process of visual perception into two phases: (1) the stage of conscious awareness of a sensory impression (apperception); and (2) the stage of associating semantic notions; i.e., the meaning the object has for us, with the content of apperception (association). In proposing the first stage he cautioned: "There remains the question whether a selective impairment of the apperceptive process can also result in the clinical picture of visual agnosia." (Translation by Jackson.[28])

Presently it is believed by many that an inability to recognize objects in the absence of a primary visual sensory deficit may occur in patients with postrolandic RH lesions. This visual processing defect is thought to arise from a failure to achieve a coherent percept in which the invariant features of an object are specifically encoded, a stage that should be achieved prior to the assignment of semantic meaning to the percept (Marr,[29] Warrington and James[30]). The difficulty in identifying pure cases of apperceptive agnosia may be due in part to the methodologic problems of establishing an intact visual ability to assign semantic meaning, when a patient has already been shown to have a defect in perceptual encoding or categorization.

When Warrington and James[30] speak of a defect in perceptual categorization, they do not mean that defective perceptual categorization is synonymous with apperceptive visual agnosia, but rather that defective perceptual categorization may represent one of several mechanisms that underlie the clinical syndrome of apperceptive visual agnosia. They, as well as many other contemporary cognitive neuropsychologists, have been careful to avoid the common earlier problem of confounding cognitive mechanisms with clinical syndromes. (For a detailed review of the terminologic and conceptual confusion often found in the study of visual agnosia, see Farah.[31])

According to Marr,[29] patients with apperceptive agnosia should be able to process visual information up to the level of a two-and-a-half-dimensional sketch, i.e., one which appreciates the contours and discontinuities of surfaces, but not up to a full three-dimensional model in which the volumetric properties of an object are specified. A study by Warrington and James[32] proposed that the perceptual categorization stage is not obligatory for visual analysis, but that the semantic categorization stage can also receive input from a precategorical visual sensory system. Their evidence for this view is reflected by three patients with postrolandic RH lesions in whom they demonstrated intact visual sensory and visual semantic knowledge but defects in visual perceptual ability. If their conclusion is correct, then the patient with apperceptive agnosia will be functionally less impaired than the patient with associative agnosia, since semantic categorization could still occur and successful interaction with the world of objects would be possible. In our own experience, this clinical situation does, indeed, occur.

Associative Agnosia

Associative visual agnosia is traditionally regarded as the inability to attach semantic meaning to visually perceived objects; thus, the ability to identify seen objects is lost. First described by Charcot[33] in 1883, Lissauer introduced the concept of a two-stage model of visual object recognition in 1890.[27] Two-task categories have generally been used to distinguish between the inability to synthesize sense data into a percept and the separation of that percept from its semantic associations: (1) the ability to match similar but unrecognized objects; and (2) the ability to draw an adequate copy of an unrecognized object.[34] Although associative visual agnosia is widely regarded as a valid clinical syndrome, there is still disagreement on the existence of a pure example, due either to objections concerning the quality of perceptual processing or, less often, to the level of preservation of the semantic system.[35]

The lesion responsible for a visual associative impairment is also disputed. Most reported cases have had left hemispheric (LH) occipitoparietal damage. However, research on split-brain cases[36] challenges the view of unilateral lesions being the sole cause, and a bilateral posterior occipitoparietal lesion has been proposed (Damasio et al.[37]). Recently a case of right hemispace associative visual agnosia was described[35] in a patient with normal visual fields, normal pursuit, and no evidence of extinction, in whom magnetic resonance imaging (MRI) demonstrated an infarct in the left prestriate cortex, and bilateral lesions in the forceps major of the corpus callosum. Although the patient could match unidentified objects presented to his right visual field, he could draw no more than a primal sketch when asked to copy them.

In Marr's model of visual processing[29] a patient's drawing reflects the level of his perceptual form representation; for Marr, the primal sketch is only the first stage in form representation. Recall that, traditionally, one of the criteria of associative agnosia is that an intact three-dimensional model of the object must be demonstrated.

In the case of Charnallet et al.,[35] since the primary visual cortex was spared bilaterally, the patient retained the ability to produce a primal sketch of unidentified objects. The fact that this patient was unable to construct a full three-dimensional representation was due, presumably, to damage in area 18 of prestriate cortex, where it is thought such visual synthesis occurs.[38] More importantly, the fact that this patient was able to assign meaning to a percept, as evidenced by his lack of visual agnosia in free vision, supports the view that a bilateral lesion is necessary for the production of an associative visual agnosia.

The traditional distinction between apperceptive and associative visual agnosia, although supported by occasional, well-described case reports, and popular for more than a century, is not a fully satisfactory classification schema, as evidenced by the lack of crisp allocation of most cases within these two clinical categories. Often presumed cases of associative agnosia have apperceptive qualities, such as the inability to match unrecognized objects presented rapidly, or the poor copying of objects. With the theory of parallel distributed processing[39] as a frame of reference, two recent examples of visual agnosia that share apperceptive and associative features were examined.[40] One patient suffered destruction of the splenium of the corpus callosum caused by carbon monoxide poisoning; the other had bilateral occipital lobe hypodensities on computed tomography (CT) resulting from MELAS, a mitochondrial encephalomyopathy with recurrent strokes and seizures. Both patients had normal visual fields and extraocular movements, yet were unable to name three of ten objects visually. Matching and three-dimensional drawing were successfully performed if patients were given enough time. The common character of their deficit was an inability to derive a global image quickly; instead they used a slow, labored, systematic examination of visual details that resulted in their eventual success in image synthesis.

These patients do not clearly fit the apperceptive-associative profile, yet they can be said to have a visual agnosia. Mendez interpreted the slow, detail-by-detail processing as evidence of a disturbance in the initial phase of visual recognition normally accomplished via parallel processing. In this model, a visual image is distributed within the pattern of activity arising from the interactions of multiple neuronal subunits. Each subunit may represent many visual images within its respective field of view that overlaps with the field of view of other subunits and, via a computational summation of subunits, results in what we see at a glance. With neuronal loss, there is loss of receptive fields and thus a decrease in resolution, which forces patients to abort parallel processing and revert to a serial analysis using a smaller field of view to preserve accuracy. Thus if given enough time, these patients can adequately match and copy by using slow serial comparisons of circumscribed details.

Although the traditional distinction between apperceptive and associative visual agnosia retains clinical validity, occasional cases reported in the literature do not fit neatly within either of these two groups. These hybrid cases demand explanation, as do the pure cases, and future research may resolve apparent contradictions by reference to emerging theories of visual processing in cognitive neuroscience.

Prosopagnosia

Prosopagnosia is the inability to recognize faces overtly, even one's own face in a mirror; the patient is capable of knowing a face is a face and can correctly report emotional expression, sex, age, and related features (beard, scar, etc.) but not the identity of the face. Recognition can be accomplished with the assistance of non-facial cues, such as voice. (For example, in an effort to recognize his wife at a party, a person with prosopagnosia asked her to wear a red ribbon in her hair.) This dramatic defect occurs in the absence of severe memory, intellectual, verbal or sensory impairment; however, most patients have other neurobehavioral deficits, including dressing apraxia, topographagnosia, unilateral spatial agnosia, achromatopsia, and poor nonverbal learning.[41, 42] Recent investigation has centered on three concerns: (1) anatomical correlates; (2) a more precise definition of the clinical impairment in face identification; and (3) the theoretical elucidation of the functional level of information processing that has gone awry; i.e., whether the problem is at a perceptual, mnestic, or configural processing level.[43]

In early neurologic reports, it had been suggested that a single right-sided medial occipitotemporal lesion was sufficient to produce prosopagnosia. However, Benson et al.[44] considered the anatomical basis of the deficit to be a lesion of the right inferior longitudinal fasciculus also affecting the splenium of the corpus callosum. Damasio et al.[45] pointed out that for persistent prosopagnosia in all but two cases reported with clinicopathologic correlation, a corresponding lesion in the LH had also been found. Yet acute unilateral right-sided lesions can produce this syndrome[41, 42]; and a case of right hemispherectomy with no radiologic evidence of left-sided damage has been shown to produce a lasting deficit.[43] Furthermore, since it is possible that bilateral lesions may be separated in time before postmortem pathologic evaluation can occur, it is still an open question whether persistent prosopagnosia requires bilateral involvement. Possibly with the improved resolution and access of MRI this debate may be settled in the future.

The study of anatomical correlations of prosopagnosia is further complicated by variations in the crispness with which the clinical syndrome is described in the literature. For this reason, current efforts have also centered on more rigorously defining the characteristics of the deficit. A patient who has apperceptive or associative visual agnosia, though unable to identify faces, should not necessarily be considered prosopagnosic. Yet nearly all patients with prosopagnosia have difficulty identifying objects in categories that have similar members; e.g., dogs, cars, etc.[43] This implies that the fundamental problem in prosopagnosia may not be in facial identification per se but in distinguishing between similar visual patterns.

Two types of functional defects, perceptual and mnestic, have been proposed to underlie the inability to recognize faces in prosopagnosia, and an attempt has been made to cluster patients within these groups. Whitely and Warrington[46] suggested that the inability to assign the same identity to two different visual representations of an object is a defect in perceptual classification. This defect was proposed as one step in a series of steps that ultimately results in recognition and occurs after a structured percept has been formed from sensory input. A disturbance in this step may be widespread or material specific; in the patient with prosopagnosia it is ideally specific for faces. The mnestic view[47] holds that an intact percept formed in the calcarine cortex is matched to a visual template stored in the inferomesial visual association cortex. Then, via limbic connections, this matched percept activates a multimodal memory store that enables identification to occur. Lesions in the white matter of the occipitotemporal cortex disrupt the process of activation of the multimodal memory store in the patient with prosopagnosia.[48]

The issue of underlying mechanisms in prosopagnosia is further complicated by evidence of covert face recognition in patients with prosopagnosia, which implies that loss of overt face recognition does not preclude the ability to recognize faces unconsciously.[48] However, the three patients with prosopagnosia in the literature with behavioral evidence of covert recognition do not have a lesion in the mesial occipitotemporal area in either hemisphere; and those with physiologic evidence of covert recognition (i.e., higher amplitude galvanic skin responses to familiar vs. unfamiliar faces) have a medial occipitotemporal lesion in only one hemisphere.[43] These patients, who are thought to have intact perceptual mechanisms, may have lost the ability to activate stored semantic information consciously.

Levine and Calvanio[42] suggested that perceptual and mnestic deficits in prosopagnosia are but two aspects of a single disorder of configural processing, which they consider to be the ability, with a single glance, to achieve an overview of an item and identify it accurately. Although the defect in configural processing may not be sufficient to prevent a patient with prosopagnosia from perceiving a face as a face, rather than as some other object, there is insufficient information to know whose face it is. Thus a patient with prosopagnosia may be capable of matching pictures of faces with a serial feature-by-feature analysis or may exhibit covert recognition of familiar faces compared with unfamiliar ones, but may not be able to achieve the next step in the process of visual synthesis. Despite preservation of some degree of perceptual discrimination, the patient lacks the perceptual overview capacity to identify the face immediately. According to this explanation, the apparent memory disorder in prosopagnosia is actually the absence of a perceptual overview or schema of how things look. It is the schema that is lost, and not that perceptual or memory skills are defective steps in a serial, template matching process. According to this theory, all patients with prosopagnosia should be unable to generate mental images because the neural network responsible for generating this schema is destroyed. Furthermore, the neural network in the basal occipitotemporal lobes is where the overlap of perceptual identification and image generation occurs. Levine et al.[49] describe image generating ability in patients with prosopagnosia and report 14 of 22 in whom the capacity to generate mental images was defective. Their contention is that the other 8, if studied properly, would also have proven to be defective.

Finally, according to Levine et al.,[49] the configural processing defect of patients with prosopagnosia is specific for features that are indistinct outside the context of the object of perception. These would include subtleties of texture, hue, and form that combine in such a unique way to allow the identification of individuals within categories that have similar members (e.g., cars, birds, faces, etc.). This category of stimuli is contrasted with categories with members that have distinct, nameable elements, such as words. Defects in the configural processing of distinct verbal elements results in alexia. These authors contend that only the left occipitotemporal area is specific for this latter type of configural processing, whereas some degree of bilateral function is required for indistinct element configural processing. Thus, according to this view, the defects in prosopagnosia and agnosic alexia are task specific rather than material specific.

MENTAL IMAGERY

Within the past 5 years, the investigation of visual imagery has moved to the forefront of research into the mechanisms of higher visual function. The application of computational models from artificial intelligence and developments within the field of functional cerebral localization have lent themselves to empirical analysis. Current research interest focuses on two issues: (1) the relation between imagery and visual perception and whether they share common neural structures and functions; and (2) the neuronal substrates of visual imagery.

Regarding the first issue, it seems that mental visual images share common neurobiological structures with visual perception, since there is no case in the literature that reports the loss of imagery without an accompanying deficit in visual perception.[50] However, caution should be used when interpreting these available cases. There are two distinct methodologies to studying imagery: verbal and visuospatial. In verbal tasks, subjects generate images from verbal cues without the need for spatial manipulation; in visuospatial tasks, they are asked to spatially manipulate objects that are imagined or presented to them visually. Goldenberg[50] suggested that there are two separate systems responsible for the processing involved in these two tasks and has found that brain damage can dissociate the ability to form images from the ability to manipulate them spatially. Prior researchers have not evaluated patients with this distinction in mind but instead have assumed that if patients cannot form images, then imagery in general is defective. It is possible that image formation is memory dependent, and that discrete brain damage only affects the ability to access visual information from long-term memory.

Farah[51] reviewed evidence for the localization of mental imagery and concluded that imagery activates the same areas as those involved in visual perception: pre-striate visual cortex, temporal cortex, and parietal cortex. Furthermore, she concluded that the generation of images from memory occurs in the left posterior hemisphere, while visuospatial manipulation of these images relies on right posterior areas. The LH, because of its proximity to language centers, should be proficient in accessing and interpreting invariant or categorical representations in the task of combining parts of an image. The right hemisphere, because of the predominance of the dorsal (spatial representational) system, should be more adept at positioning objects in a scene.[52]

On the other hand, Sergent[53] arrived at a different conclusion after she reexamined the 18 cases that Farah had used as evidence for a left posterior hemispheric preference at image generation. Sergent argued that only two of these cases, at best, could actually support Farah's conclusion. Furthermore, she asserted that split-brain data show that the right hemisphere is capable of generating detailed multipart images as well as the left (in 2 of 3 patients). In studies of healthy subjects, both hemispheres appear to be capable of generating images while the right is superior in imagery tasks in general. Neuroimaging studies of functional cerebral activity have not yet been capable of demonstrating laterality biases for image generating tasks,[54] but only that localization is dependent on the specific type of information depicted by the image or on the nature of manipulation required.

According to Sergent,[53] the most powerful objection to Farah's componential task analysis, which was devised to dissect the component operations of an imagery task to arrive at the pure step of image generation, is that to exclude patients who have visual perceptual or visual memory deficits will exclude most patients with right hemisphere lesions, since they are most likely to have problems with these functions. On the other hand, since most imaging tasks require verbal interaction, and since damage to the left occipitotemporal area usually results in language disorders, it is not surprising that patients with left hemispheric lesions will perform poorly on tasks demanding manipulation of semantic information.

THEORETICAL OVERVIEW AND CONCLUSIONS

Current trends in research on higher visual functions have emphasized a multidisciplinary approach with the application of experimental methods; inquiry has grown beyond the stage of descriptive observations toward the development of testable theories of neural and cognitive function. The picture that has emerged is that of higher visual functions dependent on interlocking sets of functional subsystems (attention, perception, comprehension, etc.) supported by a neurobiologic substrate of multiple, overlapping neural networks widely distributed throughout the brain and acting both in series and in parallel, simultaneously.

These theoretical trends were stimulated by the work of David Marr,[29] who was instrumental in developing a computational approach to theories of brain function, and vision in particular. Based on his work, Kosslyn[52] devised a theory of functional subsystems to account for seeing and imagining. The essential functions that the visual system must perform, according to Kosslyn, are recognition, mental imagery, navigation, and tracking.

At the level of visual attention,[14] the brain moves an attentional window[52] within the visual field. This window provides the central nervous system a relative coordinate system within which local, invariant (topologic) relationships required for recognition, such as shape and contour, are encoded. Localization of a stimulus in external space is determined by the location of our attentional window in its environment-centered coordinate system in relation to the position of the eyes in the head, the head on the body, and the body in space, all represented in the body-centered coordinate system.

According to Kosslyn's theory, neural modules with specific constraints act as input filters that abstract information from the stimulus located within the attentional window and encode the input into a visual buffer. Further information is retrieved from long-term memory and placed into short-term memory where it is compared to the information encoded in the visual buffer and recognition occurs when a match is made. Mental imagery uses much the same mechanism, except that no original stimulus is encoded into the visual buffer. Navigation and tracking function in a similar way by locating the attentional window in a relationship between environment- and body-centered coordinates.

These functional units come to occupy anatomical locations through what Kosslyn calls the snowball effect: as a unit develops, lateral inhibition suppresses similar functioning in adjacent ipsilateral and homologous contralateral areas, thereby strengthening the neural network. Anatomic location of function is determined by genetic influences modified by environmentally dependent or random variations.

Support for Kosslyn's theory is provided by the work of several groups,[9, 14, 16, 24, 55] elaborating on the concept of the dorsal and ventral visual system. The dorsal, tectopulvinar juxtastriate system is sensitive to low spatial frequencies mediated by the ganglionic x-system. This network has a RH predominance, notably in the inferior parietal lobe, and is concerned mostly with spatial processing. The ventral, geniculostriate-inferior temporal system is more sensitive to higher spatial frequencies mediated by the ganglionic y-system and seems to be more involved with invariant feature detection. This system is LH predominant. It is also possible that the dorsal system functions more in a preattentive, parallel, high-capacity fashion whereas the ventral system processes more at the level of conscious awareness in a serial, low-capacity manner.

Thus, when lesions cause loss of RH dorsal modules, parallel processing strategies are replaced with more serial explorations, as seen in the behavior of some patients with visual agnosia. With the loss of neuronal tissue, the brain still fulfills its function of allowing the organism to interact with its environment due to the redundancy of the system and the overlap of functional networks. For this reason, it is often difficult to localize higher functions to discrete anatomic areas.

In a critique of recent research on the higher visual functions, Sergent[53] has offered an alternative approach to interpreting available data. She argues that clinical data have not always been properly used in the development of computational hypotheses. She asserts that normal variations in functional distribution are not always taken into account, and that an assumption is often made that damaged brains will operate similarly to normal brains. Referring to a concept introduced by Goldstein,[56] she suggests that bihemispheric cooperation influences the way functions are carried out and that brain damage radically distorts the way an operation is performed. Even functions known to be carried out equally well in both hemispheres may be organized very differently in each hemisphere,[34] and to assume a strictly symmetric distribution of functional properties is inappropriate. As Vygotsky had said,[57] Sergent goes on to say that even single anatomic areas may be involved in several different functions, negating a strict one-to-one functional anatomic correlation. Natural lesions can be rather extensive, particularly when affecting the cortex, where large vascular territories are often involved. Thus, neural tissue involved in several different functions may be affected. Also, many experimental research programs include cross-modality instruments of measurement, such as using semantic devices (letters or words) in assessing visuospatial function. For these reasons, it is difficult to control for multifunctional contamination of results and to arrive at accurate interpretations when studying natural lesions.

It seems clear that the brain is a computational device comprising serial and parallel distributed processes, a network of systems operating in concert. But current experimental paradigms do not seem well suited to study system networks in the human brain, because reductionist strategies seek to control and cancel out the multiple variables that make up the totality of the system. If the whole is greater than the sum of its parts, reductionist strategies can never adequately address this totality.

REFERENCES

1. Kinsbourne M: A model for the mechanism of unilateral neglect of space. *Trans Am Neurol Assoc* 1970; 95:143–146.

2. Coslett HB, Bowers D, Heilman KM: Reproduction in cerebral activation after right hemisphere stroke. *Neurology* 1987; 37:957–962.

3. Halligan PW, Marshall JC: Laterality of motor response in visuo-spatial neglect: A case study. *Neuropsychologic* 1989; 27:1301–1307.

4. Nichelli P, Rinaldi M: Selective spatial attention and length representation in normal subjects and in patients with unilateral neglect. *Brain Cogn* 1989; 9:57–70.

5. Cappa S, Sterzi R, Vallar G, Bisiach E: Remission of hemineglect and anosognosia during vestibular stimulation. *Neuropsychologia* 1987; 25:775–782.

6. Hommel M, Peres B, Pollak P, et al: Effects of passive tactile and auditory stimuli on left visual neglect. *Arch Neurol* 1990; 47:573–576.

7. Weintraub S, Mesulam MM: Right cerebral dominance in spatial attention: Further evidence based on ipsilateral neglect. *Arch Neurol* 1987; 44:621–625.

8. Gainotti G, Giustolisi L, Nocentini U: Contralateral and ipsilateral disorders of visual attention in patients with unilateral brain damage. *J Neurol Neurosurg Psychiatry* 1990; 53:422–426.

9. Rapcsak SZ, Verfaellie M, Fleet WS, et al: Selective attention in hemispatial neglect. *Arch Neurol* 1989; 46:178–182.

10. Posner MI, Walker JA, Friedrich FA, et al: How do the parietal lobes direct covert attention? *Neuropsychologia* 1987; 25:135–145.

11. Wright MJ, Burns RJ, Geffen FM, et al: Covert orientation of visual attention in Parkinson's disease: An impairment in the maintenance of attention. *Neuropsychologia* 1990; 28:151–159.

12. Clark CR, Geffen GM, Geffen LB: Catecholamines and the covert orientation of attention in humans. *Neuropsychologia* 1989; 27:131–139.

13. Rafal RD, Posner MI, Friedman JH, et al: Orienting of visual attention in progressive supranuclear palsy. *Brain* 1988; 111:267–280.

14. Posner MI: Selective attention and cognitive control. *Trends Neural Sci* 1987; 10:13–17.

15. Reuter-Lorenz PA, Posner MI: Components of neglect from right-hemisphere damage: An analysis of line bisection. *Neuropsychologia* 1990; 28:327–333.

16. Robertson I: Anomalies in the laterality of omissions in unilateral left visual neglect: Implications for an attentional theory of neglect. *Neuropsychologia* 1989; 27:157–165.

17. Halligan PW, Marshall JC: How long is a piece of string? A study of line bisection in a case of visual neglect. *Cortex* 1988; 24:321–328.

18. Marshall JC, Halligan PW: When right goes left: An investigation of line bisection in a case of visual neglect. *Cortex* 1989; 25:503–515.

19. Weintraub S, Mesulam MM: Visual hemispatial inattention: Stimulus parameters and exploratory strategies. *J Neurol Neurosurg Psychiatry* 1988; 51:1481–1488.

20. Ishiai S, Furukawa T, Tsukagoshi H: Visuospatial processes of line bisection and the mechanisms underlying unilateral neglect. *Brain* 1989; 112:1485–1502.

21. Rizzolatti G, Riggio L, Dascola I, et al: Reorienting attention across the horizontal and vertical meridians: Evidence in favor of a premotor theory of attention. *Neuropsychologia* 1987; 25:31–40.

22. Pizzamiglio L, Cappa S, Vallar G, et al: Visual neglect for far and near extra-personal space in humans. *Cortex* 1989; 25:471–477.

23. Calvanio R, Petrone PN, Levine DN: Left visual spatial neglect is both environment-centered and body-centered. *Neurology* 1987; 37:1179–1183.

24. Farah MJ, Brunn JL, Wong AB, et al: Frames of reference for allocating attention to space: Evidence from the neglect syndrome. *Neuropsychologia* 1990; 28:335–347.

25. Shelton PA, Bowers D, Heilman KM: Peripersonal and vertical neglect. *Brain* 1990; 113:191–205.

26. Churchland PS: *Neurophilosophy: Toward a Unified Science of the Mind-Brain.* Cambridge, MIT Press, 1986.

27. Lissauer H: Ein Fall von Seelenblindheit nebst einem Beitrag zur Theorie derselban. *Arch Psychiatr Nervenkr* 1890; 21:222–270.

28. Lissauer H, translated by Jackson M: A case of visual agnosia with a contribution to theory. *Cogn Neuropsychol* 1988; 5:157–192.

29. Marr D: *Vision: A Computational Investigation into the Human Representation and Processing of Visual Information.* San Francisco, WH Freeman, 1982.

30. Warrington EK, James M: Visual object recognition in patients with right hemisphere lesion: Axes or features? *Perception* 1986; 15:355–356.

31. Farah MJ: *Visual Agnosia.* Cambridge, MIT Press, 1990.

32. Warrington EK, James M: Visual apperceptive agnosia: A clinico-anatomical study of three cases. *Cortex* 1988; 24:13–32.

33. Charcot JM: Un cas de suppression brusque et isolee de la vision mentale des objects (formes et couleurs). *Prog Med* 1883; 11:568.

34. Hecaen H, Albert ML: Visual agnosias: Disorders of visual recognition, in: Hecaen H, Albert ML (eds): *Human Neuropsychology.* New York, Wiley, 1978, pp 176–248.

35. Charnallet A, Carbonnel S, Pellat J: Right visual hemiagnosia: A single case report. *Cortex* 1988; 24:347–355.

36. Sidtis JJ, Gazzaniga MS: Competence versus performance after callosal section: looks can be deceiving, in Hellige JB (ed): *Cerebral Hemisphere Asymmetry.* New York, Praeger Publishers, 1983.

37. Damasio A, Yamada T, Damasio H, et al: Central achromatopsia: Behavioral, anatomic and psychologic aspects. *Neurology* 1980; 30:1064–1071.

38. Von Der Heydt R, Peterhans E, Baumgartner G: Illusory contours and cortical neuron responses. *Science* 1984; 224:1260–1262.

39. Rumelhart DE, McClelland JL, PDP Research Group: *Parallel Distributed Processing: Explorations in the Microstructure of Cognition,* vols 1, 2. Cambridge, MIT Press, 1986.

40. Mendez MF: Visuoperceptual function in visual agnosia. *Neurology* 1988; 38:1754–1759.

41. Landis T, Regard M, Bliestle A, et al: Prosopagnosia and agnosia for noncanonical views; an autopsied case. *Brain* 1988; 111:1287–1297.

42. Levine DN, Calvanio R: Prosopagnosia: A defect in visual configural processing. *Brain Cogn* 1989; 10:149–170.

43. Sergent J, Villemure JG: Prosopagnosia in a right hemispherectomized patient. *Brain* 1989; 112:975–995.

44. Benson DF, Segarra J, Albert ML: Visual agnosia-prosopagnosia: A clinicopathologic correlation. *Arch Neurol* 1974; 30:307–310.

45. Damasio AR, Damasio H, Tranel D: Prosopagnosia: Anatomic and physiologic aspects, in Ellis HD, Jeeves MA, Newcombe F, et al (eds): *Aspects of Face Processing.* Dordrecht, Martinus Nijhoff, 1986, pp 268–272.

46. Whiteley AM, Warrington EK: Prosopagnosia: A clinical, psychological, and anatomical study of three patients. *J Neurol Neurosurg Psychiatry* 1977; 40:395–403.

47. Damasio AR, Damasio H, Van Hoesen GW: Prosopagnosia: Anatomic basis and behavioral mechanisms. *Neurology* 1982; 32:331–341.

48. Tranel D, Damasio AR: Knowledge without awareness: An autonomic index of facial recognition by prosopagnosics. *Science* 1985; 228:1453–1454.

49. Levine D, Warach J, Farah M: Two visual systems of mental imagery: Dissociation of "what" and "where" in imagery deficits following bilateral posterior cerebral lesions. *Neurology* 1985; 35:1010–1018.

50. Goldenberg G: The ability of patients with brain damage to generate mental visual images. *Brain* 1989; 112:305–325.

51. Farah MJ: The neural basis of mental imagery. *Trends Neural Sci* 1989; 12:395–399.

52. Kosslyn SM: Seeing and imaging in the cerebral hemispheres: A computational approach. *Psychol Rev* 1987; 94:148–175.

53. Sergent J: The neuropsychology of visual image generation: Data, method and theory. *Brain Cogn,* 1990; 13:98–129.

54. Goldenberg G, Podreka I, Steiner M, et al: Regional cerebral blood flow patterns in visual imagery. *Neuropsychologia* 1989; 27:641–664.

55. Rebai TI, Mecacci L, Gadot JD, et al: Influence of spatial frequency and handedness on hemispheric asymmetry in visually steady state evoked potentials. *Neuropsychologia* 1989; 27:315–324.

56. Goldstein K: *Language and Language Disturbances.* Cambridge, MIT Press, 1948.

57. Vygotsky LS: *Thought and Language.* Cambridge, MIT Press, 1962.

PART TWO

The Ocular Motor System

CHAPTER 7

The Eyelid

Patrick A. Sibony, M.D.

*Associate Professor of Ophthalmology, Department of Ophthalmology,
State University of New York at Stony Brook Health Sciences Center School
of Medicine, Stony Brook, New York*

EYELID MOVEMENTS

There has been an increased interest in using the magnetic search coil to quantitatively analyze normal human eyelid movements. The results obtained in two recent studies[1, 2] confirm the earlier work of Becker and Fuchs.[3]

The typical spontaneous, voluntary or reflex blink consists of a rapid down-phase followed by a slower upward return to the open position. The onset of orbicularis electromyographic (EMG) activity precedes lid motion by 10 to 15 ms. For both upward and downward phases, the peak velocities consistently fall within a narrow range. Velocity is a linear function of amplitude; downphase velocities were nearly twice as fast as the up-phase. The downphase can reach maximum velocities as high as 1,700 to 1,900 degrees per second at large amplitudes. To put that in perspective, consider that the fastest eye saccades rarely exceed 1,000 degrees per second.[1–3] Based on the presence of a burst-tonic pattern of EMG activity in the levator and orbicularis oculi muscles, it has been suggested that the neural firing pattern underlying both the upward and downward phases of the blink are probably similar to that used in generating saccadic eye movements. That is the downphase results from a pulse-type firing pattern whereas the up-phase (which requires a change in final lid position) is the result of a pulse-step firing pattern.[1, 3]

The downphase of the blink is not a smooth continuous movement.[1, 4] Depending on the nature of the stimulus, the downward phase may consist of an early downward small amplitude component preceding the large-amplitude downward motion. Following glabellar tap, the early component is initiated by relaxation of the levator alone, whereas the early component following electrical stimulation of the supraorbital nerve is produced by orbicularis (R1) contraction. Thus, the relative timing of orbicularis muscle contraction and levator muscle inhibition may vary depending on the nature of the stimulus presumably reflecting the different pathways mediating each of these reflexes.[4]

The peak velocity for vertical lid saccades also increases as a function of amplitude. While the peak velocities for upward and downward lid saccades are nearly identical, the mechanisms underlying each are quite different. EMG studies have shown that upward lid saccades are consequent to a burst-tonic change in levator activity, suggesting that the premotor neurons also display a pulse-step firing pattern.[3] In contrast, downward lid saccades are not associated with orbicularis oculi activity resulting instead from levator inhibition alone. That the eyelid can generate downward movements with saccadic trajectories based purely on a passive mechanism is a notion that some have found difficult to accept.[2, 3]

To explain the downward lid saccade, various mechanisms have been proposed including gravitational forces, viscous dragging of the lid by the globe, covert periods of orbicular muscle activity, and elastic forces on the lid. Becker and Fuchs[3] and more recently Simard et al.[2] have argued that elastic forces opposing the levator muscle cannot account for the downward saccadic trajectories of the eyelid. Notwithstanding the absence of recordable orbicularis muscle EMG activity, they argue that there must be some orbicularis muscle participation. Evinger et al.[1] suggest that the eyelid is unique in possessing structures capable of drawing the eyelid down with a saccadic trajectory when the levator muscle is momentarily inhibited. These elastic forces are generated by a group of interconnected transverse ligaments consisting of Whitnalls ligament, the tarsal-canthal tendons, and Lockwoods ligament, all acting through the levator aponeurosis and the inferior retractor muscles. When the eyelid is open, tension along each of these tendinous structures increases; inhibition of the levator muscle releases this tension and draws the lid down. Manning et al.[5] found normal downward saccadic velocities in patients with orbicularis muscle weakness induced by botulinum toxin; therefore, the orbicularis oculi does not play a role in downward lid saccades.

More studies will be needed before these issues can be resolved completely. Nonetheless, the magnetic search coil is currently the best available technique to quantitatively assess eyelid motion. Whether this technique will further our understanding of different pathologic eyelid disturbances or result in practical clinical applications has yet to be determined.

Supranuclear Eyelid Movements

The location of the premotor control network responsible for the eyelid movements that accompany changes in vertical eye position are unknown. Recent studies in the European literature suggest that part of this control may originate among neurons of the periaqueductal gray, dorsal to the oculomotor nucleus—the so called supraoculomotor region.[6] A recent clinico-pathologic report is consistent with the experimental evidence. Buttner-Ennever et al.[7] describe the findings in a patient with an infiltrating midbrain astrocytoma (grade II) who developed a supranuclear downward gaze paresis and bilateral ptosis with normal horizontal and upward gaze. The tumor located primarily around the third ventricle and aqueduct involved the oculomotor nucleus, the rostral interstitial nucleus of Cajal, the subcommissural nucleus, the nucleus of Darkschewitsch, and the supraoculomotor region. While partial involvement of the central caudal nucleus, also observed in this patient, might well explain the ptosis, it is suggested that ptosis might be due to destruction of the supraoculomotor region. Precise localization based on the pathologic findings of an infiltrating tumor is, at best, quite difficult. Additional experimental and pathologic studies are needed before this issue is resolved.

In 1984, Shibutani et al.[8] showed that microstimultion of the posterior parietal association cortex of the monkey could elicit both saccades and blinks. Simultaneous unit recordings from this area showed that these neurons elicited blinks in response to visual stimuli. A clinical case consistent with these observations was described by Watson et al.[9] They observed the loss of spontaneous blinks in a patient with Balint's syndrome (with optic ataxia, a disturbance of spatial attention, psychic paralysis of gaze) due to bilateral parietal-occipital infarcts. The patient failed to blink to visual threat, photic stimulation, or loud sounds; however, corneal stimulation and glabellar tap produced normal blinks.

Apraxia of lid opening is a supranuclear disorder characterized by a transient, atonic, inability to initiate eyelid opening, not otherwise explained on the basis of a nuclear, infranuclear, or myopathic ocular motor dysfunction. This sign does not meet the operational definition of an apraxia, which assumes an intact motor system. Most cases have been described in patients with a variety of extrapyramidal diseases (e.g., progressive supranuclear palsy) or rarely bilateral or unilateral hemispheric lesions with pyramidal involvement. Two more causes have been reported: one due to a right hemispheric infarction in the distribution of the middle cerebral artery,[10] and others in patients with amyotrophic lateral sclerosis/parkinson dementia complex.[11] Esteban and Gimenez-Roldan,[12] using simultaneous EMG recordings of the levator and orbicularis muscles, showed that involuntary closure of the eyelids in these patients was due to prolonged, irregular inhibition of the normal tonic activity of the levator muscle without any consistent activity in the orbicularis oculi. The authors propose that we abandon the term apraxia and instead refer to this phenomena as blepharocolysis (from Greek *blepharon*, eyelid; and *kolysis*, inhibition).

Using videotapes to analyze lid movements, Golbe et al.[13] studied 38 patients with progressive supranuclear palsy and found a variety of eyelid movement disturbances among 10 of 38 patients studied. The abnormalities consisted of blepharospasm, apraxia of lid opening, apraxia of lid closing, slow blinks, and a reduced blink rate.

The controversy surrounding the mechanisms of oculomotor synkinesis continues. The most recent discussion was prompted by yet one more exceptional patient with a traumatic oculomotor nerve palsy followed 6 months later by partial recovery of the injured nerve and the unexpected onset of paradoxical lid elevation on the contralateral unaffected side.[14] This case is quite similar to the observations made by Lyle[15] in which experimental unilateral injury to the oculomotor nerve in monkeys results in paradoxical lid retraction on both sides. Such clinical and experimental observations are difficult to explain on the basis of misdirection alone but are not easily explained by central reorganization or ephaptic transmission either. The authors suggest that collateral axonal sprouting within the subnucleus of the inferior rectus muscle may have projected into the unaffected oculomotor nerve and terminated on the contralateral levator muscle.[14] However, it is conceivable that the contralateral nerve was subclinically injured, causing a spontaneously acquired type of oculomotor synkinesis. Since the nerves are not contiguous, ephaptic transmission is not a consideration here and how central reorganization might explain the bilaterality also seems problematic. In the final analysis, it would appear that none of these explanations seem particularly convincing.

Five cases of Guillain-Barré syndrome with lid lag were recently reported,[16, 17] adding to those previously described by Keane in 1975.[18] Whether lid lag is central in origin or explainable solely on the basis of facial paralysis is discussed in both papers.[16, 17] In those cases without facial paralysis, lid lag may well be central in origin although the more general issue of central nervous system involvement in Guillain-Barré syndrome remains an unsettled controversy.

Eyelid closure may affect eye movements in a variety of ways. For example, blinks have been shown to be associated with small and rapid downward inward movements of the eyeballs. Forced lid closure, in most cases, results in an upward deviation of the eyeballs. Blinks are known to be associated with normal horizontal saccades. In patients with abnormally slow or absent saccades, blinks may facilitate or initiate saccadic eye movements. Previous studies have shown that eyelid movements may also influence the eye movements associated with the vestibulo-ocular reflex (VOR). For example, eyelid closure will reduce the VOR gain and the duration of nystagmus during caloric testing. Two recent studies[19, 20] show that the eyelids may also affect human rotational responses as well. It has been suggested that suppression of vestibular nystagmus results from Bell's phenomena. However, vocalization will reverse the effect, suggesting instead that the level of arousal is the factor responsible for suppression.[20] Thus, to obviate this artifact, VOR testing is done best with the eyelids open.[19]

Recall that the blink reflex, elicited by supraorbital nerve stimulation, consists of two responses: a short latency, ipsilateral, oligosynaptic R1 followed by a long latency bilateral, polysynaptic R2. Paired electrical stimulation of the supraorbital nerve, delivered at variable interstimulus intervals, can be used to assess the excitability of neurons along each of these pathways. Normally, when the initial or conditioning stimulus (CS) is followed, 100 to 2,000 ms later, by the test stimulus (TS), the R2 of the TS (TS R2) is reduced compared to the R2 of the CS (CS R2). At short interstimulus intervals of 100 ms, the TS R2 is completely suppressed; as the interstimulus interval increases, the TS R2 increases in amplitude. The relationship between the TS-R2/CS-R2 (expressed as percent) vs. interstimulus intervals has been termed the recovery or excitability cycle. The R2 recovery cycle is a measure of the excitability of interneurons along the polysynaptic pathways of the blink reflex.[21–23]

Recovery cycles have been used to determine if the physiologic suppression of the TS is altered in patients with a variety of cranial dystonias. In 1985, Berardelli showed that patients with blepharospasm had a more rapid R2 recovery curve than healthy subjects because the interneurons mediating the blink were abnormally excitable.[23] These findings, recently confirmed by others,[22] have also been reported in patients with spasmodic torticollis,[22, 24] spasmodic dysphonia,[22, 25] segmental or generalized idiopathic torsion dystonia,[24] Gilles de la Tourette's syndrome,[26] parkinsonism,[21, 27] and hemifacial spasm.[28]

The reasons for the augmented excitatory responses of the long latency interneurons, even among those movement disorders without clinical signs of eyelid involvement,[23, 24] is unknown. However, indirect evidence suggests that the basal ganglia, thought to play a central role in the genesis of these movement disorders, is probably also the source of this altered level of activity among the pontomedullary polysynaptic interneurons of the blink reflex.[21–23] For example, the blink reflex is enhanced (R2 latency shortened) in patients with advanced Parkinson's disease, a condition associated with decreased dopaminergic activity, whereas, the dopaminergic hyperactivity in Huntington's chorea is associated with a diminution of the R2 component.[21] L dopa may reverse the changes in the excitability curve observed in patients with parkinsonism,[27] whereas anticholinergic agents (orophenedrine) used in Meige's syndrome had no effect on the recovery cycle.[29]

Habituation of the blink reflex elicited by supraorbital stimulation or glabellar tap is a well-recognized phenomenon. Mechanical stimulation of the corneal reflex does not show similar signs of habituation, although electrical stimulation of the cornea may. Recently, studies have shown that photic stimulation of the blink habituates in healthy subjects but fails to do so in patients with Downs syndrome.[30]

As a general rule, the short latency, oligosynaptic R1-to-supraorbital stimulation is an ipsilateral response, although a contralateral R1 can be evoked with facilitatory maneuvers such as stimulating the median nerve or contracting the orbicular muscle shortly before stimulating the supraorbital nerve. That lidocaine infiltration of the contralateral supraorbital nerve fails to eliminate this response indicates the contralateral R1 occurs on a central basis. However, some contralateral responses are the result of peripheral stimulation alone if, for example, the stimulating electrode is moved toward the midline. In this case the response is abolished by lidocaine block.[31]

The blink reflex was studied in 14 patients with prolonged coma (33 days to 5.9 years). There were no abnormalities of the blink reflex among those patients who later recovered, whereas a variety of abnormal responses (absence of one or more responses, a shorter R1 latency, lower R2 amplitudes) were noted among the non-recovery group.[32]

Tanaka et al.[33] studied the blink reflex in 80 healthy neonates and 12 neonates with neurologic abnormalities. They showed that synaptic connections of the blink reflex are established by 32 weeks. Among the healthy neonates, R1 latency decreased proportionately with increasing age, presumably reflecting myelination of the pontine pathways between ages 32 to 42 weeks. During active sleep, the R1 was consistently present, whereas the R2 was suppressed on the ipsilateral side and absent on the contralateral side. Among those with neurologic problems, the presence of prolonged latencies or suppressed responses that persisted more than 3 months generally had a poorer prognosis. There was generally a more favorable outlook among neonates with normal responses or those with early correction of abnormal responses.

Robinson et al.[34] have recently shown that the time neonates spend with their eyelids closed is related to gestational age and the ambient level of light. The amount of time spent with eyelids closed increases from 24 weeks to peak at 28 weeks and then declines thereafter. These changes in the proportion of time spent with open or closed lids are related to the development of the blink reflex and the onset of circadian rhythms.

The effect of general anesthesia on the blink reflex was studied in ten patients undergoing elective surgical procedures.[35] The blink reflex was absent during halogenated volatile inhalational anesthesia and did not return until well after the end-tidal anesthetic levels were nil. Recovery of consciousness and the ability to complete volitional blinks often preceded the return of any reflex blink activity. In some patients, reflex blinks were still diminished 2 to 3 hours after cessation of anesthesia even though the patients were fully oriented and corneal and glabellar reflexes were clinically normal. The authors suggest that the blink reflex might provide an objective measure of subtle central nervous system dysfunction after inhalational anesthesia.

There is a considerable amount of evidence to suggest that blink rates can be influenced by central dopaminergic activity. Bartko et al.[36] showed that 4 hours after the administration of an intramuscular (IM) test dose of haloperidol, 15 of 18 patients showed a decrease in blink rate. The response in the blink rate correlated with the subsequent therapeutic response to the drug. Peripheral factors such as visual threat or direct stimulation of the trigeminal afferent fibers can also affect the blink rate. The blink rate may be influenced by the imminent break-up of the tear film, since blink rates decrease after instillation of topical anesthetic.[37]

BLEPHAROSPASM

The diagnosis, treatment, and pathophysiology of blepharospasm and cranial dystonias were reviewed in several publications.[21–23, 38] An epidemiologic study from the Mayo clinic[39] shows that the most common dystonia was torticollis (incidence: 10.9 per 10^6; prevalence: 88.6 per 10^6) followed by blepharospasm (incidence, 4.6; prevalence, 17.2), Meige's syndrome (incidence, 3.3; prevalence, 68.9), spasmodic dysphonia (incidence, 2.7; prevalence, 51.7), and writers cramp (incidence, 2.7; prevalence, 68.9). The presence of thyroid disease, autoimmune disorders, and sympathomimetic use were present in several of the patients, but the small numbers in this study made it impossible to assess their significance. Two of the patients with oromandibular dystonia were found to have lacunes in the brain stem, basal ganglia, and thalamus, once again confirming the impression that focal lesions may cause dystonias in a small number of patients.

Grandas et al.[40] reviewed 264 patients with blepharospasm and found that 14% had a coexisting disorder such as Parkinson's disease, progressive supranuclear palsy, exposure to neuroleptic drugs, and in rare cases multiple system atrophy or structural brain stem. Janati[41] described two new cases of blepharospasm associated with olivopontocerebellar atrophy. There are no consistent pathologic findings present among patients with various cranial dystonias as shown in one autopsy study on four patients with cranial dystonia. One patient had a brain stem angioma, the other three had no identifiable abnormalities of the brain.[42] In the Grandas et al. study,[40] a family history of blepharospasm or dystonia was found in 10% of patients. Blepharospasm was the only dystonic feature in 22%; other associated involuntary movements especially in the oromandibular area occurred in 78%. Blepharospasm usually preceded oromandibular dystonia, which in turn preceded torticollis, leading the authors to suggest that there may be a somatotopic progression in many patients with dystonia. Periods of remission lasting 1 month to 6 years were observed in 11% of the patients.[40] During sleep, patients with blepharospasm or Meige's syndrome still show persistent spasms, although the frequency and severity were significantly curtailed.[43]

Elston et al.[44] noted that over half of 272 patients (57%) with cranial dystonias gave a history of ocular symptoms (dryness, irritation, photophobia) at the onset of blepharospasm. One hundred and seventy (of the 272 patients) had documented ophthalmologic examinations, 40% of which showed demonstrable abnormalities of the ocular surface or eyelids such as blepharitis, keratitis sicca, and a variety of other unilateral and bilateral conditions (e.g., dysthyroid orbitopathy, zoster, contact lens keratopathy, Fuchs' dystrophy, etc). The association between dry eye symptoms and the cranial dystonias remains unclear but has been observed by others. Elston et al.[44] discuss the relationship between local eye disease and cranial dystonia. It seems unlikely that these ocular conditions cause the dystonia but perhaps instead trigger the condition in patients already predisposed toward developing this dystonia.

Eye-winking tics of childhood are exaggerated contractions of the orbicularis muscle that can, to a certain degree, be voluntarily controlled. They usually increase in frequency when the child is bored, tired, or anxious and disappear after months or years. Excessive intermittent blinking in childhood in the absence of any associated ocular or systemic condition is generally a self-limited benign process.[45] When it occurs in adulthood it may be the forme fruste for a cranial dystonia. Elston et al.[46] describe a family in which different members in three generations had eye-winking tics and/or blepharospasm. The authors suggest that eye-winking tics, excessive blinking, and blepharospasm may be age-related manifestations of the same fundamental abnormality.

Immunologic mechanisms have in the past been suggested as a possible cause of blepharospasm based on its rare association with a variety of autoimmune disorders, including lupus, myasthenia, and thyroid disease.[39, 47, 48] A case of torticollis and blepharospasm were described in a patient with lupus.[48] The association of thyroid disease in patients with dystonia has been noted in the past; however, Grandas et al.[47] based on their large series show that the association is not statistically significant and in fact may be fortuitous in that both diseases show a preponderance of affected women.

Despite the recent successes of botulinum in the treatment of blepharospasm, there continue to be attempts to treat this problem pharmacologically.[49, 50] In one double blind placebo controlled single-dose challenge design,[49] patients with blepharospasm and Meige's syndrome were treated with intravenous (IV) biperiden, clonazepam, haloperidol, and lisuride. Significant improvements were noted in blepharospasm rating scales in response to biperiden and clonazepam with a trend toward improvement with lisuride. The hazards of abrupt withdrawal of trihexyphenidyl were emphasized in a patient who developed acute worsening of dystonia and severe respiratory distress.[51]

HEMIFACIAL SPASM

Over the last 10 years, there has been widespread acceptance of the notion that hemifacial spasm is due to microvascular compression (MVC) of the facial nerve at the root entry zone. One of the strongest pieces of evidence for the validity of this concept has been the surgical success obtained with microvascular decompression. Adams[52] critically reviewed the evidence for MVC and concludes that significant gaps still remain in our understanding. The reservations, expressed by Adams,[52] do not discredit the entire concept of MVC; however, they raise a number of important questions that need to be addressed by the proponents of this theory. For example, the issue of what precisely constitutes vascular compression remains unclear. Is arterial notching of the nerve a prerequisite or can venules without notching also result in MVC? How does one account for the asymptomatic patient with vessels that compress the nerve and why is it that some patients, without evident compression, develop hemifacial spasm? How is it that improvement may occur with mild manipulation of the facial nerve alone? Neurophysiologic studies, often cited in support of the concept, are fraught with potential artifacts, according to Adams.[52] For example, the effects of very slight movements can substantively alter latencies and amplitudes.

Based on an analysis of the blink reflex and recovery cycle, Valls-sole and Tolosa[28] have shown that the excitability of both the ipsilateral facial motor neurons and brain stem interneurons along the polysynaptic pathways are increased in patients with hemifacial spasm.

Synaptic jitter is an electrophysiologic phenomenon characterized by small variations in latency between the presynaptic stimulus and postsynaptic response. Jitter can be used to estimate the number of synapses in a reflex arc; the greater the jitter, the greater the number of synapses. The low jitter observed in patients with hemifacial spasm was thought to provide further evidence for an ephaptic mechanism in the genesis of hemifacial spasm.[53]

Friedman et al.[54] present a family in which hemifacial spasm involving the left side occurred in five members through three generations. Blink reflex recordings in one case showed bilateral R1.

Several retrospective studies have attempted to determine just how uncommon tumors are in the genesis of hemifacial spasm. In a survey based on the responses from a group of investigators using botulinum injections (only half responded), Sprik and Wirtschafter[55] found that nine of 1,656 (.54%) patients with hemifacial spasm were found to have a tumor, but only one half of these patients actually underwent radiographic studies. Digre et al.[56] found 2 unsuspected tumors among 46 patients with hemifacial spasm studied retrospectively. Epidermoid tumors are among the more common mass lesions associated with hemifacial spasm but are still quite unusual. Of 18 patients selected for the presence of an epidermoid, only three (17%) had signs resembling hemifacial spasm.[57] Among 429 patients with hemifacial spasm, none had mass lesions. The authors combined both groups to estimate the incidence of epidermoid tumors in hemifacial spasm and found an incidence of .7%. While these studies may be faulty in an epidemiologic sense, it nonetheless seems clear that the presence of a mass lesion in patients with hemifacial spasm is rare (probably somewhere between .4% to 4.3%). In the absence of any atypical features, it could reasonably be argued that computed tomography (CT) is unnecessary in patients with typical, isolated hemifacial spasm.[57]

There seems little question, however, about the need for CT or magnetic resonance imaging (MRI) in hemifacial spasm with atypical features of any kind. For example, those patients with epidermoid tumors invariably had associated findings attributable to dysfunction of adjacent neural structures (e.g., headaches, other cranial neuropathies, cerebellar signs, and exacerbation with positional changes).[57] Perkin and Illingworth[58] discuss the association of hemifacial spasm with facial pain in three patients, one of whom had a cholesteatoma. A cerebellar arteriovenous malformation (AVM) with hemifacial spasm was associated with a bruit and vertigo.[59]

Hemifacial spasm in children (ages 3, 5, 12 years old) was found to be due to: occlusion of the straight sinus with large collateral vessels at the base of the brain; an intrinsic mass located in the lower pons and extending into the cerebellar vermis, compressing the fourth ventricle; and an intrinsic mass invading the cerebellar vermis and cerebellar peduncle.[60] According to Odkvist et al.,[61] the patients with hemifacial spasm may in some cases exhibit vestibular-ocular motor symptoms including nystagmus, asymmetric calorics, vertigo, abnormal saccades, and square waves. The authors suggest that whatever causes hemifacial spasm also seems to have subtle effects on the eighth cranial nerve or brain stem as well. While the authors argue that radiographic studies should be performed in patients with associated vestibular signs and symptoms, they failed to mention the results of radiographic studies in their series.

BOTULINUM

After an exhaustive study involving 292 investigators in 27 foreign countries treating at least 4,222 patients with strabismus and 4,340 patients with blepharospasm in over 20,000 treatment sessions, the Food and Drug Administration has finally approved the widespread use of botulinum toxin. The American Academy of Ophthalmology concurred.[62] One can only hope that the health insurance companies will shortly follow suit, since many patients are now responsible for bearing the cost of this effective but relatively expensive drug. The use of botulinum to treat a variety of problems has been reviewed recently in a number of papers throughout the medical literature.[62-71]

Several recent studies[63-65] have confirmed what has already been well established: that botulinum is an effective, safe form of therapy in the treatment of essential blepharospasm with most patients responding for an average duration of about 12 to 14 weeks. While some patients may sporadically fail to respond, repeated injections sometimes at the same dose or with increasing doses will result in the desired effect in most patients afflicted with blepharospasm, Meige's syndrome, and hemifacial spasm.[63-65]

In an attempt to limit the common side effects of botulinum injections, Scott[72] has begun to experiment with botulinum antitoxin. Immediate injection of antitoxin after botulinum was found to block the effects of botulinum on the levator and the orbicular muscles. Delays of up to 5 hours enhanced the effect of the antitoxin, whereas antitoxin administered up to 21 hours after botulinum was not as effective. The occurrence of ptosis and vertical diplopia following botulinum injection at small doses is a limiting factor in the treatment of patients with blepharospasm. Scott suggests that antitoxin injections to the levator muscle might allow an increase in the dose of botulinum to the orbicular muscle, thereby increasing the duration of effect and reducing the side effects in certain patients. No systemic allergic reactions to the antitoxin have been observed.

Gonnering,[73] confirming the results of previous studies, showed the absence of antibody formation in 38 patients treated for blepharospasm, Meige's syndrome, and hemifacial spasm who were given a mean cumulative dose of 140 units. It remains to be seen if the lack of antibody formation is also true for patients receiving substantially higher doses needed in the treatment of spasmodic torticollis. The presence of antibodies might be expected to lead to an increase in the dose of botulinum to attain therapeutic results with repeated injections.

Repeated injections appear to be well tolerated and safe.[63, 64, 67] Dutton and Buckley[63] found that the mean reduction in spasm intensity did not decline with repeated treatments (between 1 and 14) nor was there any tendency toward increasing or decreasing duration of effect. Their data suggest that there is no tolerance effect after 3 years of use. While Kraft[64] found a slight tendency toward decreasing duration of effect over one to six treatment sessions, the difference was small. Biglan has been able to extend the duration of action for up to 3 to 4 months with higher doses. Despite these higher doses, only 7% of their patients developed ptosis. They were able to avoid the complications by changing the sites of injection. Instead of injecting into the medial and lateral portion of the palpebral orbicular muscle, they placed one injection at the midline near the lid margin of the upper and lower lid. Three additional injections were placed near the orbicularis raphe lateral to the orbital rim. In contrast, using the standard injection sites. Dutton and Buckley[63] found that increasing the dosage (from 12.5 units to 75 units) had no significant effect on the duration of action.

Certain groups of patients may show a tendency toward increased or decreased durations of effect. For example it seems that the more severe the spasms, the shorter the duration.[63, 64] Patients with hemifacial spasm tend to respond 2 to 3 weeks later on the average than patients with blepharospasm.[63–65, 73]

The data concerning duration of effect have been difficult to interpret since there are no uniform or objective criteria by which to determine exactly when treatment should be reinstituted. Thresholds for repeat injection among different physicians vary and in some cases may be influenced by the demands of the patient. Some patients will insist on repeat injection at the earliest sign of recurrence, others can wait until they return to preinjection levels of severity. Perhaps patients with unilateral hemifacial spasm may be better able to tolerate the early signs of recurrence than patients with oromandibular dystonia who have bilateral symptoms.

The optimum location of injection sites is still an issue to be settled. There seems to be general agreement that the center of the upper lid is to be avoided because of a higher tendency to develop visually significant ptosis.[63, 64] The advantages of avoiding injections in the lower eyelid have been previously emphasized to obviate any effects on the inferior oblique muscle and to avoid lower lid ectropion.[74] Biglan et al.[65] however showed that the centers of the upper and lower lids can be injected (using higher dosages) if the additional lateral injections lie outside the orbital rim.

The common and usually well-tolerated side effects of botulinum including ptosis, lagophthalmos, dry eye, and diplopia have been well described in the past and confirmed in these more recent studies. Mention was already made of the relatively low incidence of ptosis in Biglan's series.[65] Some of the more recent reports have included side effects not previously described; whether these were directly related to the botulinum is in many cases unclear. For example, in the Dutton series[63] there were five cases of numbness of the nose or lower face (possibly related to direct mechanical injury to sensory nerves), one patient complained after two treatment sessions of generalized weakness lasting 2 weeks, three patients complained of generalized pruritis, and another reported nausea of 3 weeks duration. Haug et al.[75] attempt to link a case of Guillain-Barré syndrome to botulinum injections administered 11 months earlier.

Botulinum has been used with variable degrees of success in patients with a variety of other conditions including spasmodic torticollis, oromandibular dystonia, spasmodic dysphonia,[76-78] orbicularis myokymia,[79] and spastic sequelae of facial paralysis.[70, 80] For those ophthalmologists who venture beyond the confines of the orbicular muscle, it is good to realize patients with spasmodic torticollis require substantially higher doses of botulinum and that one of the important complications of higher doses is laryngeal paralysis with dysphonia and dysphagia.[81, 82]

FACIAL NERVE

The *American Journal of Otology* has published a series of reviews on the facial nerve, the product of the Facial Nerve Study Group, whose aim was to disseminate practical information on management of selected facial nerve problems. The series is a concise and up-to-date reference source on the embryology, anatomy, prognostic testing, and pathophysiology of the facial nerve.[83-86]

In an attempt to a avoid surgical tarsorrhaphy for those patients with facial paralysis for which topical lubricants have failed, the physician can inject botulinum into the levator muscle to induce a protective ptosis. The effect usually lasts weeks to months. Diamond[87] provides us with another option: application of cyanoacrylate adhesive to both lid margins. The effect lasts a mean of 9 days and seems to be well tolerated by the patient.

Improvement in soft tissue contrast, ease of multiplanar imaging, and the absence of ionizing radiation are features that have led to the increased use of MRI as a useful adjunct to CT in the evaluation of facial neuropathies. MRI in conjunction with gadolinium contrast and a surface coil is capable of demonstrating the entire length of the facial nerve.[88, 89] It has proven to be quite useful in evaluating mass lesions in the cerebellopontine angle (CPA), the intratemporal portion of the facial nerve, in determining the presence of foraminal extension of tumors, and in distinguishing central fascicular lesions from peripheral lesions.[88-92] Because temporal bone fractures usually have multiple signals of increased intensity, MRI has been less helpful in patients with traumatic facial neuropathies.[88]

Two MRI studies on Bell's palsy showed diffuse enhancement throughout the length of the facial nerve: in 1 patient, hyperintense signals were confined to the brain stem and labyrinthine segment of the nerve; in another case of mild paralysis, there was no enhancement.[88, 92] In another study[93] of 18 patients with Bell's palsy, 5 exhibited abnormal signals in the central nervous system including the brain stem and the white matter of the subcortex or cerebral hemispheres. Only 2 of the 18 cases were localized to the pons ipsilateral to the paretic facial nerve. These findings only serve to emphasize, once again, that Bell's palsy affects a heterogeneous group of patients. Many questions remain about the prognostic and therapeutic implications of MRI findings in patients with Bell's palsy.

The goals of acoustic neuroma surgery have changed considerably over the past 75 years. An appalling mortality rate of 80% seen in the early stages of its development have fallen to less than 5% with the introduction of microsurgical techniques and modern anesthesia. The remaining issues now focus on functional preservation of facial movements and hearing. Success rates clearly have been shown to be related to the size of the tumor, making early detection of critical importance. The advent of improved radiographic and electrophysiologic diagnostic techniques have led to earlier diagnosis, improvement in the surgical morbidity, a diminution in the duration of symptoms, and reduction in size of the tumor at presentation.[94]

More recently the interdisciplinary discussion continues to focus on the relative merits of various surgical approaches to the CPA, specifically the translabyrinthine technique[95–99] vs. the suboccipital approach.[100–103] In the past, the use of either technique was based on tumor size; most preferring the suboccipital route for larger tumors.[103] This approach for many still holds, particularly among neurosurgeons; however, among both neurosurgeons[95] and otolaryngologists,[96–99] the recent literature suggests that even large tumors can be removed through the translabyrinthine route.[95, 96] While mortality rates for both procedures are similar (1.5% to 3%), proponents of the translabyrinthine approach have cited the advantages of a direct approach to the CPA through the temporal bone, improved exposure through bone without retracting the cerebellum (a requisite in suboccipital surgery), the greater likelihood of preserving the seventh cranial nerve function, less overall morbidity, and shorter hospital stays. However, deafness is an inevitable consequence of the translabyrinthine approach.[95–99] The suboccipital approach is preferred by some because postoperative facial nerve function is comparable and visualization of the medial surface of the tumor and contiguous brain stem is desirable.[103] While preservation of hearing is often cited by proponents of the suboccipital approach, the numbers of patients likely to come out of surgery with functional hearing is quite small.[95, 96] Most patients have already lost any useful hearing prior to surgery. Since excellent results have been reported for each of these surgical techniques, it would appear that the experience of the surgeon would be more important than the technique itself.[95]

It has been suggested that 9% of patients with recurrent facial neuropathies have tumors of the facial nerve prompting some to suggest that transmastoid decompression should be performed in these patients even in the absence of radiographic evidence of tumor. In an attempt to resolve the controversy surrounding this recommendation, Pitt et al.[104] reported on a group of patients with recurrent Bell's palsy. Among 1,980 patients with facial neuropathy, 7.1% had a recurrence. Fifteen percent of patients with one recurrence had a second recurrence; the chance of subsequent recurrences increases with each successive episode. The incidence of diabetes mellitus among the entire group of patients was 31.5%. None of the patients with ipsilateral recurrences had evidence of a tumor.

Facial paralysis in patients with a vestibular schwannoma is generally regarded a late finding; however, Wexler et al.[105] described a patient who presented with the rapid onset of a facial nerve palsy initially thought to represent a Bell's palsy. Two recent reports review the clinical, diagnostic, and therapeutic features of intratemporal facial nerve neuromas.[106, 107] Odonoghue's[106] series included 48 patients, and King et al. described 14 primary facial nerve tumors involving the petrous segment of the nerve. The most common presenting symptom was hearing loss, followed by a progressive facial paresis usually preceded by facial twitching.[106, 107] Occasionally tumors may present with recurrent facial paralysis.[104] The tumor is sometimes visible behind the tympanic membrane. Intracranial extension can result in elevation of the intracranial pressure; rarely, the tumor may extend out through the stylomastoid foramen into the parotid gland. Diagnosis can be confirmed with CT; more recent experience with MR imaging has been discussed. Some of the factors that play into the decision to intervene surgically include the fact that biopsy or excision will inevitably result in facial weakness, that prognosis for substitution or grafting procedures is poor among patients with prolonged paralysis, and the possibility that some cases may progress slowly or remain static for many years.[106, 107] Moreover, it may be difficult to distinguish traumatic neuromas from facial nerve tumors.[108]

There still remains some controversy surrounding the value of decompression procedures especially for recurrent facial neuropathies.[109] Graham and Kartush[110] claim that there may be a role for decompression in a certain subset of patients with Melkersson-Rosenthal syndrome, although the evidence that decompression for Bell's palsy or recurrent idiopathic facial paralysis is lacking.

The triad of recurrent orofacial swelling predominantly affecting the lips, intermittent facial nerve palsy and lingua plicata are the features that define the Melkersson-Rosenthal syndrome.[111, 112] Greene and Rogers[111] described the clinical features in 36 patients. The complete triad was present in only 25% of patients. Orofacial involvement was the dominant feature present in all patients and the forme fruste in nearly half. Lingua plicata and facial nerve paralysis were each present among half the patients in the series. Biopsy specimens of the lip confirmed the classic finding of noncaseating granulomas. Laboratory studies were not helpful, although in one case the patient had an elevated angiotensin-converting enzyme level.[113] Melkersson-Rosenthal syndrome has been associated with a variety of disorders in the past including hyperhidrosis, acroparesthesia, migraine, retrobulbar optic neuritis, paresis of the medial rectus muscle, and Crohn's disease. A recent report describes a patient with seronegative oligoarthritis.[112] The suggestion that these patients merely represent a sarcoid variant has been disputed by some who have found consistently normal levels of angiotensin-converting enzyme, negative Kveim tests, and normal calcium levels. Treatment with numerous modalities including antibiotics, steroid injections, danazol, clofazamine, and facial nerve decompression have met with limited success. A case report documents success with prednisone and methotrexate.[113]

Devriese et al.[114] retrospectively studied 1,235 patients with Bell's palsy. The patients' ages ranged from 20 to 40 years, and the ratio of men to women was 53:47. The distribution differed in men and women; women showed a slight bimodal distribution with peaks between ages 20 to 30 years and again between 60 and 70 years. Bell's palsy was more common in the last 3 months of the year, suggesting a seasonal effect. Associated conditions occurred in about 25% of patients. Hypertension was present in 13% and diabetes mellitus was noted in 2.5%. Their series was almost evenly divided between patients treated with prednisone and those not treated; however, the results of steroid treatment were uninterpretable because patients were selected for treatment based on "complete or almost complete loss of function." Recovery of normal function occurred in 59%; 35% had slight residual dysfunction. The single most important prognostic factor was the age of the patient; older patients had poorer outcomes.[114, 115]

Two more case reports describing the histopathologic findings in facial paralysis showed the presence of inflammatory infiltration of the nerve. In one case due to zoster ophthalmicus, a biopsy of the labyrinthine segment was performed 1 year after the original event.[116] The case described by Liston and Kleid[117] obtained from a 70-year-old patient who died from an aortic aneurysm 1 week after onset showed diffuse inflammatory infiltration, myelin breakdown, and edema. These findings are similar to many of the previous reports on Bell's palsy and zoster, although there are as many pathologic reports showing the absence of inflammation. A recent study by Jonsson et al.[118] showing elevated serum interferon levels in patients with Bell's palsy provides further circumstantial evidence for a viral etiology in Bell's palsy.

Fifteen percent of patients who have had Bell's palsy will have residual hypokinetic and hyperkinetic sequelae.[119] The therapeutic armamentarium, discussed in several reports, includes the use of EMG rehabilitation, oculinum, and various surgical techniques, including gold implants, nerve grafts, and muscle transfer procedures.[119–123]

Among 43 consecutive patients from Sweden with facial paralysis, 6 patients (14%) had evidence of borreliosis (Lyme disease). Diagnosis was based on a constellation of clinical findings (erythema migrans, arthralgias, polyneuropathy, meningeal symptoms) and laboratory abnormalities (serologic studies, abnormal cerebrospinal fluid [SFC] fluid). Four of the 6 had abnormal CSF.[124]

Rare causes of facial paralysis were described including: infanticidal intracranial insertion of a stylet,[125] acquired immunodeficiency syndrome,[126–128] leukemic infiltration of the tympanic cavity,[129] intratemporal hemangioma,[130] dural cavernous angioma eroding the tegmen tympani,[131] benign parotid masses (Warthin tumor, abscess),[132] metastasis to the internal auditory canal,[133] ethylene glycol intoxication,[134] and cutaneous squamous cell carcinoma.[135]

Cranial nerve palsies have been associated with a variety of craniofacial and limb malformations although the distinction between many of these syndromes is confusing. These entities have been grouped together and referred to as "terminal transverse defects with orofacial manifestations" (TTM-OFM) because of their tendency to spare proximal limb structures. Among the entities included in this group of developmental anomalies is Möbius' syndrome. A review of 24 patients with TTM-OFM shows that ocular motility findings range from abduction deficiencies (Möbius' syndrome) to complete horizontal gaze palsies (Duane's syndrome). Unilateral facial and abducens palsies also occur. The varied patterns of motility deficits in association with similar systemic anomalies suggest that there are common factors underlying all these entities.[136]

Falco[137] reported that among 44,000 births, there were 92 recorded cases of congenital facial nerve palsies, 91% of which were associated with forceps delivery. They found that forceps delivery, birth weight of 3,500 g or more, and primiparity were all significant risk factors for the acquired facial palsy. Recovery was complete in 90%.

The use of retroauricular facial nerve block to obtain eyelid akinesia may be associated with a variety of unintended side effects including dysphonia, laryngospasm, and lateral vocal cord paralysis. Hyaluronidase should probably be avoided, particularly in thin patients because of the proximity of the facial nerve to the vagus, glossopharyngeal, and accessory nerves.[138]

In summary, the important controversial areas in the facial nerve remain unresolved. Still no controlled prospective study on the value of steroids in Bell's palsy exists; although many physicians will administer steroids, the enthusiasm for surgical decompression is waning, and the cause of Bell's palsy continues to elude us.

PTOSIS

The presence of an isolated unilateral ptosis is rarely a sign of an oculomotor palsy. However, there were several recent publications[139–142] describing patients with an isolated ptosis due to aneurysmal or pituitary compression of the third nerve. Such cases serve to emphasize the importance of careful history and examination because in many instances there were additional clues. For example, some of these patients gave a history of headache,[139, 142] fluctuation in the degree of ptosis,[140, 141] a mildly dilated but reactive pupil,[142] or an incomitant phoria.[140]

With partially opacified contact lenses to simulate ptosis; Meyer et al. showed that for each millimeter of ptosis there was a loss of 8 degrees in the superior Goldmann visual field (II3e).[143]

The recognition of aponeurotic ptosis was emphasized in the neurologic literature by Deady et al.,[144] who described five patients misdiagnosed with Horner's syndrome, ocular myasthenia, or ocular myopathy because of the coincidental presence, in some cases, of physiologic anisocoria or subjective improvements after tensilon. In one patient, who happened to have physiologic anisocoria with divergent strabismus, angiography was recommended; fortunately, the patient refused. The signs of associated aponeurotic ptosis include the presence of intact levator muscle function, an elevated lid crease, and thinning of the upper lid above the tarsal plate. Some patients may have had a history of trauma, ocular surgery, eyelid edema, chronic contact lens wear, and occasionally a history of worsening at the end of the day.

In contrast to the aponeurotic forms of ptosis, simple congenital ptosis has been shown to be myopathic in origin. While the lid crease may be abnormal or absent in both involutional or congenital ptosis, levator muscle function can help distinguish the two. With aponeurotic defects, levator muscle function is usually normal, whereas in congenital ptosis, levator muscle impairment correlates directly with the degree of ptosis. Histologically, congenital ptosis showed myopathic changes in the levator muscle characterized by a decrease in the number of striated fibers, hyalin degeneration, vacuolization, proliferation of sarcolemmal nuclei, an increase in endomysial collagen, and loss of cross-striations. These findings differ from those seen with denervation or disuse. In contrast, patients with aponeurotic defects have shown a high proportion of striated fibers within the levator muscle.[145]

Harrad et al.[146] retrospectively studied 300 cases of congenital ptosis taken from a series of 424 consecutive cases of ptosis. The causes included simple congenital ptosis ($n = 216$), trigemino-oculomotor synkinesis ($n = 31$), blepharophimosis ($n = 35$), congenital III nerve palsy ($n = 6$), cyclic third nerve spasms ($n = 2$), neurofibromatosis, and seven miscellaneous causes (Duane's syndrome, craniofacial dysostosis, Horner's syndrome, and others). Amblyopia was present in 37 of 216 patients (14%) and was due to strabismus (54%), astigmatism (16%), anisometropia (5%), and multifactorial causes (10%). Only 5 patients of the 37 (14%) developed amblyopia as a result of stimulus deprivation.

Joubert's syndrome is a rare disorder characterized by episodic tachypnea, nystagmus, ataxia, psychomotor retardation, and agenesis of the cerebellar vermis. Appleton et al.[147] described a patient with Joubert's syndrome, restricted eye movements, and ptosis due to congenital ocular fibrosis and histidinemia. The significance of these associated findings are unknown. The syndrome of blepharophimosis, ptosis, and epicanthus inversus was reviewed.[148] The rare association of aniridia with various degrees of ptosis was reported in a family pedigree with eight affected members across four generations.[149] Yet four more new or unknown syndromes were reported in which ptosis was but one of many developmental anomalies.[150–154]

Berlin et al.[155] reviewed their experience with levator aponeurotic surgery in 140 patients (174 eyelids). An acceptable result at 6 weeks, defined as a lid level within 1 mm of the desired level, was achieved in 74% of patients. However, the long-term success rate decreased because of a drop in lid position 2 to 4 months postoperatively in some patients possibly because of resorption of polygalactin sutures used in all their cases. They suggest that nonabsorbable sutures might offer better long-term results.

It has been suggested that the results of the Fasanella-Servat procedure on ptosis was the result of resecting Müller's fibers, among other structures of the lid. However a recent study examining resected specimens shows that the effectiveness of the Fasanella-Servat procedure does not depend on removing significant amounts of Müller's fibers, because the absence of smooth muscle in resected specimens had no effect on outcome. Instead the authors suggest that improvement results from a combination of factors including the amount of vertical lamellar shortening of the tarsus, scarring, and the plication effect of Müller's fibers and the aponeurosis on the tarsus.[156] These findings nonetheless do not negate the beneficial effects and comparable success rates obtained by selectively resecting 6 to 9 mm of conjunctiva and Müller's fibers (Putterman procedure) to correct mild-to-moderate ptosis of 3 mm or less.[157]

The surgical experience in Iowa treating ptosis due to third nerve palsy was described retrospectively by Malone and Nerad.[158] A survey of 10 responding members of the Ptosis Research Society shows that among 298 cases of congenital ptosis, 18% required repeat surgery; among 501 cases of acquired ptosis, 12% required repeat surgery. Only 2% in each category underwent a third procedure.[159] Spoor and Kwitko[160] describe a modified approach to the frontalis muscle sling by suturing fascia lata directly to the tarsus and frontalis muscle through an eyelid crease and brow incision. Transposition of the levator muscle to the frontalis muscle was used to treat two cases of ptosis due to the Marcus-Gunn phenomenon. Experiments in monkeys show that the transposed levator muscle takes on electrophysiologic and histochemical properties of the frontalis muscle after surgery.[161]

MISCELLANEOUS

Small[162, 163] has recently emphasized the distinction between lower eyelid retraction and cicatricial ectropion. Cicatricial ectropion results from tightening of the anterior skin muscle lamella and is corrected by releasing the anterior traction with an incision below the lower lid margin and bridging the gap with a graft. Some of the causes include trauma, burns, blepharoplasty, scleroderma, and topical fluorouracil. Lower lid retraction, in contrast, results from downward traction of all layers of the lid (anterior skin, orbicular muscle, as well as the inferior retractor muscles, which include the capsulopalpebral ligament, inferior tarsal muscle, and orbital septum) and is caused commonly by Graves' orbitopathy, anophthalmos, surgery, trauma, facial nerve paralysis, and dermatitis. He describes a procedure to correct lower lid retraction without a graft. The lower lid is repaired by releasing the retractor muscles from their tarsal attachments. A lateral canthoplasty and lower lid prezygomatic flap anchored to the orbital periorbita support the released lid.[163]

Small also described a new approach to the treatment of upper lid retraction in thyroid orbitopathy by sectioning the levator muscle proximal to Whitnalls ligament and using adjustable sutures to position the upper lid.[164]

A morphometric histologic study[164, 165] has shown that unlike other extraocular muscles in Graves disease that usually show signs of inflammation and fibrosis, the levator muscle instead shows thickening of the muscle sheath, expansion of the extracellular space, and muscle hypertrophy. There were surprisingly few, if any, signs of inflammation in most of the patients studied. Small suggests that the levator muscle, unlike the ocular-rotatory muscles that become fibrotic and restricted, retains its function and in fact becomes hyperactive, causing lid retraction. In contrast, Weetman[166] did find signs of lymphocytic infiltration consisting mostly of T cells in the levator muscle, although no mention was made of muscle fiber size.

Small's well-documented findings challenge many of our common notions on the reasons for upper lid retraction in thyroid orbitopathy that at different times has attributed upper eyelid retraction to increased sympathetic tone, inferior rectus muscle restriction, or fibrotic retraction of the levator muscle. Proptosis alone can cause an apparent lower lid retraction but does not cause upper lid retraction. Freuh[167] questions Small's contention that hypertrophy alone can account for lid retraction, suggesting instead that this may be a secondary phenomena in response to either an increased weight on the levator muscle due to thickening of the levator aponeurosis or increased resistance due to thickening of the muscle sheath.

The gray line of the eyelid has in the past been attributed to represent the mucocutaneous junction, the orifices of the meibomian glands, or the edge of the tarsus. Wulc et al. showed that the gray line actually represents the surface marking of the superficial marginal portion of the orbicular muscle. They point out that the gray line is not seen in all patients. It is more evident in young healthy patients and becomes more distinct with lid closure as the muscle contracts. It may be obscured in darkly pigmented individuals and in patients with blepharitis.[168]

Facial myokymia was described in a patient with syringobulbia. Histopathologic examination of the brain stem following pulmonary embolism disclosed a syrinx involving the spinal cord and lower half of medulla, but nothing to suggest direct involvement of the facial nucleus or nerve. The authors hypothesize that interruption of aberrant corticobulbar fibers in the medulla disinhibited a rhythmic neural generator in the facial nucleus.[169]

REFERENCES

1. Evinger C, Manning KA, Sibony PA: Eyelid movements: Mechanisms and normal data. *Invest Ophthalmol Vis Sci,* 1991; 32:387–400.
2. Simard R, Guitton D, Beraja R, et al: Upper eyelid movements measured with search coil in magnetic field technique during blinks and vertical saccades. *Invest Ophthalmol Vis Sci,* in press.

3. Becker W, Fuchs AF: Lid-eye coordination during vertical gaze changes in man and monkey. *J Neurophysiol* 1988; 4:1227–1252.

4. Snow B, Frith RW: The relationship of eyelid movement to the blink reflex. *J Neurol Sci* 1989; 91:179–189.

5. Manning KA, Evinger CE, Sibony PA: Eyelid movements before and after botulinum therapy in patients with lid spasms. *Ann Neurol,* 1990; 28:653–660.

6. Schmidtke K, Buttner-Ennever JA, Horn AKE: Premotor control of eyelid movements in monkey. *Eur J Neurosc Suppl* 1988; p 168.

7. Buttner-Ennever JA, Acheson JF, Buttner U, et al: Ptosis and supranuclear downgaze paralysis. *Neurology* 1989; 39:385–389.

8. Shibutani H, Sakata H, Hyvarinen J: Saccade and blinking evoked by microstimulation of the posterior parietal association cortex of the monkey. *Exp Brain Res* 1984; 55:1–8.

9. Watson RT, Rapcsak Z: Loss of spontaneous blinking in a patient with Balint's syndrome. *Arch Neurol* 1989; 46:567–570.

10. Johnston JC, Rosenbaum DM, Piccone CM, et al: Apraxia of eyelid opening secondary to right hemispheric infarction. *Ann Neurol* 1989; 25:622–624.

11. Lepore FE, Steele JC, Cox TA, et al: Supranuclear disturbances of ocular motility in Lytico-Bodig. *Neurology* 1988; 38:1849–1853.

12. Esteban A, Gimenez-Roldan S: Involuntary closure of eyelids in parkinsonism: Electrophysiological evidence for prolonged inhibition of the levator palpebrae muscles. *J Neurol Sci* 1988; 85:333–345.

13. Golbe LI, Davis PH, Lepore FE: Eyelid movement abnormalities in progressive supranuclear palsy. *Movement Disord* 1989; 4:297–302.

14. Guy J, Engel HM, Lessner AM: Acquired contralateral oculomotor synkinesis. *Arch Neurol* 1989; 46:1021–1023.

15. Lyle DJ: Experimental oculomotor nerve regeneration. *Am J Ophthalmol* 1966; 61:1239–1243.

16. Tan E, Cansu T, Kirkali P, et al: Lid lag and the Guillain-Barre syndrome. *J Clin Neuroophthalmol* 1990; 10:121–123.

17. Neetens A, Smet H: Lid lag in Guillain-Barre-Strohl syndrome. *Arch Neurol* 1988; 45:1046–1047.

18. Keane J: Lid lag in Guillan Barre syndrome. *Arch Neurol* 1975; 32:478–479.

19. Wall C, Furman JMR: Eyes open vs eyes closed: Effect on human rotational responses. *Ann Otolaryngol Rhinol Laryngol* 1988; 98:625–629.

20. Weismann BM, Ekelman BL, DiScenna AO, et al: Effect of eyelid closure and vocalization upon the vestibulo-ocular reflex during rotational testing. *Ann Otolaryngol Rhinol Laryngol* 1989; 98:548–550.

21. Kimura J: Blink reflex in facial dyskinesia. *Adv Neurol* 1988; 49:39–63.

22. Tolosa E, Montserrat L, Bayes A: Blink reflex studies in focal dystonias: Enhanced excitability of brainstem interneurons in cranial dystonia and spasmodic torticollis. *Movement Disord* 1988; 3:61–69.

23. Berardelli A, Rothwell JC, Day BL, et al: The pathophysiology of cranial dystonia. *Adv Neurol* 1988; 50:525–535.

24. Nakashima K, Rothwell JC, Thompson PD, et al: The blink reflex in patients with idiopathic torsion dystonia. *Arch Neurol* 1990; 47:413–416.

25. Cohen LG, Ludlow CL, Warden M, et al: Blink reflex excitability recovery curves in patients with spasmodic dysphonia. *Neurology* 1989; 39:572–577.

26. Smith SJM, Lees AJ: Abnormalities of the blink reflex in Gilles de la Tourette syndrome. *J Neurol Neurosurg Psychiatry* 1989; 52:895–898.

27. Iriarte LM, Chacon J, Madrazo J, et al: Blink reflex in dyskinetic and nondyskinetic patients with Parkinson's disease. *Eur Neurol* 1989; 29:67–70.

28. Valls-Sole J, Tolosa ES: Blink reflex excitability cycle in hemifacial spasm. *Neurology* 1989; 39:1061–1066.

29. Rossi B, Vignocchi G, Siciliano G, et al: Effects of anticholinergic agents on the excitability of the blink reflex in Meige syndrome. *Eur Neurol* 1989; 29:281–283.

30. Gandhavadi B, Melvin JL: Habituation of optically evoked blink reflex in mentally retarded adults. *J Mental Defic Res* 1989; 33:1–11.

31. Soliven B, Meer J, Uncini A, et al: Physiologic and anatomic basis for contralateral R1 in blink reflex. *Muscle Nerve* 1988; 11:848–851.

32. Sazbon L, Solzi P, Steinvil Y, et al: Blink reflex in patients in prolonged comatose state. *Electromyogr Clin Neurophysiol* 1988; 28:151–158.

33. Tanaka J, Mamaki T, Yabuuchi H: Prognostic value of electrically elicited blink reflex in neonates. *Arch Neurol* 1989; 46:189–194.

34. Robinson J, Moseley MJ, Thompson JR, et al: Eyelid opening in preterm neonates. *Arch Dis Childhood* 1989; 64:943–948.

35. Marelli RA, Hillel AD: Effects of general anesthesia on the human blink reflex. *Head Neck* 1989; 11:137–149.

36. Bartko G, Herczeg I, Zador G: Blink rate response to haloperidol as possible predictor of therapeutic outcome. *Biol Psychiatry* 1990; 27:113–115.

37. Collins M, Seeto RM, Campbell L, et al: Blinking and corneal sensitivity. *Acta Ophthalmol* 1989; 67:525–531.

38. Jordan DR, Patrinely JR, Anderson RL, et al: Essential blepharospasm and related dystonias. *Surv Ophthalmol* 1989; 34:123–132.

39. Nutt JG, Muenter MD, Aronson A, et al: Epidemiology of focal and generalized dystonia in Rochester, Minn. *Movement Disord* 1988; 3:188–194.

40. Grandas F, Elston J, Quinn N, et al: Blepharospasm: A review of 264 patients. *J Neurol Neurosurg Psychiatry* 1988; 51:767–772.

41. Janati A, Metzer S, Archer RL, et al: Blepharospasm associated with olivopontocerebellar atrophy. *J Clin Neuro-ophthalmol* 1989; 9:281–284.

42. Gibb WRG, Lees AJ, Marsden CD: Pathological report of four patients presenting with cranial dystonias. *Movement Disord* 1988; 3:211–221.

43. Silvestri R, Domenico PD, DiRosa AE, et al: The effect of nocturnal physiological sleep on various movement disorders. *Movement Disord* 1990; 5:8–14.

44. Elston JS, Marsden CD, Grandas F, et al: The significance of ophthalmological symptoms in idiopathic blepharospasm. *Eye* 1988; 2:435–439.

45. Vrabec TR, Levin AV, Nelson LB: Functional blinking in childhood. *Pediatrics* 1989; 83:967–970.

46. Elston JS, Granje FC, Lees AJ: The relationship between eye winking tics, frequent eye blinking and blepharospasm. *J Neurol Neurosurg Psychiatry* 1989; 52:477–480.

47. Grandas F, Elston J, Quinn N, et al: Letters to the editor. *Movement Disord* 1990; 5:89.

48. Rajagopalan N, Humphrey PRD, Bucknall RC: Torticollis and blepharospasm in systemic lupus erythematosus. *Movement Disord* 1989; 4:345–348.

49. Ransmayr G, Kleedorfer B, Dierckx RA, et al: Pharmacological study in Meiges syndrome with predominant blepharospasm. *Clin Neuropharmacology* 1988; 11:68–76.

50. Fasanella RM, Aghajanian GK: Treatment of benign essential blepharospasm with cyproheptadine. *N Engl J Med* 1990; 322:778.

51. Roldan-Giminez S, Mateo D, Martin M: Life threatening cranial dystonia following trihexyphenidyl withdrawal. *Movement Disord* 1989; 4:349–353.

52. Adams CBT: Microvascular compression: An alternative view and hypothesis. *J Neurosurg* 1989; 57:1–12.

53. Saunders DB: Ephaptic transmission in hemifacial spasm: A single fiber EMG study. *Muscle Nerve* 1989; 12:690–694.

54. Friedman A, Jamrozik Z, Bojakowski J: Familial hemifacial spasm. *Movement Disord* 1989; 4:213–218.

55. Sprik C, Withschafter JD: Hemifacial spasm due to intracranial tumor: An international survey of botulinum toxin investigators. *Ophthalmology* 1988; 95:1042–1045.

56. Digre KB, Corbett JJ, Smoker WRK, et al: CT and hemifacial spasm. *Neurology* 1988; 49:1111–1113.

57. Auger RG, Piepgaras DG: Hemifacial spasm associated with epidermoid tumors of the cerebellopontine angle. *Neurology* 1989; 39:577–580.

58. Perkin GD, Illingworth RD: The association of hemifacial spasm and facial pain. *J Neurol Neurosurg Psychiatry* 1989; 52:663–665.

59. Yang PJ, Higashida RT, Halbach VV, et al: Intravascular embolization of a cerebellar arteriovenous malformation for treatment of hemifacial spasm. *AJNR* 1989; 10:403–405.

60. Flueler U, Taylor D, Hing S, et al: Hemifacial spasm in infancy. *Arch Ophthalmol* 1990; 108:812–815.

61. Odkvist LM, Thell J, Essen C: Vestibulo-oculomotor disturbances in trigeminal neuralgia and hemifacial spasm. *Acta Otolaryngol (Stockh)* 1988; 105:570–575.

62. American Academy of Ophthalmology (Ad Hoc Committee on Ophthalmic Procedures Assessment; original draft by Scott A): Botulinum toxin therapy of eye muscle disorders: Safety and effectiveness. *Ophthalmology: Instrument and Book Issue* 1989, pp 37–41.

63. Dutton JJ, Buckley EG: Long term results and complications of boutulinum A toxin in the treatment of blepharospasm. *Ophthalmology* 1988; 95:1529–1534.

64. Kraft SP, Lang AE: Botulinum toxin injections in the treatment of blepharospasm, hemifacial spasm and eyelid fasciculations. *Can J Neurol Sci* 1988; 15:276–280.

65. Biglan AW, May M, Bowers RA: Management of facial spasm with Clostridium botulinum toxin, type A (Oculinum)? *Arch Otolaryngol Head Neck Surg* 1988; 114:1407–1412.

66. Kraft SP, Lang AE: Cranial dystonia, blepharospasm, hemifacial spasm: clinical features and treatment including the use of botulinum toxin. *Can Med Assoc J* 1988; 139:837–844.

67. Pittar G, Dunlop DB, Dunlop C: Who needs botulinum toxin. *Med J Aust* 1988; 149:232–233.

68. Kennedy RH, Bartley GB, Flanagan JC, et al: Treatment of blepharospasm with botulinum toxin. *Mayo Clin Proc* 1989; 64:1085–1090.

69. Borodic GE, Cozzolino D: Blepharospasm and its treatment, with emphasis on the use of botulinum. *Plast Reconstr Surg* 1989; 83:546–554.

70. Elston JS: Botulinum toxin therapy for involuntary facial movement. *Eye* 1988; 2:12–15.

71. Tolosa E, Marti MJ, Kulisevsky J: Botulinum toxin injection therapy for hemifacial spasm. *Adv Neurol* 1988; 49:479–491.

72. Scott AB: Antitoxin reduces botulinum side effects. *Eye* 1988; 2:29–32.

73. Gonnering RS: Negative antibody response to long term treatment of facial spasm with botulinum toxin. *Am J Ophthalmol* 1988; 105:313–315.

74. Reifler DM: The effect of omitting botulinum toxin from the lower eyelid blepharism (letter). *Am J Ophthalmol* 1988; 106:637-638.

75. Haug BA, Dressler D, Prange HW: Polyradiculoneuritis following botulinum toxin therapy. *J Neurol* 1990; 237:62–63.

76. Blitzer A, Brin MF, Greene PE, et al: Botulinum toxin injection for the treatment of oromandibular dystonia. *Ann Otol Rhinol Laryngol* 1989; 98:93–96.

77. Jankovic J: Blepharospasm and oromandibular-laryngeal-cervical dystonia: A controlled trial of botulinum A toxin therapy. *Adv Neurol* 1988; 50:583–591.

78. Gelb DJ, Lowenstein DH, Aminoff MJ: Controlled trial of botulinum toxin injections in the treatment of spasmodic torticollis. *Neurology* 1989; 39:80–84.

79. Jordan DR, Anderson RL, Thiese SM: Intractable orbicularis myokymia: Treatment alternatives. *Ophthalmic Surg* 1989; 20:280–283.

80. Clark RP, Berris CE: Botulinum toxin: A treatment for facial asymmetry caused by facial nerve paralysis. *Plast Reconst Surg* 1989; 84:353–355.

81. Koay CE, Alun-Jones T: Pharyngeal paralysis due to botulinum toxin injection. *J Laryngol Otol* 1989; 103:698–699.

82. Brin MF, Fahn S, Moskowitz C, et al: Localized injections of botulinum toxin for the treatment of focal dystonia and hemifacial spasm. *Adv Neurol* 1988; 50:599–608.

83. Jarsdoerfer RA: Facial nerve manual: Embryology of the facial nerve. *Am J Otol* 1988; 9:423–426.

84. Malone B, Maisel RH: Facial nerve manual: Anatomy of the facial nerve. *Am J Otol* 1988; 9:494–504.

85. Huges GB: Facial nerve manual: Prognostic tests in acute facial palsy. *Am J Otol* 1989; 10:304–311.

86. Pillsbury HC III: Facial nerve manual: Pathophysiology of facial nerve disorders. *Am J Otol* 1989; 10:405–412.

87. Diamond JP: Temporary tarsorrhaphy with cyanoacrylate adhesive for seventh nerve palsy. *Lancet* 1989; 335:1039.

88. Millen SJ, Daniels DL, Meyer G: Gadolinium enhanced magnetic resonance imaging in facial nerve lesions. *Otolaryngol Head Neck Surg* 1990; 102:26–33.

89. Daniels DL, Czervionke LF, Millen SJ, et al: MR imaging of facial nerve enhancement in Bell's palsy or after temporal bone surgery. *Radiology* 1989; 171:807–809.

90. Schwaber MK, Zealear D, Nettervilled JL, et al: The use of magnetic resonance imaging with high resolution CT in the evaluation of facial paralysis. *Otolaryngol Head Neck Surg* 1989; 101:449–458.

91. Wortham DG, Teresi LM, Lufkin RB, et al: Magnetic resonance imaging of the facial nerve. *Otolaryngol Head Neck Surg* 1989; 101:295–301.

92. LaBagnara J Jr, Jahn AF, Habif DV, et al: MRI findings in two cases of acute facial paralysis. *Otolaryngol-Head-Neck-Surg* 1989; 101:562–565.

93. Jonsson L, Hemmingsson A, Thomander L, et al: Magnetic resonance imaging in patients with Bell's palsy. *Acta Otolaryngol* 1989; 468:403–405.

94. Glascock ME, Levine SC, McKennan KX: The changing characteristics of acoustic neuroma patients over the last 10 years. *Laryngoscope* 1987; 97:1164–1167.

95. Hardy DG, Macfarlane R, Baguley D, et al: Surgery for acoustic neurinoma. *J Neurosurg* 1989; 71:799–804.

96. Thomsen J, Tos M, Harmsen A: Acoustic neuroma surgery: Results of translabyrinthine tumour removal in 300 patients. Discussion of choice of approach in relation to overall results and possibility of hearing preservation. *Br J Neurosurg* 1989; 3:349–360.

97. Mercke U, Harris S, Sundbarg G: Translabyrinthine acoustic neuroma surgery as performed by the otoneurosurgical group at Lund University Hospital. *Acta Otolaryngol (Stockh)* 1988; 452:34–37.

98. Tos M, Thomsen J: The translabyrinthine approach for the removal of large acoustic neuromas. *Arch Otorhinolaryngol* 1989; 246:292–296.

99. Tos M, Thomsen J, Harmsen A: Results of translabyrinthine removal of 300 acoustic neuromas related to tumour size. *Acta Otolaryngol* 1988; 452:38–51.

100. Symon L, Bordi LT, Compton JS, et al: Acoustic neuroma: A review of 392 cases. *Br J Neurosurg* 1989; 3:343–348.

101. Bentivoglio P, Cheeseman AD, Symon L: Surgical management of acoustic neuromas during the last five years. Part I. *Surg Neurol* 1988; 29:197–204.

102. Bentivoglio P, Cheeseman AD, Symon L: Surgical management of acoustic neuromas during the last five years. Part II. *Surg Neurol* 1988; 29:205–209.

103. Ditullio MV, Malkasian D, Rand RW: A critical comparison of neurosurgical and otolaryngol approaches to acoustic neuromas. *J Neurosurg* 1978; 48:1–12.

104. Pitt DB, Adour KK, Hilsinger RL: Recurrent Bells palsy: An analysis of 140 patients. *Laryngoscope* 1988; 98:535–540.

105. Wexler DB, Fetter T, Gantz BJ: Vestibular schwannoma presenting with sudden facial paralysis. *Arch Otolaryngol Head Neck Surg* 1990; 116:483–485.

106. O'Donoghue GMN, Brackmann DE, House JW, et al: Neuromas of the facial nerve. *Am J Otol* 10:49–54.

107. King TT, Morrison AW: Primary facial nerve tumors within the skull. *J Neurosurg* 1990; 72:1–8.

108. Snyderman C, May M, Berman MA: Facial paralysis: Traumatic neuromas vs facial nerve neoplasms. *Otolaryngol Head Neck Surg* 1988; 98:53–59.

109. May M: Management of recurrent facial paralysis (the facial nerve). *Am J Otol* 1988; 9:256–267.

110. Graham MD, Kartush JM: Total facial nerve decompression from recurrent facial paralysis: An update. *Otolaryngol Head Neck Surg* 1989; 101:442–444.

111. Greene RM, Rogers RS: Melkersson-Rosenthal syndrome: A review of 36 patients. *J Am Acad Dermatol* 1989; 21:1263–1270.

112. Eggelmeijer F, Ten Bruggenkate CM, Calame JJ, et al: Melkersson-Rosenthal syndrome in a patient with seronegative oligoarthritis. *Clin Exp Rheum* 1989; 7:431–434.

113. Leicht S, Youngberg G, Modica L: Melkersson-Rosenthal syndrome: Elevations in serum angiotensin converting enzyme and results of treatment with methotrexate. *South Med J* 1989; 82:74–76.

114. Devriese PP, Schumacher T, Scheide A, et al: Incidence, prognosis and recovery of Bell's palsy: A survey of about 1,000 patients. *Clin Otolaryngol* 1990; 15:15–27.

115. Smith IM, Heath JP, Murray JAM, et al: Idiopathic facial (Bell's) palsy: A clinical survey of prognostic factors. *Clin Otolaryngol* 1988; 13:17–23.

116. Jackson GC, Johnson GD, Hyams VJ, et al: Pathologic findings in the labyrinthine segment of the facial nerve in a case of facial paralysis. *Ann Otol Rhinol Laryngol* 1990; 99:327–329.

117. Liston SL, Keid S: Histopathology of Bell's palsy. *Laryngoscope* 1989; 99:23–26.

118. Jonsson L, Alm G, Thomander L: Elevated serum interferon levels in patients with Bells palsy. *Arch Otolaryngol Head Neck Surg* 1989; 115:37–40.

119. May M, Croxson GR, Klein SR: Bell's palsy: Management of sequelae using EMG rehabilitation, botulinum toxin and surgery. *Am J Otol* 1989; 3:220–229.

120. Harrison DH: Current trends in the treatment of established unilateral facial palsy. *Ann R Coll Surg Engl* 1990; 22:94–98.

121. Mackinnon SE, Dellon AL: A surgical algorithm for the management of facial palsy. *Microsurgery* 1988; 9:30–35.

122. Sobol SM, Alward P: Early gold weight lid implant for rehabilitation of faulty eyelid closure with facial paralysis: An alternative to tarsorraphy. *Head Neck* 1990; 12:149–153.

123. Clark RP, Berris CE: Botulinum toxin: A treatment for facial assymetry caused by facial nerve paralysis. *Plast Reconstr Surg* 1989; 84:353–356.

124. Bjerkhoel A, Carlsson M, Ohlsson J: Peripheral facial palsy caused by the borrelia spirochete. *Acta Otolaryngol* 1989; 108:424–430.

125. Notermans NC, Gosskens RHJM, Tulleken CAF, et al: Cranial nerve palsy as a delayed complication of attempted infanticide by insertion of a stylet through the fontanel. *J Neurosurg* 1990; 72:818–820.

126. Langford-Kuntz A, Reichart P, Phole HD: Impairment of cranio-facial nerves due to AIDS: Report of 2 cases. *Int J Oral Maxillofac Surg* 1988; 17:227–229.

127. Wechsler AF, Ho DD: Bilateral Bells palsy at the time of HIV seroconversion. *Neurology* 1989; 39:747–748.

128. Belec L, Gherardi R, Georges AJ, et al: Peripheral facial paralysis and HIV infection: Report of four African cases and review of the literature. *J Neurol* 1989; 236:411–414.

129. Kurabayashi H, Miyawki S, Naruse T, et al: Bilateral tympanic cavity infiltration with effusion in a patient with acute myeloblastic leukemia. *Blut* 1989; 58:45–46.

130. Lo WWM, Brackmann DE, Shelton C: Facial nerve hemangioma. *Ann Otol Rhinol Laryngol* 1989; 98:160–161.

131. Possati E, Giuliano G, Ferracini R, et al: Facial nerve palsy secondary to dural cavernous angioma of the middle cranial fossa eroding the tegmen tympani. *Neurosurgery* 1988; 23: 245–247.

132. DeLozier HL, Spinella MJ, Johnson GD: Facial nerve paralysis with benign parotid masses. *Ann Otol Rhinol Laryngol* 1989; 98:644–647.

133. Moloy PJ, del Junco R, Porter RW, et al: Metastasis from an unknown primary presenting as a tumor in the internal auditory meatus. *Am J Otol* 1989; 10:297–300.

134. Palmer BF, Eigenbrodt EH, Henrich WK: Cranial nerve deficit: A clue to the diagnosis of ethylene glycol poisoning. *Am J Med* 1989; 87:91–92.

135. Cloustan PD, Sharpe DM, Corbett AJ, et al: Perineural spread of cutaneous head and neck cancer: Its orbital and central neurologic complications. *Arch Neurol* 1990; 47:73–77.

136. Miller MT, Ray V, Owens P, et al: Mobius and Mobius-like syndromes (TTV-OFM, OMLH). *J Pediatr Ophthal Strabismus* 1989; 26:176–188.

137. Falco NA, Eriksson E: Facial nerve palsy in the newborn: Incidence and outcome. *Plast Reconstr Surg* 1990; 85:1–4.

138. Lindquist TD, Kopietz LA, Spigelman AV, et al: Complications of Nadbath facial nerve block and a review of the literature. *Ophthalmic Surg* 1988; 4:272–273.

139. Good EF: Ptosis as the sole manifestation of compression of the oculomotor nerve by an aneurysm of the posterior communication artery. *J Clin Neuroophthal* 1990; 10:59–61.

140. Yen MY, Liu JH, Jaw SJ: Ptosis as the early manifestation of pituitary tumor. *Br J Ophthalmol* 1990; 74:188–191.

141. Small KW, Buckley EG: Recurrent blepharoptosis secondary to a pituitary tumor. *Am J Ophthalmol* 1988; 106:760–761.

142. Bartleson JD, Trautmann JC, Sundt TM: Minimal oculomotor nerve paresis secondary to unruptured intracranial aneurysm. *Arch Neurol* 1986; 43:1015–1020.

143. Meyer DR, Linberg J, Pwell SR, et al: Quantitating the superior visual field loss associated with ptosis. *Arch Ophthalmol* 1989; 107:840–843.

144. Deady JP, Morrell AJ, Sutton GA: Recognising aponeurotic ptosis. *J Neurol Neurosurg Psychiatry* 1989; 52:996–998.

145. Sutula FC: Histological changes in congenital and acquired blepharoptosis. *Eye* 1988; 2:179–184.

146. Harrad RA, Graham CM, Collin JRO: Amblyopia and strabismus in congenital ptosis. *Eye* 1988; 2:625–627.

147. Appleton RE, Chitayat D, Jan JE, et al: Jouberts syndrome associated with congenital ocular fibrosis and histidinemia. *Arch Neurol* 1989; 46:579–582.

148. Oley C, Baraitser M: Blepharophimosis, ptosis, epicanthu inversus syndrome (BPES syndrome). *J Med Genet* 1988; 25:47–51.

149. Cohen SM, Nelson LB: Aniridia with congenital ptosis and glaucoma: A family study. *Ann Ophthalmol* 1988; 20:53–57.

150. Baraitser M, Winter RM: Iris coloboma, ptosis, hypertelorism, and mental retardation: New syndrome. *J Med Genet* 1988; 25:41–43.

151. Carnevale F, Krajewska G, Fischetto R, et al: Ptosis of eyelids, strabismus, diastasis recti, hip defect, cryptorchidism, and developmental delay in two sibs. *Am J Med Genet* 1989; 33:186–189.

152. Tsukahara M, Azuno Y, Kajii T: Type A1 brachydactyly, dwarfism, ptosis, mixed partial hearing loss, microcephaly and mental retardation. *Am J Med Genet* 1989; 33:7–9.

153. Mehta L, Lewis I, Patton MA: Unkonwn syndrome: Congenital heart disease, ptosis, ypodontia, and craniosynostosis. *J Med Genet* 1989; 26:664–666.

154. Shephard RC, Goudie DR, Tolmie JL: Unknown syndrome: Noonan-like craniofacial features, digital anomalies and premature birth. *J Med Genet* 1989; 26:470–472.

155. Berlin AJ, Vestal KP: Levator aponeurosis surgery: A retrospective review. *Ophthalmology* 1989; 96:1033–1037.

156. Buckman G, Jakobiec FA, Hyde K, et al: Success of the Fasanella-Servat operation independent of Muller's smooth muscle excision. *Ophthalmology* 1989; 96:413–418.

157. Guyuron B, Davies B: Experience with the modified Putterman procedure. *Plast Reconstr Surg* 1988; 82:775–780.

158. Malone TJ, Nerard JA: The surgical treatment of blepharoptosis in oculomotor nerve palsy. *Am J Ophthalmol* 1988; 105:57–64.

159. Brown BZ: Ptosis revision. *Int Ophthalmol Clin* 1989; 4:217–218.

160. Spoor TC, Kwitko GM: Blepharoptosis repair by fascia lata suspension with direct tarsal and frontalis fixation. *Am J Ophthalmol* 1990; 109:314–317.

161. LeMagne JM: Transposition of the levator muscle and its reinnervation. *Eye* 1988; 2:189–192.

162. Small RG: The tight retracted lower eyelid. *Trans Am Ophthalmol Soc* 1989; 87:362–383.

163. Small RG, Scott M: The tight retracted lower eyelid. *Arch Ophthalmol* 1990; 108:438–444.

164. Small RG: Upper eyelid retraction in Graves ophthalmopathy: A new surgical technique and a study of the abnormal levator. *Trans Am Ophthalmol Soc* 1989; 86:725–793.

165. Small RG: Enlargement of the levator palpebrae superioris muscle fibers in Graves ophthalmopathy. *Ophthalmology* 1989; 96:424–430.

166. Weetman AP, Cohen S, Gatter KC, et al: Immunohistochemical analysis of the retrobulbar tissues in Graves ophthalmopathy. *Clin Exp Immunol* 1989; 75:222–227.

167. Frueh BR: Eyelid retraction in Graves eye disease (letters). *Ophthalmology* 1989; 96:1574–1575.

168. Wule AE, Dryden RM, Khatchaturian R: Where is the gray line? *Arch Ophthalmol* 1987; 105:1092–1098.

169. Riaz G, Campbell WW, Carr J, et al: Facial myokymia in syringobulbia. *Arch Neurol* 1990; 47:472–474.

CHAPTER 8

Development and Maintenance of Ocular Alignment

Ronald J. Tusa, M.D., Ph.D.

Assistant Professor, Departments of Neurology and Ophthalmology, The Johns Hopkins University School of Medicine, Baltimore, Maryland

David S. Zee, M.D.

Professor, Departments of Neurology and Ophthalmology, The Johns Hopkins University School of Medicine, Baltimore, Maryland

Of all the eye movement disorders, those disturbing binocularity most commonly cause patients to consult a physician. Most patients with lesions within the smooth pursuit or optokinetic systems do not notice any visual disturbance unless they develop impaired motion perception[1] or their slow phase movements are in the direction opposite to the target.[2] Likewise, most patients with saccadic deficits do not seek medical attention unless they develop extremely dysmetric or slow saccades, or saccadic oscillations such as opsoclonus. On the other hand, nearly all patients with ocular misalignment or deficits in vergence have symptoms. A small degree of ocular misalignment can result in visual blurring, diplopia, poor depth perception, or a sense of strain or fatigue.

In this chapter, we will review some newer ideas and information about vergence eye movements and the mechanisms by which we maintain normal ocular alignment throughout life. These areas of ocular motility should not be solely the

Reprinted from *Current Neuro-ophthalmology*®, vol. 3.
Copyright 1991, Mosby–Year Book, Inc.

province of the strabismus surgeon, as a variety of neurologic and neuro-ophthalmologic disorders are associated with ocular misalignment and deficits in vergence.

BINOCULAR VISION AND SENSORY FUSION

When viewing a point in space with the eyes aligned, there is a set of points in space called the *horopter,* which is imaged on corresponding retinal elements. These points all have zero *retinal disparity.* The horopter passes through the fixation point and is concave toward the observer. *Panum's fusional area* defines that part of space encompassing the horopter where binocular vision is preserved, yet also contains points that have a certain degree of retinal disparity. Objects lying outside Panum's fusional area normally result in diplopia. Panum's fusional area can be quantified with Julesz random dot stereograms. For stationary images, the images must come within 6 to 12 degrees of arc of each other for fusion to take place. Once fusion has taken place, the two retinal images can be separated by as much as 2 degrees before losing fusion.[3, 4] *Sensory fusion* is the ability to visually fuse the two retinal images together. *Stereopsis* is the three-dimensional perception obtained when separate images, differing only in the relative horizontal direction, are viewed from each eye. It is useful to subdivide stereopsis into different degrees. *Local stereopsis* (or fine stereopsis) is the point-by-point matching of disparate stimuli within Panum's fusional area. *Global stereopsis* is the perception of a surface with a recognizable form based on the use of local stereopsis.[5] *Coarse stereopsis* is the perception of depth in the presence of diplopia, which uses retinal disparity cues outside Panum's fusional area. Coarse stereopsis provides sensory cues for fusional vergence eye movements. *Depth perception* depends on stereopsis and monocular cues including overlay of contours, relative size of objects, and motion parallax.

FUNCTIONAL DESCRIPTION OF VERGENCE EYE MOVEMENTS

Vergence has four components: *tonic vergence,* which determines the baseline alignment of the visual axes in darkness; *accommodative vergence,* induced by visual blur; *fusional vergence,* induced by retinal disparity; and *proximal vergence or nearness,* induced by a sense of target distance, which is based on a number of sensory cues including perspective and looming.[6, 7] In this section, we will primarily describe current concepts of fusional vergence. Fusional vergence probably has two functional components. One primarily uses large disparities (coarse stereopsis) to initiate the vergence response, and the other uses small disparities (local stereopsis) within the limits of Panum's fusional area to sustain fusion.[8]

Amplitude of Vergence Eye Movements

Fusional amplitudes can be measured with a continuous rotary prism or a prism bar placed in front of one eye. The prism power at which the patient reports diplopia is the *breakpoint of fusion* and reflects the fusional amplitude of the subject. Fusional amplitudes are subdivided into *convergence amplitude* and *divergence amplitude*. Table 1 lists the average convergence and divergence amplitudes of 218 individuals with normal vision and no strabismus.[9] Fusional amplitude does not change with age.[10] Another important measurement is the *recovery point of fusion*, which is the prism power at which single vision is reestablished. The recovery point is usually 2 to 4 prism diopters (Δ) less than that at the breakpoint.[11]

In patients with large phorias, the fusional amplitude is equal to the fusional breakpoint plus the degree of inherent misalignment at the distance at which fusion is measured. For example, suppose a patient has sufficient fusional amplitude to overcome a 20Δ exophoria for a distant target (6 m). If the convergence breakpoint is 5Δ, then the convergence amplitude is really 25Δ. The *fusional reserve* for convergence, at this distance, though, is only 5Δ. Similarly, if the divergence breakpoint is 30Δ, then the true divergence amplitude is only 10Δ. Fusional amplitudes are relatively unaffected by the change in the phoria induced by wearing a displacing prism.[12] Unfortunately, there is little information about fusional amplitudes in patients with neurologic disorders.

Velocity of Vergence Eye Movements

It is traditionally taught that vergence eye movements are slow. They take up to a second for completion, when tested in a laboratory setting using isolated retinal-disparity stimuli under dichotic viewing conditions (each eye sees a different image). Vergence movements are much faster, however, when tested under more natural conditions using, for example, real targets, or if the subject moves himself toward a stationary target.[13] Occasionally, disjunctive (oppositely directed) saccades occur in response to stimuli that call for pure vergence movements without any conjugate change.[14] These disjunctive saccades increase the speed with which the vergence change is accomplished.

TABLE 1.

Average Vergence Amplitudes

Distance	Convergence Amplitude (Δ)	Divergence Amplitude (Δ)
Far (6 m)	14.10	5.82
Near (25 cm)	38.02	16.47

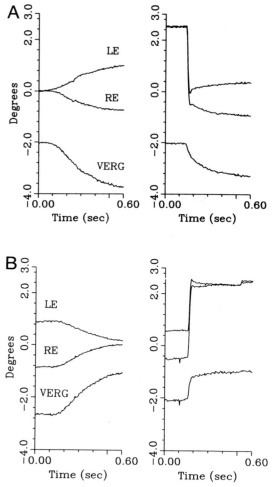

FIG 1.
Vergence response to a 2-degree step change in target vergence, with and without a saccade. **A,** convergence; **B,** divergence. The vergence component is faster by several-fold when conjoined with a saccade. *LE* = left eye; *RE* = right eye; *VERG* = vergence response. (From Leigh KJ, Zee DS: *The Neurology of Eye Movements.* Philadelphia, FA Davis, 1991.)

Perhaps the most important, and the most natural, circumstance in which the velocity of the vergence change is increased is when the target of interest changes its position across the visual field as well as in depth. A combined version and vergence movement is required, and the vergence component is faster by several-fold when conjoined with a saccade (Fig 1). The mechanism for this facilitation is unknown, though it suggests that the movements of each eye do not simply reflect the sum of separate commands from the conjugate (version) and the vergence systems. Rather, there appears to be a nonlinear interaction between version and vergence; whether this occurs in central premotor structures, in the ocular motor neurons, in the muscles themselves, or in all three, is unknown.

INTERACTIONS BETWEEN ACCOMMODATION AND VERGENCE

The synkinetic relationship between accommodation (A) of the lens and accommodative-linked convergence (AC) can be expressed as a ratio (AC/A). The units of AC/A are prism diopters of vergence/sphere diopters of accommodation. The normal range of the AC/A ratio is 3 to 5.[15] Not only is convergence (C) causally linked to accommodation, but accommodation (A) is linked to vergence (convergence-linked accommodation; CA). This relationship also can be expressed as a ratio (the CA/C ratio, expressed in sphere diopters of accommodation per prism diopter of vergence).

It is still unclear how accommodative vergence and fusional vergence drives interact. Maddox believed that accommodative vergence was the main contribution to vergence, but was aided by fusional vergence.[6] Others, however, have argued that fusional vergence is the most important contributor to ocular alignment and that accommodative vergence of the lens is predominantly linked to fusional vergence.[16] In this view, the role of blur is to serve as the stimulus for the fine-tuning of accommodation. Other stimuli—sense of nearness, size, texture, looming—may be also important for stimulating vergence under conditions of natural viewing. Recent models have addressed the interactions between vergence and accommodation. These will be dealt with below after discussing *phoria adaptation.*

One may ask if the AC/A or CA/C ratios are genetically fixed, or if they can be modified by environmental factors. If subjects wear periscopic spectacles to simulate an increase in the interocular separation, both the AC/A and the CA/C ratios can be changed.[17, 18] Such a mechanism would be necessary to optimize visual function as the interpupillary distance increases during growth, or to assure an accurate response when accommodation or vergence becomes fatigued.

NORMAL DEVELOPMENT

Stereopsis develops at about 3 months of age based on recording visual tracking eye movements by Julesz patterns[19] and visual-evoked potentials elicited by a dynamic random-dot correlogram.[20] Lack of binocularity before this age does not appear to be due to ocular misalignment, but rather to immature binocular vision.[21]

Normally, the lens can change refraction by 10Δ (focal length 10 cm to infinity). Infants as young as 2 months can alter their accommodation in the appropriate direction for changing target distances.[22] Three to 4 months after birth, infants can accurately accommodate over a 4Δ range at 4.6Δ/sec.[22, 23] Healthy newborns are hyperopic ($+2\Delta \pm 2\Delta$). They become increasingly hyperopic for the first 6 months, and then less so thereafter.[24]

In the first month of life, vergence movements in response to approaching and receding targets are in the appropriate direction, but the range and accuracy are low.[23, 25] Over the course of 3 months, the precision of vergence responses improves rapidly. These vergence eye movements may be primarily driven by accommodation cues since infants less than 6 months of age do not make appropriate refixation saccades or vergence movements when a prism is placed in front of one eye.[23] By 6 months of age, however, fusional responses become adultlike.[26]

At birth, only 30% of infants (out of 3,000 examined) have normal ocular alignment, 67% are exotropic, and less than 1% are esotropic.[27] Over the next 6 to 8 months, the exotropia is corrected in most subjects, while 0.1% of the infants develop persistent esotropia.

ADAPTIVE MECHANISMS TO MAINTAIN OCULAR ALIGNMENT

Most research in ocular motor learning has focused on conjugate adaptive mechanisms, especially those of the saccadic and vestibular systems. Recall that Hering's law of equal innervation dictates that any attempt to increase the innervation to a weak muscle in one eye must be accompanied by a commensurate increase in innervation to the yoke muscle of the other eye. This is the basis for *conjugate adaptation*. Usually, however, muscle weakness is unilateral and asymmetric so that adaptive corrections are *disconjugate* and must vary with the position of the eye in the orbit. We will discuss various types of *disconjugate adaptation*.

Adaptation to Unilateral Muscle Weakness

Viirre et al.[28] surgically weakened a horizontal rectus muscle in one eye of monkeys and then demonstrated a seemingly monocular recalibration, provided that the animal was exposed to binocular vision and that the degree of muscle weakening was relatively small. Animals with severe muscle weakening exhibited little monocular adaptation. When the normal eye was patched, though, these animals exhibited, as expected, a strong conjugate adaptation.

These results suggest that a crucial determinant for disconjugate plasticity might be the degree to which animals or humans can use their eyes together. Patients with a large deviation; e.g., complete ocular motor palsy, might not undergo disconjugate adaptation (or monocular recalibration) if they do not have the experience of using the eyes together. We studied a patient with a complete sixth cranial nerve paralysis who had surgery so that he could fuse images when his eyes were near the primary position.[29] After binocular vision for 7 days, his phoria became relatively comitant over a 20-degree range of positions near the primary one. On the other hand, after prolonged monocular viewing, his phoria became noncomitant. Again, the process of binocular viewing was probably the crucial stimulus to disconjugate adaptation. The relative roles of the sensory input, retinal disparity, and the attendant motor response, fusion, remain to be clarified. Orbital proprioceptors, too, may play a role in this disconjugate, position-dependent adaptation.

Adaptation of Tonic Vergence (Phoria Adaptation) and AC/A Ratios

If retinal disparity is introduced by placing a prism in front of one eye, the subject's phoria changes by an amount equal to the power of the prism. There is no tropia if the new retinal disparity is within the fusional amplitude. Nevertheless, the residual retinal disparity during fixation *(fixation disparity),* or steady-state vergence error during binocular viewing, is increased though diplopia will not occur if the retinal disparity is still within Panum's fusional area. In a matter of minutes, though, the subject undergoes *phoria adaptation* (also called prism adaptation). Then, both the phoria and the residual retinal disparity during fusion revert to their preprism values when measured with the prism on. There has been a resetting of the alignment of the two visual axes by an amount equivalent to the prismatic demand.[30] The rate and the amount of phoria adaptation depend on the strength of the prism and the fusional amplitudes of the subject.[31]

Accommodation also has an adaptive mechanism.[32] By opening the visual feedback loop, one can measure the tonic level of accommodation; i.e., the accommodative phoria. Using appropriate lenses, one can show that the tonic level of accommodation can also be adaptively readjusted, independent of any change in retinal disparity.

Schor[33, 34] has developed a model for phoria adaptation that incorporates both accommodation and vergence (Fig 2). The fast fusional system uses retinal disparity as its error signal, and the slow fusional adaptive system uses the motor output of the fast fusional system as its error signal. The fast fusional vergence system appears to use an imperfect, leaky integrator with a time constant of 10 to 15 seconds. This is the vergence position integrator (to be described). The slow fusional adaptive system also uses a leaky integrator but with a much longer time constant (minutes or longer). Thus, in time, the slow fusional mechanism takes over much of the load of keeping the eyes aligned by resetting the level of tonic vergence. In this way, the residual retinal disparity during fusion is reduced to its preprism value. Thus, phoria adaptation resets the resting position of the eyes toward the original phoria and thereby restores the dynamic range (or *fusional reserve*) in which fast fusional vergence can function. Sustained accommodation may also

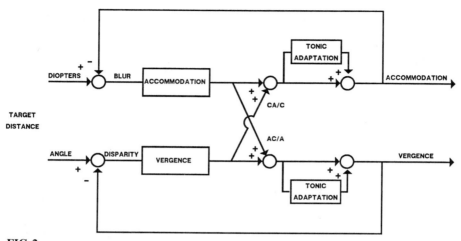

FIG 2.

Block diagram illustrating the interactions between accommodation and vergence. The AC/A ratio and the tonic vergence level are thought to be adapted by tonic adaptation circuits in the accommodation and vergence loop, respectively. AC/A is the accommodation vergence cross-link and CA/C is the vergence accommodation cross-link. (Adapted from Schor CM: *Am J Optom Physiol Opt* 1985; 62:369–374.)

play a role in phoria adaptation in humans,[35] though this is less certain in monkeys. Monkeys do not increase their level of tonic vergence following a period of increased accommodative convergence induced by viewing through a negative lens.[36]

Adaptation to Spectacle-Corrected Anisometropia

A special case of phoria adaptation is that required for an anisometropic spectacle correction. Anisometropia requires a corrective lens of a different power for each eye. Corrective spectacle lenses have a prismatic effect that results in the relative displacement of an image of an object from its actual position. Because the spectacles are fixed with respect to the eyes, they cause a rotational magnification effect that changes the amount the eye must rotate to fix on a target at a given point in space. The rotational magnification effect contrasts with the linear magnification effect that describes the relative size of an image of an object. Contact lenses have a small linear but no rotational magnification effect. The prismatic effect of a spectacle lens is roughly proportional to both its power and the distance from its optical center and will therefore increase continuously toward the lens periphery. Since, with an anisometropic correction, the prismatic effect of each spectacle lens is different, the retinal disparity of the images of a given object will change as a function of gaze position. Accordingly, ocular alignment must change as a function of orbital position to retain fusion.

When subjects begin wearing an anisometropic spectacle correction, their phoria (as measured while wearing their spectacle correction) soon reverts to the preadaptation state in all positions of gaze.[37] Thus, the resting ocular alignment varies with the position of the eye in the orbit. This would be a way to assure concomitancy while wearing glasses; ocular alignment would be correct in all orbital positions. However, to achieve fusion promptly on changing gaze, a subject wearing an anisometropic spectacle correction must be able to change the alignment of the visual axes during the saccade.

This capability has been studied in both healthy subjects and in patients who are changing from contact to spectacle lenses or vice versa.[38-40] An animal model to study this phenomenon has also been developed with laterally displacing prisms of different powers and orientations in different portions of field of gaze.[41] In these studies, it was found that during every saccade, the two eyes no longer travelled together. Near the onset of horizontal saccades, the eyes began to diverge or converge, whichever was appropriate to the induced prismatic effect of the optical combination. (Note that healthy subjects show a transient divergence followed by convergence during horizontal saccades. Adaptive changes were superimposed on this inherent propensity to diverge.) By the end of each saccade, the eyes had achieved most of the realignment necessary to assure bifoveal fixation. If the intrasaccadic vergence change was not enough, the eyes might continue to diverge or converge as necessary so that correct ocular realignment was achieved within a few hundred milliseconds after the end of the saccade.

It is important to note that the intrasaccadic and postsaccadic vergence movements occurred under both binocular and monocular viewing conditions. In other words, the subjects appeared to have learned to preprogram intrasaccadic and postsaccadic disconjugate movements that, once learned, occurred independently of retinal disparity cues.

Subjects wearing the anisometropic spectacle corrections also showed appropriate adaptive changes in vertical alignment, which, when the degree of anisometropia was large, exceeded the vertical fusional amplitude. This finding implies that the adaptive mechanism can either use retinal disparity or the attempt to fuse as a stimulus for adaptation, but does not need complete fusion per se.

Another observation was made in one patient[39] regarding the effect of the spectacles, per se, on the adaptive response. Under monocular viewing conditions, simply putting on the spectacles led to an increase in the level of intrasaccadic vergence above that when viewing monocularly without any glasses. This finding emphasizes the potential importance of context in eliciting adaptive responses. It was as if the central nervous system anticipated the need for more intrasaccadic vergence whenever the glasses were put on.

One other feature emerged from these studies. Relatively brief exposures to a new binocular viewing condition could lead to exceedingly fast adaptive changes. In one instance, an anisometropic subject, who had been exclusively wearing contact lenses for over a week, needed just several minutes of binocular viewing through his old spectacles to induce a considerable reversion toward the prior state of disconjugate adaptation (up to 1.25 degrees of vergence change during monocular viewing).[39]

The exact mechanisms underlying both the static and the dynamic changes in ocular alignment that occur with spectacle-corrected anisometropia are not known. Presumably, it is the retinal disparity that occurs at the end of saccades, or perhaps the retinal-disparity driven vergence effort to overcome it, that is the cue to readjust the relative innervation to the eyes during the saccade. Schor et al.[42] have shown that retinal disparity, per se, does not induce disconjugate adaptation unless it is closely linked with the saccade. Furthermore, pursuit and saccades can be differentially adapted if the disconjugate stimulus is presented during one or the other type of movement.

Motor learning itself could be an independent adjustment of the innervation to the two eyes, or perhaps, in the case for saccades, a manifestation of an interaction between saccade and vergence eye movements. Recall that even under normal circumstances, changes in ocular alignment are facilitated when vergence movements are combined with an ongoing saccade. Whatever the precise mechanisms, such a disconjugate adaptive capability is exceedingly important. It will make adjustments not only for acquired abnormalities but also for the small inherent asymmetries in ocular muscle strength and in orbital mechanical properties that exist in all humans.

NEURAL SUBSTRATE

Binocular Vision and Stereopsis

A neural pathway from retina to parietal cortex mediates perception of depth, including stereopsis. This pathway overlaps that which mediates motion perception, but is separate from that which mediates perception of color and shape, which involves temporal cortex.[43, 44] This anatomic segregation of different perceptual functions provides the substrate for selective deficits following focal cortical lesions and may account for the segregation of certain congenital defects; e.g., congenital esotropia and latent nystagmus, that are associated with impaired stereopsis and motion perception.[45, 46]

The major input for depth is mediated by large-cell, β-retinal ganglion neurons. These neurons receive converging input from all three types of cone receptors, and so they are color-nonspecific. These neurons in turn project to the magnocellular layers of the dorsal lateral geniculate nucleus (layers 1 and 2), which in turn project to layer 4Cα in cortical area V1 (striate cortex). Further processing of depth is mediated by extrastriate cortex (Fig 3). This consists of a pathway from layer 4B of V1 directly to the middle temporal (MT) area and indirectly to MT via

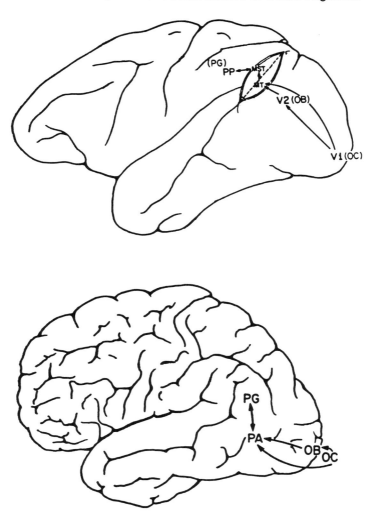

FIG 3.
Lateral view of the monkey brain *(top)* and human brain *(bottom)* illustrating the location and connections of cortical areas believed to be involved in stereopsis. The location of the cortical areas in the monkey brain are based on electrophysiologic studies. These electrophysiologically defined areas best correspond to the cytoarchitectonically defined areas of Von Bonin and Bailey,[110] which are enclosed in parentheses. The location of the cortical areas in the human brain are based on the cytoarchitectonic-mapping studies of Von Economo,[111] which correspond to the cytoarchitectonically defined areas in the monkey. *PP* = posterior parietal; *MST* = medial superior temporal area; *MT* = middle temporal area; *V2* = prestriate cortex; *V1* = striate cortex. PG, OB, and OC are abbreviations for German terms originally used by Von Economo.[111]

the thick cytochrome oxidase stripe regions of prestriate cortex (V2). Area MT in turn projects to the medial superior temporal (MST) area, which in turn projects to posterior parietal (PP) cortex. The human brain may contain areas homologous to these cortical areas (see Fig 3).[47]

The majority of neurons in V1 and V2 in the monkey are binocularly driven, and many of these (84%) are sensitive to retinal disparity.[48] Binocular neurons that are not tuned to retinal disparity have been called *flat neurons*. Those that are retinal-disparity tuned include: *tuned neurons,* which are selective over the range of Panum's fusional area (± 6 degrees of arc); *far neurons,* which give excitatory responses to objects farther then the points of fixation, and inhibitory responses to nearer objects; and *near neurons,* which have the opposite behavior. Tuned neurons may mediate local (or fine) stereopsis, whereas the far and near neurons may mediate coarse stereopsis and fusional vergence.[48]

At successive stages of the cortical pathway from V1 to PP cortex, neurons receive increasing amounts of converging excitatory (and inhibitory) input both from within the same hemisphere and from the fellow hemisphere. As a result, the receptive fields of neurons at more successive stages increase in size. In addition, most neurons within V1, V2, and MT in one hemisphere only process information in the contralateral visual field and a few degrees into the ipsilateral visual field, whereas neurons in MST and PP process information in the entire visual field. As a consequence of this converging input, cells at more successive stages process more complex features of depth.[49] For example, cells in V1 and V2 primarily encode local stereopsis for stationary stimuli; cells in MT encode the three-dimensionality of moving objects, but only in the frontoparallel plane; cells in areas MST encode motion and depth of objects in three-dimensional space, including objects moving toward or away from the animal, objects rotating in space and motion parallax; and area PP encodes visual motion and depth encountered during movement through the environment (optic flow).[50-52]

Neural Elements for Vergence

Studies of the oculomotor nucleus have shown that medial rectus motoneurons are segregated into different groups. Three different aggregates of medial rectus motoneurons have been identified: subgroup A, located ventral and rostral; subgroup B, located dorsal and caudal; and subgroup C, located dorsomedial and rostral. The last, subgroup C, comprises the smallest cell bodies and can be labeled independently of the other subgroups by selective injections of radioactive tracer into the outer (orbital) layer of the medial rectus muscle.[53]

Since the outer layer of the ocular muscles contains smaller muscle fibers, which are more likely involved in generating slower eye movements, it is tempting to speculate that the neurons in subgroup C have a selective function, perhaps in vergence. Nevertheless, there is no physiologic evidence to support this hypothesis.

Motor Commands for Vergence.—Neurophysiologic studies in monkeys have shown that almost all oculomotor neurons subserving the medial rectus and the majority of neurons in the abducens nucleus discharge for both conjugate (version) and disjunctive (vergence) eye movements.[54, 55] Near, and perhaps within, the oculomotor nucleus there are some neurons that appear to discharge exclusively for vergence. Whether or not these are a subpopulation of medial rectus motoneurons or oculomotor interneurons has yet to be established. Even though most of the motoneurons subserving the lateral and medial recti carry both version and vergence signals, the sensitivity of individual neurons to changes in eye position varies according to whether the eye position was reached by a version or by a vergence movement.[54] In other words, there is evidence that different neurons play relatively smaller or larger roles in conjugate vs. vergence eye movements.

Premotor Commands for Vergence.—Neurons involved specifically in the control of vergence, and presumably projecting to ocular motoneurons, have been found in the mesencephalic reticular formation, 1 to 2-mm dorsal and dorsolateral to the oculomotor nucleus.[56, 57] Three main types of neurons can be found: those that discharge in relation to vergence angle (vergence tonic cells [VTN]); to vergence velocity (vergence burst cells [VBN]); and to both vergence angle and velocity (vergence burst-tonic cells [VBTN]). Figure 4 illustrates possible ways in which these different types of neurons might be interconnected.

Most vergence tonic cells increase their discharge directly in relation to the angle of convergence; they change their firing rate 10 to 30 ms before any detectable eye movements. A second, smaller group of cells increases the rate of discharge with divergence. The activity of both of these types of cells is unaffected by the direction of conjugate gaze.

Vergence burst cells exhibit a burst of activity, before and during vergence, that is linearly related to the velocity of the vergence movement.[58] For most of these cells, the number of spikes within each burst, i.e., the integral of the rate of discharge, is correlated with the amplitude of the movement. These cells have been called vergence burst neurons, in analogy to the saccadic burst neurons that discharge in relation to saccade velocity. There are both convergence and divergence burst neurons; the former are more abundant.

Vergence burst-tonic cells combine vergence position and vergence velocity information in their output—the burst is related to vergence velocity and the tonic firing rate to vergence angle. Most of these burst-tonic vergence cells are next to the dorsolateral portion of the oculomotor nucleus but some are further away, about 5-mm dorsal and 5-mm lateral to the oculomotor nucleus.

Less is known about the pathways to and from these midbrain vergence neurons. The role of abducens and oculomotor interneurons (each of which has projections to the other nucleus) in generating the vergence command is also unknown. Clinically, lesions in the medial longitudinal fasciculus (MLF) do not impair the ability to make vergence movements. The MLF does, however, carry activity related to vergence.[55] Furthermore, monkeys with a lidocaine-induced internuclear ophthalmoplegia show an increased AC/A ratio, implying that the MLF actually carries signals that inhibit convergence.[59]

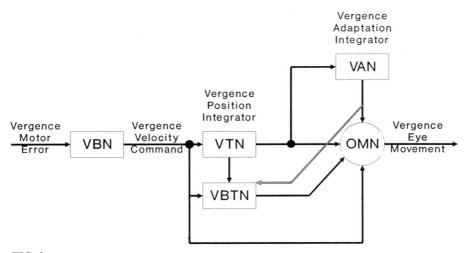

FIG 4.
Hypothetical scheme of brain stem circuitry involved in the generation of vergence eye movements. Vergence burst neurons *(VBN)*, vergence tonic neurons *(VTN)*, and vergence burst-tonic neurons *(VBTN)* have all been found in the region of the oculomotor nucleus *(OMN)*. It is possible that activity on VTN arises from neural integration (by a vergence position integrator) of the activity from VBN. VBN are presumably driven by a vergence motor error signal. Activity on VBTN may arise from a combination of inputs from VBN and VTN. There is probably also a vergence adaptation integrator (equivalent to tonic adaptation in Fig 2), which modulates the tonic level of spontaneous activity feeding onto the OMN. This adaptation circuit may use a separate pool of neurons, which we have labeled vergence adaptation neurons (VAN). They may project directly to OMN or to VBTN. Most probably do not project to VTN.[62]

Premotor inputs to the vergence system from the cerebral hemispheres are even less understood. Patients with nondominant parietal lobe lesions may have impaired stereopsis, but the pathways from parietal cortex to the midbrain vergence centers are not known.

Premotor Signals for Vergence

The organization of vergence premotor neurons has many parallels with that of the saccadic system so that it will be useful to compare the functional roles of these various types of neurons in the generation of saccadic and vergence movements.[40, 60] Both the saccadic system and the vergence system must provide the appropriate position-coded information to hold the eyes at the end of each movement, in a particular orbital position for the former and at a particular vergence angle for the latter. Since the eyes are held reasonably well in position even when the lights are turned off, immediate visual feedback cannot account for the perseveration of tonic activity in the dark. One way to attain the necessary position information is to integrate, in the mathematical sense, the prior velocity command that brought the eyes to their present position. Models for generating conjugate eye movements incorporate such a velocity-to-position integrator. Models of the vergence system have also incorporated an integrator to explain vergence input-output relationships.[61] This vergence position integrator is presumably distinct from the conjugate position integrator, though careful testing for vergence activity from premotor neurons that carry eye position signals during conjugate movements has not been reported.

It has been suggested that the source of input to the vergence integrator is the output of the vergence burst cells.[58] The vergence tonic cells may carry the output of the vergence integrator. The vergence burst-tonic cells seem to combine both vergence velocity and vergence position information. A parsimonious interpretation of these observations is that the vergence system uses a direct (velocity) pathway from vergence burst neurons in parallel with a vergence integrator (position) pathway, and that the combined signal may be the input to the ocular motoneurons (see Fig 4). The finding that ocular motoneurons discharge not only in relation to the angle of vergence but also to the velocity of vergence is consonant with this idea.

Disconjugate Adaptation

The anatomic substrate underlying phoria and other types of disconjugate adaptation is not known. Mays and Tello[62] used monkeys to show that with phoria adaptation many, but not all, of the vergence tonic neurons (VTN, see Fig 4) show a downward shift of the line relating discharge rate to vergence angle. This finding implies that the resetting of vergence tone associated with phoria adaptation may reflect input directly from a set of hypothetical vergence adaptation neurons (VAN, see Fig 4) onto motoneurons or perhaps upon vergence burst-tonic neurons (VBTN, see Fig 4). Patients with cerebellar lesions occasionally show a decrease in phoria adaptation,[63] but in most cases it is normal.[64] Monkeys with floccular lesions can still adapt their tonic vergence to prisms and their AC/A ratio to periscopic spectacles.[36] It may be that the deep cerebellar nuclei are related to disconjugate adaptation, since lesions in the deep nuclei produce unequal saccades.[65]

DISORDERS

Stereoanomalies

Some individuals have normal fine or local stereopsis, but have impaired coarse stereopsis consistent with selective loss of far or near retinal-disparity neurons in cortical areas V1 and V2 (see previous section on binocular vision and sensory fusion). Two anomalies have been described. A selective inability to localize stimuli presented with large (>0.5 degrees) uncrossed disparities, and a selective inability to localize stimuli presented with large crossed disparities.[66] Individuals with these stereoanomalies also are unable to diverge or converge to these stimuli when tachistoscopically presented.[67]

Patients with right parietal lobe lesions have normal local or fine stereopsis in both visual hemifields; i.e., they are able to detect local disparities on a point-to-point basis for images within Panum's fusional area. In contrast, they have impaired global stereopsis; i.e., they are not able to use these local disparities to perceive a surface in depth, consequently, they have difficulty perceiving objects in three-dimensional space using binocular cues alone.[68, 69] These data are consistent with the concept that global stereopsis depends on local stereopsis mediated by striate and prestriate cortex in both hemispheres converging onto a perceptive mechanism mediated in right parietal cortex. Fusional vergence may be impaired in patients with right parietal lesions.[70]

Strabismus

Phoria is an inherent misalignment of the eyes, which is kept in check by the fusional mechanism. The degree of phoria largely reflects the level of tonic vergence, which depends on the output of the slow adaptive fusional mechanism (VAN, see Fig 4), and any residual activity from the vergence position integrator (VTN and VBTN, see Fig 4). The level of accommodation also will influence the phoria via accommodative-driven vergence (see Fig 2). At what level accommodative vergence is combined with fusional vergence is not known, but the VTN and VBTN presumably also carry vergence signals driven by accommodation.

Tropia or strabismus is a misalignment of the visual axes that cannot be overcome by the fusional mechanisms. Strabismus affects about 2% of the population.[71] Tropias may occur if the phoria is very large, or if the range of the fusional mechanism is small. Strabismus has been divided into several types based on presumed etiologies.[72] We will describe the more common types.

Congenital or Infantile Esotropia.—Congenital esotropia is one of the most common types of strabismus. It is not present at birth, but develops before the age of 6 months.[73] It is usually constant and large angle.

Ideas regarding the cause of congenital esotropia have their origins in two classic rival hypotheses, sensory and motor, which were originally proposed by Worth[74] and Chavasse.[75] In the sensory hypothesis, the primary defect is believed to be a congenital abnormality in sensory fusion, leaving the motor vergence system without regulation. The motor hypothesis maintains that the sensory capacity to stimulate fusion is initially intact, but the primary problem is motor fusion (or vergence). The resultant strabismus then leads to a secondary loss of binocularity in cortical neurons. A current hypothesis is that congenital esotropia develops as a result of a loss of binocular vision combined with an exuberant convergence mechanism, which is really a combination of the classic sensory and motor hypotheses.[76]

To what extent patients with congenital esotropia have global stereopsis is controversial. Those who have used dynamic random-element stereograms have reported no stereopsis in individuals between the ages of 3 to 36 months, even if the strabismus is surgically corrected at an early age.[45, 77] Those who have used static stereograms have reported stereopsis in 20% to 40% of individuals.[78] The difference in the results may be due to the presence of monocular cues in the static stereograms.[79] Fusional vergence eye movements do occur in patients with congenital esotropia, but they are very slow.[80] It has been suggested that these slow movements are induced by the tonic adaptation circuit within the vergence circuit (see Fig 2), and that the fast component of the vergence circuit is absent or defective.[80]

Some investigators have found changes in eye muscle proprioceptors in congenital esotropia and have suggested that a disturbance in ocular proprioception may play an important role in the pathogenesis of this disorder.[81, 82] Proprioceptive information may act with visual input in developing binocularly activated neurons in visual cortex.[83] Whether changes in muscle proprioceptors in congenital esotropia mediate the defect or are a consequence of the strabismus is still unclear.

Congenital esotropia is associated with latent or manifest latent nystagmus (LN) 25% of the time, and dissociated vertical deviation (DVD) 42% to 44% of the time.[84, 85] Nearly all patients with LN or DVD have early onset strabismus.[85, 86] LN is a conjugate jerk nystagmus that occurs during infancy and persists throughout life. It is revealed by monocular eye patching. The slow phases of the nystagmus are directed temporal-to-nasal with respect to the viewing eye. LN is hypothesized to be due to a nasal-temporal velocity bias in the optokinetic nystagmus (OKN) system[87, 88] or in the smooth pursuit system[46, 87] induced during monocular viewing. Other causes for LN have been suggested, including defective egocentric localization and an eye muscle proprioceptive imbalance.[89, 90]

Accommodative or Refractive Esotropia.—Accommodative esotropia develops after the age of 6 months and usually between the ages of 2 and 3 years. The delayed onset may be to an immature accommodative response.[91] In addition, it develops gradually and usually presents as an intermittent strabismus.

Accommodative esotropia occurs in the presence of an uncorrected hyperopia and an inadequate motor fusion (insufficient fusional divergence). Because of the hyperopia, excessive accommodation occurs, which leads to excessive convergence. The excessive accommodation leads to an esotropia only when the amplitude of fusional divergence is not large enough to overcome the large esophoria.

Misalignment Due to Abnormal Vergence-Accommodation Interactions.—Duane[92] suggested that strabismus is due to an imbalance between active convergence and divergence mechanisms. He classified esotropia into convergence excess (deviation greater at near) and divergence insufficiency (deviation greater at far). Similarly, he classified exotropias into divergence excess and convergence insufficiency. Deviations that were the same both at near or far were classified as mixtures of divergence excess and convergence insufficiency (basic exotropia).

Convergence excess (high AC/A ratio) can occur at any age, but usually between 6 months and 7 years of age. The deviation is larger at near than far. It can occur in patients with emmetropia, hypermetropia, or myopia. It is due to an abnormal synkinesis between accommodation and accommodative convergence. The effort to accommodate elicits an abnormally high accommodative convergence response. If fusional vergence can cope with the increased convergence tone (i.e., the vergence amplitude is greater than the induced retinal disparity), only an esophoria occurs, otherwise esotropia becomes manifest. Abnormally high AC/A ratios occur in 46% of children with esotropia.[93]

Convergence insufficiency (low AC/C ratio) is associated with an exodeviation at least 15Δ larger during fixation at near than at far. Such individuals lack adequate convergence when they accommodate and may develop exotropia if they have a poor fusional mechanism.

Schor and Horner[94] have proposed that convergence insufficiency and excess may have their basis in alterations in the strength of the cross-linkages between accommodation and convergence or in the sensitivity of the slow adaptive mechanisms for vergence and accommodation. Convergence insufficiency may be due to a low AC/A ratio, whereas convergence excess may be due to a high AC/A ratio.

Patients with unusually high AC/A ratios and convergence excess usually have a poor ability to adaptively adjust their level of tonic accommodation (and a robust adaptation of tonic vergence), while patients with unusually low AC/A ratios and convergence insufficiency usually have a poor ability to adaptively adjust their level of tonic vergence (and a robust adaptation of tonic accommodation). High AC/A ratios are usually associated with low CA/C ratios and vice versa. Such an analysis of vergence disorders has not yet been applied to patients with acquired neurologic disorders.

Brain Trauma.—Because of the high incidence of congenital strabismus in patients with intracranial lesions, cerebral palsy, and mental retardation, some have suggested that congenital strabismus may be secondary to brain trauma or perinatal ischemia.[95-98] Paralytic strabismus frequently acquires the characteristics of comitant strabismus over the course of weeks to months (spread of comitance) due to overaction and contracture of the antagonist muscles and perhaps adaptive mechanisms related to orbital-position-dependent phoria adaptation.

Ocular Misalignment Due to Visual Deprivation.—Patients with uniocular visual loss have an 80% chance of developing strabismus.[99] If visual loss occurs before the age of 5 years, either esotropia or exotropia occur. Strabismus usually persists even if normal visual acuity is restored.[99-101] In contrast, if visual loss occurs after the age of 5 years, exotropia usually occurs, and normal ocular alignment may be restored if the visual impairment is corrected. This has been best documented in patients with acquired cataracts.[102]

What are the possible mechanisms for irreversible, deprivation-induced strabismus during the first 5 years of life, and what determines whether exotropia or esotropia develops? Human subjects patched during infancy do not develop normal binocularity.[103] Monkeys reared with 4 to 8 weeks of monocular, binocular, or alternating monocular eyelid suture during infancy have a persistent loss of binocularly driven cells in striate cortex.[104–106] As a result of this loss of binocularity, neither humans nor monkeys would be expected to develop normal fusion. They would, therefore, lack the major sensory system used to detect ocular misalignment (the role of proprioception in maintaining ocular alignment is unclear).

The age that visual deprivation was initiated within the critical period may determine which type of strabismus (exotropia or esotropia) develops. This is suggested by a series of studies in monkeys. If monkeys receive 50 days of visual deprivation beginning within 24 hours of birth, persistent exotropia always occurs.[107] In contrast, if monkeys receive visual deprivation for 3 to 7 months beginning at 3 to 14 days of age, esotropia primarily occurs.[108, 109] As previously stated, most normal newborns have significant exotropia at birth, which is corrected, and sometimes overcorrected, over the course of the next 6 months.[27] Therefore, if visual deprivation occurs within the first several days of birth, the infants may be left with a persistent exotropia. This may be due to a lack of development of convergence mechanisms. If deprivation occurred at a later time, it may result in esotropia by allowing vergence tone to increase without binocular visual feedback.

REFERENCES

1. Zihl J, Von Cramon D, Mai N: Selective disturbance of movement vision after bilateral brain damage. *Brain* 1983; 106:313–340.

2. Kelly BJ, Rosenberg ML, Zee DS, et al: Unilateral pursuit-induced congenital nystagmus. *Neurology* 1989; 39:414–416.

3. Fender DH, Julesz B: Extension of Panum's fusional area in binocularly stabilized vision. *J Opt Soc Am* 1967; 57:819–830.

4. Piantinada TP: Stereo hysteresis revisited. *Vis Res* 1986; 26:431–437.

5. Julesz B: *Foundations of Cyclopean Perception.* Chicago, University of Chicago Press, 1971, p 406.

6. Maddox EE: The Clinical Use of Prisms. Bristol, John Wright and Sons, 1893.

7. Wick B, Bedell HE: Magnitude and velocity of proximal vergence. *Invest Ophthalmol Vis Sci* 1989; 30:755–760.

8. Jones R, Stephens GL: Horizontal fusional amplitudes. *Invest Ophthalmol Vis Sci* 1989; 30:1638–1642.

9. Berens C, Losey CC, Hardy LH: Routine examination of the ocular muscles and non-operative treatment. *Am J Ophthalmol* 1927; 10:910–918.

10. Mellick A: Convergence. An investigation into the normal standards of age groups. *Br J Ophthalmol* 1949; 33:755–763.

11. Tait EF: Fusional vergence. *Am J Ophthalmol* 1949; 32:1223–1230.

12. Stephens GL, Jones R: Horizontal fusional amplitudes after adaptation to prism. *Ophthalmol Physiol Opt* 1990; 10:25–28.

13. Erkelens CJ, Van der Steen J, Steinman RM, et al: Ocular vergence under natural conditions. *Proc R Soc Lon (Biol)* 1989; 236:417–465.

14. Levi L, Zee DS, Hain TC: Disjunctive and disconjugate saccades during symmetrical vergence. *Invest Ophthalmol Vis Sci* 1987; 28:332.

15. Ogle KN, Martens TG, Dyer JA: *Oculomotor Imbalance in Binocular Vision and Fixation Disparity.* Philadelphia, Lea & Febiger, 1967, p 372.

16. Semmlow JL, Hung G: The near response: Theories of control, in Schor CM, Ciuffreda KJ (eds): *Vergence Eye Movements: Basic and Clinical Aspects.* Stoneham, Mass, Butterworth, 1983, pp 175–195.

17. Judge SJ, Miles FA: Changes in the coupling between accommodation and vergence eye movements induced in human subjects by altering the effective interocular separation. *Perception* 1985; 14:617–629.

18. Miles FA, Judge SJ, Optican LM: Optically induced changes in the couplings between vergence and accommodation. *J Neurosci* 1987; 7:2576–2589.

19. Fox R, Aslin RN, Shea SL, et al: Stereopsis in human infants. *Science* 1980; 207:323–324.

20. Braddick O, Atkinson J: The development of binocular function in infancy. *Acta Ophthalmol* 1983; 157:25–35.

21. Birch EE, Gwiazda J, Held R: The development of vergence does not account for the onset of stereopsis. *Perception* 1983; 12:331–336.

22. Howland HC, Dobson V, Sayles N: Accommodation in infants as measured by photorefraction. *Vision Res* 1987; 27:2141–2152.

23. Aslin RN: Motor aspects of visual development in infancy, in Salapatek P, Cohen L (eds): *Handbook of Infant Perception.* London, Academic Press, 1987, pp 43–113.

24. Banks MS: The development of visual accommodation during early infancy. *Child Dev* 1980; 51:646–666.

25. Slater AM, Findlay JM: Binocular fixation in the newborn baby. *J Exp Child Psychol* 1975; 20:248–273.

26. Aslin RN: Development of binocular fixation in human infants. *J Exp Child Psychol* 1977; 23:133–150.

27. Archer SM, Sondhi N, Helverston EM: Strabismus in infancy. *Ophthalmology* 1989; 96:133–137.

28. Viirre E, Cadera W, Vilis T: Monocular adaptation of the saccadic system and vestibulo-ocular reflex. *Invest Ophthalmol Vis Sci* 1988; 29:1339–1347.

29. Zee DS, Optican LM: Studies of adaptation in human ocular motor disorders, in Berthoz A, Melvill Jones G (eds): *Reviews of Oculomotor Research, Adaptive Mechanisms in Gaze Control,* vol 1. London, Elsevier, 1985, pp 165–176.

30. Sethi B: Vergence adaptation: A review. *Doc Ophthalmol* 1986; 63:247–263.

31. Sethi B, North RV: Vergence adaptive changes with varying magnitudes of prism-induced disparities and fusional amplitudes. *Am J Optom Physiol Opt* 1987; 64:263–268.

32. Schor CM, Johnson CA, Post RB: Adaptation of tonic accommodation. *Ophthalmol Physiol Opt* 1984; 4:133–137.

33. Schor CM: The relationship between fusional vergence eye movements and fixation disparity. *Vision Res* 1979; 19:1359–1367.

34. Schor CM: Models of mutual interactions between accommodation and convergence. *Am J Optom Physiol Opt* 1985; 62:369–374.

35. Schor CM, Kotulak JC: Dynamic interactions between accommodation and convergence are velocity sensitive. *Vision Res* 1986; 26:927–942.

36. Judge SJ: Optically-induced changes in tonic vergence and AC/A ratio in normal monkeys and monkeys with lesions of the flocculus and ventral paraflocculus. *Exp Brain Res* 1987; 66:1–9.

37. Henson DB, Dharamshi BG: Oculomotor adaptation to induced heterophoria and anisometropia. *Invest Ophthalmol Vis Sci* 1982; 22:234–240.

38. Erkelens CJ, Collewijn H, Steinman RM: Asymmetrical adaptation of human saccades to anisometropia spectacles. *Invest Ophthalmol Vis Sci* 1989; 30:1132–1145.

39. Oohira A, Zee DS, Guyton DL: Disconjugate adaptation to long-standing, large-amplitude spectacle-corrected anisometropia. *Invest Ophthalmol Vis Sci,* 1991; 32:1693–1703.

40. Zee DS, Levi L: Neurological aspects of vergence eye movements. *Rev Neurol (Paris)* 1989; 145:613–620.

41. Oohira A, Zee DS: Disconjugate ocular motor adaptation in rhesus monkey, in Shimazu H, Shinoda Y (eds): *Vestibular and Brain Stem Control of Eye, Head and Body Movements.* New York, Springer-Verlag, in press.

42. Schor CM, Gleason J, Horner D: Selective nonconjugate binocular adaptation of vertical saccades and pursuits. *Vision Res* 1990; 30:1827–1844.

43. Livingstone M, Hubel D: Segregation of form, color, movement, and depth: Anatomy, physiology, and perception. *Science* 1988; 240:740–749.

44. Maunsell JHR, Newsome WT: Visual processing in monkey extrastriate cortex. *Ann Rev Neurosci* 1987; 10:363–401.

45. Dobson V, Sebris SL: Longitudinal study of acuity and stereopsis in infants with or at-risk for esotropia. *Invest Ophthalmol Vis Sci* 1989; 30:1146–1158.

46. Tychsen L, Lisberger SG: Maldevelopment of visual motion processing in humans who had strabismus with onset of infancy. *J Neurosci* 1986; 6:2495–2508.

47. Tusa RJ, Zee DS: Cerebral control of smooth pursuit and optokinetic nystagmus, in Lessell S, van Dalen JTW (eds): *Current Neuro-ophthalmology,* vol 2. Chicago, Year Book Medical Publishers, 1989, pp 115–146.

48. Poggio GF, Poggio T: The analysis of stereopsis. *Ann Rev Neurosci* 1984; 7:379–412.

49. Allman J, Miezin F, McGuinness E: Stimulus specific responses from beyond the classical receptive field. *Ann Rev Neurosci* 1985; 8:407–430.

50. Maunsell JHR, Van Essen DC: Functional properties of neurons in middle temporal visual area of the macaque monkey. *J Neurophysiol* 1983; 49:1148–1167.

51. Sakata H, Shibutani H, Ito Y, et al: Parietal cortical neurons responding to rotary movement of visual stimulus in space. *Exp Brain Res* 1986; 61:658–663.

52. Tanaka K, Hikosaka K, Saito H-A, et al: Analysis of local and wide-field movements in the superior temporal visual areas of the macaque monkey. *J Neurosci* 1986; 6:134–144.

53. Buttner-Ennever J, Akert K: Medial rectus subgroups of the oculomotor nucleus and their abducens internuclear input in the monkey. *J Comp Neurol* 1981; 197:17–27.

54. Mays LE, Porter JD: Neural control of vergence eye movements: Activity of abducens and oculomotor neurons. *J. Neurophysiol* 1984; 52:743–761.

55. Gamlin PDR, Gnadt JW, Mays LE: Abducens internuclear neurons carry an inappropriate signal for ocular convergence. *J Neurophysiol* 1989; 62:70–81.

56. Mays LE: Neural control of vergence eye movements: Convergence and divergence neurons in midbrain. *J Neurophysiol* 1984; 51:1091–1108.

57. Judge SJ, Cumming BG: Neurons in the monkey midbrain with activity related to vergence eye movement and accommodation. *J Neurophysiol* 1986; 55:915–930.

58. Mays LE, Porter JD, Gamlin PDR, et al: Neural control of vergence eye movements: Neurons encoding vergence velocity. *J Neurophysiol* 1986; 56:1007–1021.

59. Gamlin PDR, Gnadt JW, Mays LE: Lidocaine-induced unilateral internuclear ophthalmoplegia: Effects of convergence and conjugate eye movements. *J Neurophysiol* 1989; 62:82–95.

60. Leigh RJ, Zee DS: *The Neurology of Eye Movements.* Philadelphia, FA Davis, 1991.

61. Krishnan VV, Stark L: Model of the disparity vergence system, in Schor CM, Ciuffreda KJ

(eds): *Vergence Eye Movements: Basic and Clinical Aspects.* Woburn, Mass, Butterworth, 1983, pp 349–371.

62. Mays LE, Tello CA: Neurophysiological correlates of convergence and its tonic adjustment, in Keller E, Zee DS (eds): *Adaptive Processes in Visual and Oculomotor Systems,* Oxford, Pergamon, 1986, pp 143–150.

63. Milder DG, Reinecke RD: Phoria adaptation in prisms. *Arch Neurol* 1983; 40:339–342.

64. Hain TC, Luebke A: Phoria adaptation in patients with cerebellar lesions. *Invest Ophthalmol Vis Sci* 1990; 31:1394–1397.

65. Vilis T, Snow R, Hore J: Cerebellar saccadic dysmetria is not equal in the two eyes. *Exp Brain Res* 1983; 51:343–350.

66. Richards W: Stereopsis and stereoblindness. *Exp Brain Res* 1970; 10:380–388.

67. Jones R: Anomalies of disparity detection in the human visual system. *J Physiol* 1977; 265:621–640.

68. Hamsher K de S: Stereopsis and unilateral brain disease., *Invest Ophthalmol Vis Sci* 1978; 17:336–343.

69. Vaina LM: Selective impairment of visual motion interpretation following lesions of the right occipito-parietal area in humans. *Biol Cybern* 1989; 61:347–359.

70. Fowler S, Munro N, Richardson A: Vergence control in patients with lesions of the posterior parietal cortex. *J Physiol (London)* 1989; 417:92.

71. Asbury T, Eggers HM: Strabismus, in Vaughn D, Asbury T, Tabbara RF (eds): *General Ophthalmology.* Englewood Cliffs, NJ, Prentice-Hall, Lange Medical Publications, 1980, pp 206–227.

72. von Noorden GK: *Binocular Vision and Ocular Motility.* St Louis, CV Mosby Co, 1990, pp 285–426.

73. Nixon RB, Helveston EM, Miller K, et al: Incidence of strabismus in neonates. *Am J Ophthalmol* 1985; 100:798–801.

74. Worth C: *Squint: Its Causes, Pathology, and Treatment.* Philadelphia, Blakiston, 1903, pp 59–62.

75. Chavasse FB: *Worth's Squint: Or the Binocular Reflexes and the Treatment of Strabismus,* ed 7. Philadelphia, Blakiston, 1939, pp 519–521.

76. Archer SM, Sondhi N, Helverston EM: Strabismus in infancy. *Ophthalmology* 1989; 133–137.

77. Archer SM, Helveston EM, Miller KK, et al: Stereopsis in normal infants and infants with congenital esotropia. *Am J Ophthalmol* 1986; 101:591–596.

78. Rogers GL, Bremer DL, Leguire LE, et al: Clinical assessment of visual function in the young child: A prospective study of binocular vision. *J Pediatr Ophthalmol Strabismus* 1986; 23:233–235.

79. Cooper J, Feldman, J: Depth perception in strabismus (letter). *Br J Ophthalmol* 1981; 65:510.

80. Campos EC, Bolzani R, Gualdi G, et al: Recording of disparity vergence in comitant esotropia. *Doc Ophthalmol* 1989; 71:69–76.

81. Corsi M, Sodi A, Salvi G, et al: Morphological study of extraocular muscle proprioceptor alterations in congenital strabismus. *Ophthalmologica* 1990; 200:154–163.

82. Martinez AJ, Biglan AW, Hiles DA: Structural features of extraocular muscles of children with strabismus. *Arch Ophthalmol* 1980; 98:533–539.

83. Maffei L, Fiorentini A: Role of oculomotor proprioception in the visual system of the cat, in Lennerstrand G, von Noorden GK, Campos EC (eds): *Strabismus and Amblyopia.* New York, Plenum Press, 1988, pp 337–343.

84. von Noorden GK: A reassessment of infantile esotropia: XLIV Edward Jackson Memorial Lecture. *Am J Ophthalmol* 1988; 105:1–10.

85. Helveston EM: Dissociated vertical deviation: A clinical and laboratory study. *Trans Am Ophthalmol Soc* 1980; 78:734–779.

86. Dell'Osso L, Traccis S, Abel LA: Strabismus-A necessary condition for latent and manifest latent nystagmus. *Neuro Ophthalmol* 1983; 3:247–257.

87. Kommerell G: Ocular motor phenomena in infantile strabismus, in Kennard C, Ciffford Rose F (eds): *Physiological Aspects of Clinical Neuro-Ophthalmology,* London, Chapman and Hall, 1988, pp 357–376.

88. Schor CM: Subcortical binocular suppression affects the development of latent amd optokinetic nystagmus. *Am J Optom Physiol Opt* 1983; 60:481–502.

89. Dell'Osso LF, Schmidt D, Daroff RB: Latent, manifest latent, and congenital nystagmus. *Arch Ophthalmol* 1979; 97:1877.

90. Ishikawa S: Latent nystagmus and its etiology, in Reinecke RD (ed): *Strabismus: Proceedings of the Third Meeting of the International Strabismological Association.* New York, Grune and Stratton, 1978, pp 203–214.

91. Haynes H, White B, Held R: Visual accommodation in human infants. *Science* 1965; 148:528.

92. Duane A: A new classification of the motor anomalies of the eye, based upon physiologic principles. *Ann Ophthalmol Otol* part I, Oct 1896; part II, Jan 1897.

93. Parks MM: Abnormal accommodative convergence in squint. *Arch Ophthalmol* 1958; 59:364–380.

94. Schor C, Horner D: Adaptive disorders of accommodation and vergence in binocular dysfunction. *Ophthalmol Physiol Opt* 1989; 9:264–268.

95. Hiles DA, Wallar PH, McFalane F: Current concepts in the management of strabismus in children with cerebral palsy. *Ann Ophthalmol* 1975; 7:789–797.

96. Black PD: Ocular defects in children with cerebral palsy. *Br Med J* 1980; 1:487–488.

97. Bankes JLK: Eye defects of mentally handicapped children. *Br Med J* 1974; 2:533–535.

98. Frandsen AD: Occurrence of squint: A clinical-statistical study on the prevalence of squint and associated signs in different groups and ages of the Danish population. *Acta Ophthalmol (Copenh)* 1960; 62:1–158.

99. Sidikaro Y, von Noorden GK: Observations in sensory heterotropia. *J Pediatr Ophthalmol Strabismus* 1982; 19:12–19.

100. Tytla ME, Maurer D, Lewis TL, et al: Contrast sensitivity in children treated for congenital cataract. *Clin Vision Sci* 1988; 2:251–264.

101. Grossman SA, Peyman G: Long-term visual results after pars plicate lensectomy-vitrectomy for congenital cataracts. *Br J Ophthalmol* 1988; 72:601–606.

102. Lyle TK: The importance of orthoptic investigation before contact lens fitting in unilateral aphakia-A preliminary report. *Trans Ophthalmol Soc UK* 1953; 73:387–398.

103. Awaya S, Sugawara M, Miyake S: Observations in patients with occlusion amblyopia. Results of treatment. *Trans Ophthalmol Soc UK* 1979; 99:447–454.

104. Blakemore C, Vital-Durand F, Garey LJ: Recovery from monocular deprivation in the monkey. I. Reversal of physiological effects in the visual cortex. *Proc R Soc Lond* 1981; 213:399–423.

105. LeVay S, Wiesel TN, Hubel DH: The development of ocular dominance columns in normal and visually deprived monkeys. *J Comp Neurol* 1980; 191:1–51.

106. Wiesel TN, Hubel DH: Ordered arrangement of orientation columns in monkeys lacking visual experience. *J Comp Neurol* 1974; 158:307–318.

107. Tusa RJ, Repka MX, Smith CB, et al: Early visual deprivation results in persistent strabismus and nystagmus in monkeys. *Invest Ophthalmol Vis Sci* 1991; 32:130–137.

108. Quick MW, Tigges M, Gammon JA, et al: Early abnormal visual experience induces strabismus in infant monkeys. *Invest Ophthalmol Vis Sci* 1989; 30:1012–1017.

109. Regal DM, Boothe R, Teller DY, et al: Visual acuity and visual responsiveness in dark-reared monkeys *(Macaca nemestria)*. *Vision Res* 1976; 16:523–530.

110. Von Bonin G, Bailey P: *The Neocortex of Macaca Mulatta*. Urbana, Ill, University of Illinois Press, 1947, p 163.

111. Von Economo CF: *The Cytoarchitectonics of The Human Cerebral Cortex*. London, Oxford Medical Publications, 1929.

CHAPTER 9

Nystagmus, Saccadic Intrusions/Oscillations and Oscillopsia

L.F. Dell'Osso, Ph.D.

Professor, Departments of Neurology and Biomedical Engineering, Case Western Reserve University School of Medicine, Director, Ocular Motor Neurophysiology Laboratory, Veterans Administration Medical Center, Cleveland, Ohio

Understanding the pathophysiology of ocular oscillations necessitates differentiation between those involving only the slow system and those that are purely saccadic. Oscillations containing both saccades and slow phases require identification of both the causative phase (i.e., that which takes the eyes away from their intended direction) and the corrective phase. Modern recording methods have made these determinations possible and thereby clarified the underlying ocular motor mechanisms responsible for many oscillations. Table 1 lists 47 types of nystagmus (two of which were not in the previous volumes) along with many other terms found in the literature to describe them; similarly, Table 2 lists 16 saccadic oscillations and intrusions (one of which has been renamed since the previous volume) with other descriptive terms. The tables evolved from those that appeared in previous biannual volumes on this subject.[1-5]

The definitions and categorizations used herein result from applying criteria derived from accurate ocular motility recordings. They differentiate between nystagmus and saccadic oscillations and, as a result, some eye movements originally described with the word "nystagmus," are really saccadic oscillations. Most oscilla-

TABLE 1.

Forty-seven Types of Nystagmus*

Acquired	Flash-induced	Pursuit after-
"fixation"	flicker-induced	induced
Anticipatory	induced	Pursuit-defect†
induced	Gaze-evoked	Pseudospontaneous
Arthrokinetic	deviational	induced
induced	gaze-paretic	Rebound
somatosensory	"neurasthenic"	Reflex
Associated	"seducible"	Baer's
induced	"setting-in"	See-Saw
Stransky's	Horizontal	Somatosensory
Audiokinetic	Induced	induced
induced	provoked	Spontaneous
Bartel's	Intermittent vertical	Stepping around
induced	Jerk	apparent/real
Bruns'	Latent/Manifest latent	induced
Centripetal	monocular "fixation"	somatosensory
Cervical	unimacular	Torsional
neck torsion	Lateral medullary	rotary
vertebral-basilar artery	Lid	Uniocular
insufficiency	Miner's†	Upbeat
Circular/Elliptic/Oblique	occupational	Vertical
alternating windmill	Muscle-paretic	Vestibular
circumduction	myasthenic	a(po)geotropic/geotropic
diagonal	Optokinetic	alternating current
elliptic	induced	Bechterew's
gyratory	"kinetic"	caloric/caloric-after
oblique	"optic"	compensatory
radiary	optomotor	electrical/faradic/galvanic
Congenital	panoramic	head-shaking
"fixation"	"railway"	induced
hereditary	sigma	L-
Convergence	"train"	labyrinthine
Convergence-evoked	Optokinetic after-	perverted
Dissociated	induced	pneumatic/compression
disjunctive	post-optokinetic	positional/alcohol
Downbeat	reverse post-optokinetic	positioning
Drug-induced	Pendular	postrotational
barbiturate	talantropia	pseudocaloric
bow tie	Periodic/Aperiodic alternating	rotational/perrotary
induced	alternans	secondary phase
Epileptic	Physiologic	
ictal	end-point	
	fatigue	

*Synonyms and other terms are indented under either the preferred or the more inclusive designation; some nystagmus types may be acquired or congenital; quoted terms are erroneous or nonspecific.
†May not exist.

TABLE 2.

Sixteen Types of Saccadic Intrusions and Oscillations*

Bobbing/Dipping
  inverse bobbing
  reverse bobbing
Convergence-retraction "nystagmus"
  "nystagmus" retractoris
Double saccadic pulses
  (single/multiple)
  saccadic intrusions/oscillations
Dynamic overshoot
  "quiver"
Dysmetria
Flutter
  microflutter
Flutter dysmetria
Macro saccadic oscillations
Myoclonus
  laryngeal "nystagmus"
  "lightning eye movements"
  pharyngeal "nystagmus"
Opsoclonus
  "dancing eyes"
  "lightning eye movements"
  saccadomania
Psychogenic flutter
  hysterical flutter
  hysterical "nystagmus"
  "ocular fibrillation"
  "ocular shuddering"
  psychological "nystagmus"
  voluntary flutter
  voluntary "nystagmus"
	Saccadic lateropulsion
	  ipsipulsion
	  contrapulsion
	Saccadic pulses/pulse trains
	  abduction "nystagmus"
	  ataxic "nystagmus"
	  saccadic intrusions/oscillations
	  stepless saccades
	Square-wave jerks/oscillations
	  Gegenrucke
	  hopping nystagmus
	  "lightening eye movements"
	  myoclonus
	  saccadic intrusions/oscillations
	  Zickzakbewegungen
	Square-wave pulses (single/bursts)
	  Kippdeviationen/"Kippnystagmus"
	  "macro square-wave jerks"
	  "pendular macro-oscillations"
	  saccadic "nystagmus"
	  saccadic oscillations/intrusions
	Superior oblique myokymia

*Synonyms and other terms are indented under either the preferred or the more inclusive designation; quoted terms are erroneous or nonspecific.

tions were named before the benefits of accurate recordings. Quotation marks are used for those oscillations that are *not* truly nystagmus or for purely subjective clinical terms found in the literature that are inadequate, not clearly defined, or have been misapplied. Since these ambiguous or erroneous terms do not convey accurate information about the basic nature of the movement, their use is not recommended in scientific communications. In those cases where historical precedence supports their continued usage (e.g., abduction "nystagmus" and convergence-retraction "nystagmus"), the quotation marks show that these are non-nystagmic oscillations (i.e., saccadic). The best names describe the mechanism thought to be responsible for the eye movement (e.g., saccadic pulse); such terms maximize the information carried to the reader and clearly describe a movement by its well-defined component parts. The use of amplitude-related terms has proven to be misleading when later work has uncovered the same oscillation at a different amplitude; terms like "micro," "mini" or "macro" do not imply a different mechanism and should not be used in the primary name of an oscillation (see the suggestion to substitute "square-wave pulses" for the misleading "macro square-wave jerks"). This does not preclude their use in describing a specific case where the oscillation may be smaller or larger than is normally seen. There is a great deal of idiosyncratic difference in ocular motor oscillations, and low-amplitude oscillations seen in "healthy" subjects may actually be preclinical signs of later, larger oscillations.

NYSTAGMUS

The word "nystagmus" is derived from the Greek word νησταγμος meaning drowsiness, which in turn is derived from νησταξειν meaning to nod in one's sleep. It should be noted that this nodding oscillation is generated and sustained by the slow downward drifting of the head; the upward head jerks are corrective (i.e., they serve to restore upright head posture). In keeping with this original definition, nystagmus is defined as follows: a biphasic ocular oscillation containing slow eye movements (SEM) that are responsible for its genesis and continuation. Fast eye movements (saccades), if they are present, serve a corrective function and do not represent the basic ocular motor dysfunction. The two phases of ocular nystagmus are approximately equal in amplitude. It was once suggested that the term for pendular oscillations should be "talantropia" (from the Greek word ταλαντροπια for oscillating) to distinguish it from jerk nystagmus,[6] but this terminology did not become popular. This section contains discussions of each nystagmus type in which significant work has been done in the past 2 years; they are in alphabetical order. For more detailed descriptions of other types, the reader is referred to the aforementioned previous volumes.

A study of the effects of sampling frequency, analog filtering, and A/D conversion bits on the accuracy of velocity determinations of fast and slow phases of nystagmus concluded that 400 Hz, 70 Hz, and 12 bits were the respective requirements of these variables.[7] This is a complicated issue and there are problems associated with over-sampling as well as under-sampling that are not immediately obvious. It has been our experience that a 200-Hz sampling frequency, 100-Hz analog filtering and 12 bit A/D conversion is more than adequate for slow phase velocities; in fact, many times we cut the differentiator bandwidth to 21 to 24 Hz with no difference in slow phase velocities. For saccadic velocities, the higher sampling rate is required. Given the usual need to limit the size of computer data arrays per trial, it is probably better to sample the position signal at 200 Hz to include all of the frequencies of interest and later interpolate the data arrays to effectively double that sampling rate before differentiating.

Anticipatory Nystagmus

Anticipatory SEM are predictive movements that occur prior to either ramp or step target motions. When these movements are interspaced with saccades in the opposite direction, anticipatory nystagmus results.[8] Boman and Hotson recently showed that with a continuously visible target, prior to the initiation of ramp motion, an anticipatory nystagmus was produced that restricted eye position and velocity errors. However, prior to ramp termination, this nystagmus was not produced and slow eye velocities changed by as much as 6 degrees/sec.

Circular/Elliptic/Oblique Nystagmus

Traccis et al. reported the successful treatment of an acquired pendular elliptical nystagmus in multiple sclerosis using isoniazid and base-out prisms.[9] The drug abolished the nystagmus and relieved oscillopsia (OSOP) in two patients but was ineffective in the third in whom the base-out prisms were used. By careful questioning of these three patients, it was discovered that the OSOP associated with circular-elliptic nystagmus, unlike that of horizontal, vertical, diagonal, or torsional nystagmus, is in the *same* direction as the eye motion. Comparison was made to linear nystagmus where the retinal image motion is the same as eye motion and the perceived motion is opposite to the retinal image motion and to torsional nystagmus where the retinal image motion is in the opposite direction to eye motion and the perceived motion is in the same direction as the retinal image motion. In circular or elliptic nystagmus, both the retinal image and perceived motion are in the same direction as the eye motion. Therefore, a clockwise nystagmus (as seen from the *subject's* point of view) produces a clockwise OSOP and vice versa.

Congenital Nystagmus

We studied the accuracy and cycle-to-cycle repeatability of the foveation periods in congenital nystagmus (CN) since visual acuity is directly related to these indices.[10] During a 5-second interval of fixation, the standard deviation of mean horizontal foveal position was ±13 minarc (±5 minarc vertical) and mean foveation time was 59 ms. There were 1-second intervals of fixation with standard deviations of 0 minarc. Position and velocity histograms reflected the increase in data about the zero position and velocity points caused by the foveation periods of the waveforms. We applied phase-plane analysis to the CN waveforms and demonstrated beat-to-beat overlap in the position and velocities during the foveation periods. Contrary to the notion that CN was due to poor fixation reflexes, we concluded that the fixation reflexes in subjects with CN were remarkably strong and accurate despite the large oscillation always present. Even in albinos, where the fovea is not normal, CN foveation periods were found to approximate those of normal foveas.[11] In a study of various indices of CN waveforms, the highest correlations were found to be between: (1) foveation time and the maximum rate of the histogram indicating the rate of duration of the eye in each spatial position; (2) amplitude and intensity; and (3) mean slow-phase velocity and intensity.[12] Visual acuity correlated best with foveation time. Bedell et al. found foveation-period variations similar to ours (13 to 67 minarc horizontally and 8 to 20 minarc vertically).[13] They attributed the vertical variation to crosstalk from the horizontal CN. Based on their finding of a correlation between the variations in the horizontal and vertical meridians in both idiopaths and albinos, they correctly concluded that CN is a *motor* and not a *sensory* disorder in *both* populations (see previous volumes for discussions of this issue). They further concluded that subjects with nystagmus might also exhibit *normal* ocular motor behavior under certain conditions; smooth pursuit or the vestibuloocular reflex (VOR) perhaps?

The accuracy, repeatability, and duration of the foveation periods are the most critical features of CN waveforms' effect on visual acuity. As a result of our studies of the dynamics of the foveation periods in CN, I developed a nystagmus foveation function (NFF) that should function as a sensitive indicator of the gaze angle of best acuity in an individual and a means of correlating waveform characteristics and acuity between subjects, something that CN intensity cannot do. This function is formed by the quotient of the product of foveation period per cycle and CN frequency in the numerator and the product of the standard deviations of the mean foveation-period position and velocity in the denominator. Preliminary data for one subject have demonstrated the direct relation between the value of the NFF and the gaze and convergence angles of best acuity. For a discussion of the importance of the foveation periods and the suppression of OSOP, see the section on oscillopsia in this chapter.

Abadi and Worfolk studied the relationship between visual acuity and the duration of low velocity in CN slow phases.[14] They found a significant correlation between the duration of slow-phase velocities below 10 degree/sec and acuity. Although this was a somewhat cruder measure of the foveation periods, it does illustrate their importance in acuity. This paper contains velocity histograms of various waveforms and their effect on good foveation. Other researchers also found a correlation between acuity and foveation-period duration[15] or variability.[13] As expected, this latter study did not find a correlation in albinos, whose acuity is limited by afferent defects. One study of acuity and several waveform variables did not find a correlation between patients.[16] This does not mean that correlations do not exist in specific individuals; experience has proven that damping CN and increasing foveation-period duration *will* improve acuity if it is not limited by afferent defects. The reason for the variability in the results of these studies is probably due to the intercorrelations of several variables and it is for this reason that the

NFF described earlier should yield better results. The NFF contains *all* the motor variables relevant to acuity. A study on the use of telescopic aids for low-vision patients (with and without nystagmus) showed that head motion was an important factor in preserving the stable retinal images necessary for good acuity.[17]

We studied the foveation periods of an individual with CN during smooth pursuit and VOR and demonstrated near unity gains for both over target velocities ranging from a few degrees per second to 215 degrees/sec and for rotations in the normal range.[18] We also demonstrated, using phase-plane analysis, that both smooth pursuit and VOR were normal during foveation periods. By subtracting the target position and velocity from those of the eye, we reconstructed the retinal error phase planes during pursuit and VOR and showed them to virtually duplicate the phase plane of eye movement during fixation of a stationary target. Thus, by two unrelated methods, we proved that these subsystems were *normal* in CN and that hypotheses or models claiming deficits in either of them as the cause of CN were invalid.

In a study of smooth pursuit, VOR, and optokinetic nystagmus (OKN) in individuals with CN, Kurzan and Büttner confirmed the hypothesis that the measured waveforms are caused by a shift in the static neutral zone to a new position (the dynamic neutral zone).[19] In agreement with our observations, they found that even low stimulus velocities cause large shifts in the neutral zone and higher velocities caused an increased shift. They also confirmed that this shift has no measurable latency. Given their verification of the neutral-zone shift, they concluded that smooth pursuit was *normal* and that retinal slip velocity is adequately utilized for the generation of smooth pursuit eye movements in individuals with CN. Lueck et al. studied a patient who presented with episodes of OSOP with smooth pursuit and OKN responses that exhibited nystagmus slow phases in the direction opposite to the stimulus.[20] Several different mechanisms for the etiology of this nystagmus were discussed; in my opinion, this was a rare form of CN that is related to those previously reported by Rosenberg et al. and discussed in the last volume.[21] This patient exhibited a jerk left CN in far left gaze and when tracking from the right to the left. Thus, his neutral zone, which was in left gaze when fixating stationary targets, shifted to the right so that the jerk left CN was superimposed on leftward pursuit movements. This case is the missing link between normal CN (where the nystagmus is present while viewing stationary targets and the neutral zone can easily be seen to shift during pursuit) and those cases previously recorded (where there was no nystagmus during fixation of stationary targets and a shift in neutral zone with pursuit caused the nystagmus to become manifest). The pursuit-induced neutral zone shift was the explanation I offered for the mechanism involved in producing the CN in the two patients previously reported and that explanation is supported by this more recent patient. In a study of smooth pursuit in several cases of hereditary CN, Takahashi demonstrated smooth pursuit during the foveation periods in his subjects.[22] The finding that there was a distinct difference in the CN of the male subjects from that of the female subjects during pursuit has neither been reported before nor noted in our data.

Finding an animal model for CN has proved to be an elusive goal. Tusa et al. described the strabismus and nystagmus found in monkeys due to early visual deprivations.[23] They studied three rhesus and three cynomolgus monkeys who had monocular eyelid suture within 24 hours of birth and reverse suture at age 25 days that was continued for another 25 days. At 50 days of age, when both eyelids were opened, the monkeys had 20 to 30 diopters of exotropia and nystagmus that persisted for the duration of the study (1 year). The cynomolgus monkeys developed a monocular 8 to 10 Hz pendular nystagmus in the eye sutured first; the rhesus monkeys developed a conjugate nystagmus with both jerk and pendular components. The slow phases often had increasing velocity profiles, and the rhesus monkeys had a superimposed latent component on the nystagmus. Certain characteristics of the nystagmus corresponded to human CN, others did not, and the difference in the two species of monkeys is troublesome. There are apparently species differences in the types of nystagmus that result from visual deprivation and extending this model to humans is difficult. More study of the nystagmus induced in these monkeys is required before some of these findings might be useful in understanding the mechanisms involved in CN in humans where visual deprivation is not the primary cause.

I have hypothesized that there are basically two oscillations that are the foundations for all of the CN waveforms: pendular and an increasing-velocity slow phase jerk nystagmus. The variations found in the waveforms described are a result of the individual's fixation subsystem attempting to maintain target foveation for as long as possible before the slow phase causes the eyes to accelerate away from the target. Thus, the foveation periods are created. A recent study of the evolution of CN waveforms in infants supports this hypothesis.[24] The authors found that CN often starts with a large triangular waveform at 1 to 4 months of age and evolves into a smaller amplitude, higher frequency pendular waveform that subsequently might give way to a jerk waveform by 7 months to 1½ years of age. Unfortunately, the low bandwidth of the electro-oculographic (EOG) signals may have prevented identification of small foveating or braking saccades. Despite this, the figures do indicate the possible presence of these small saccades in even the earliest waveforms. The time course of the waveform evolution was found to parallel that of the sensitive period of visual development. Thus, the attempt to see would develop and increase the nystagmus frequency along with foveation periods. After 6 months of age, the triangular waveforms are virtually nonexistent (in agreement with adult data) and replaced by pendular or jerk waveforms. The authors attributed this to the development of fusional convergence.

Also addressed in this paper was the issue of the name, "congenital," in CN. It is well recognized that many cases of CN do not appear until the first weeks or months of life although it must be remembered that several have been documented *at birth*. Eye movement recordings have shown that there are many forms of nystagmus present in infancy, so-called "infantile nystagmus." CN is one form of infantile nystagmus but so are latent/manifest latent nystagmus (LMLN), spasmus nutans, and others. Therefore, it would increase confusion to rename CN, a specific type of nystagmus, with the general description "infantile nystagmus." Neither the literal translation of CN nor the exact moment that CN appears is important here; what is important in differentiating CN from the other forms of infantile nystagmus. The argument that the term "congenital" is inappropriate has also been raised in describing congenital esotropia.[25] Actually, Gresty et al. documented six patients in whom CN emerged in later life.[26] The age of onset in these patients ranged from 12 to 30 years, and the nystagmus was proven to be CN by recordings. These patients make accurate ocular motility recordings indispensable in the diagnosis of nystagmus. They exhibited the null shift with pursuit and OKN that is a characteristic of CN. One of the subjects had a brother with CN, making his a hereditary CN that appeared late in life. The presence of foveation periods in these late-onset CN waveforms proves that the ability to suppress an acceleration of the eyes off target is part of our normal ocular motor arsenal and not something developed in early life by those with CN.

Several papers have appeared that emphasize the associated sensory defects found in individuals with CN.[27–29] Some have stressed the high percentage of patients with CN and these defects, but this may reflect the authors' patient population more than the CN population in general. Whatever the numbers, two things are clear: (1) physicians do have to look for any sensory defects that may be present in an individual with CN and treat them; (2) no matter what the sensory defects are, the CN is still a *motor* instability and it remains erroneous to classify CN as consisting of sensory and motor subtypes or to state that CN is a disorder indicative of "a primary disturbance of the ocular motor or visual sensory systems," the primary disturbance responsible for CN is in the ocular *motor* system.

In some families, CN is hereditary, as can be seen by its presence in more than one member. However, when information about other members of the family is unavailable or if the individual with CN is the only known member of the family to have this disorder, one still cannot rule out heredity as a mode of transmission. Shallo-Hoffmann et al. studied the eye movements of family members of subjects with CN.[30] In each of five families, abnormalities of seemingly nonaffected members were demonstrated; in four, saccadic instabilities were found and in the fifth, a CN waveform. Increased frequency of square-wave jerks (SWJ) and square-wave oscillations (SWO) were seen in family members. This is a curious finding since CN is due to a SEM instability, not saccadic. Neither the reason why unaffected family members would demonstrate saccadic instabilities nor the relationship of such instabilities to CN is clear. The results of this study suggest that, in isolated cases of CN, the presence of saccadic instabilities in family members might be indicative of hereditary CN. Hereditary vertical pendular CN was documented in two sisters.[31] Nystagmus has been reported with many other hereditary conditions, but these reports usually do not contain accurate eye movement records and preclude the identification of the nystagmus as CN.[32–38] In one report of three patients with congenital absence of conjugate horizontal eye movements and nystagmus, recordings did show a pendular nystagmus in two of the three.[39]

One area that has received much attention and is the result of some confused ideas about the etiology of CN is the subject of individuals with albinism. Most, but not all, albinos also have CN. Apkarian et al. showed that *all* albinos exhibit asymmetry in the monocular visual evoked potential (VEP).[40] However, not all albinos demonstrate nystagmus and therefore the link between aberrant projections and organization of the ocular motor system in non-albinos with CN is in question. They found no crossed projections in a non-albino with nystagmus. Apkarian et al. devised a decisive test for human albinism and reported a case of albinism with LMLN.[41] Apkarian and Spekreijse also reported another non-albino with nystagmus who had no crossed fibers.[42] In fact, Apkarian has tested at least 14 patients with CN and has found *none* with optic pathway misrouting (personal communication, 1990). In a study of 18 albinos, 5 of whom had no noticeable nystagmus, all showed global stereopsis.[43] These findings are interesting when contrasted with the investigations in albino animal models where a paucity of binocularly driven cortical neurons is found in visual areas 17, 18, and 19. Other studies have also verified that albinos demonstrate VEP asymmetries whereas those with idiopathic CN do not.[44, 45] Thus, since electrophysiologic evidence has proven that individuals with CN do *not* have crossed fibers, hypotheses and models that rely on crossed fibers and "reversed" pursuit have no basis in fact.

Rosenberg and Jabbari suggested that a horizontal grating stimulus might be used where the conventional check stimulus for VEP produces poor results due to horizontal nystagmus. In a paper on the recognition and management of albinism, Abadi and Pascal described twin girls who had similar CN waveforms but whose fast phases were in opposite directions. In this paper, the authors stated that all forms of albinism are characterized by nystagmus; this appears to be in contradiction to the studies mentioned earlier. As a final note on albinism and CN, it has been suggested that although acuity is primarily limited in albinism by retinal factors, reducing the CN can lead to an improvement.[46]

We are beginning studies of the effects of afferent (cutaneous) stimulation of the ophthalmic division of the trigeminal nerve on CN, based on our observations of the effects of contact lenses.[47] Our preliminary results show this to be a robust response.[48] We documented 50% decreases in CN amplitude with pressure, vibration, or electrical stimulation. We hypothesized that the afferent stimulation was affecting the proprioceptive calibration of the extraocular muscles since these fibers travel in the trigeminal nerve. These results infer that there is a strong effect on eye movement by changing the proprioceptive bias to the extraocular muscles despite the absence of a classical stretch reflex.

Hatayama et al. examined several patients with and without base-out prisms.[49] Unfortunately, they used bitemporal EOG to record the eye movements. Four of the five patients showed a damping of the CN waveform during fixation in primary position. However, only three of the five showed an increase in acuity and one of the three was the patient in whom no damping of the CN was seen. The use of base-out prisms will usually damp CN and, more importantly, increase foveation time. However, to improve acuity, -1.00 spheres must be added to the refraction of pre-presbyopic patients to negate the effect of the accommodation accompanying the prism-induced convergence. It was not clear if this spherical correction was added to the refraction of these patients. I would anticipate that, had this been done, the acuity would have increased in more of the patients. For those interested in accurate head posture measurement with minimal artifact, an apparatus has recently been described.[50] It is my opinion that head posture is not a good way to measure CN gaze-angle nulls preoperatively or postoperatively. There is too much error that can be introduced by the subject. It is best to fix the head and measure the CN at known gaze angles.

Castanera studied the length-tension diagrams of the medial rectus muscle after the Faden operation.[51] He compared two techniques and found that primary length and spring constant were unchanged with a bridge suture technique whereas a marked stiffening appeared with the original technique. It would be interesting to know which of these techniques results in the greater damping of CN. Sendler et al. described the results of 26 patients with CN who underwent the artificial divergence operation.[52] Seventeen patients showed significant improvement after the procedure; in three, the procedure had to be combined with the Kestenbaum procedure, and in 6 patients where the affect of artificial divergence (tested with a base-out prism) did not damp the nystagmus, the Kestenbaum procedure was used. All patients had good binocular function. This study suggests that artificial divergence alone or in combination with other procedures may have a significant damping effect on CN. In support of this, our recordings have shown that, in patients where both convergence and gaze angle induce nulls, the convergence null is almost always a better one. In a study in rhesus monkeys, Gamlin et al. found that there was some degree of co-contraction of the lateral and medial rectus muscles during convergence eye movements.[53] This finding may be the mechanism by which CN is damped during convergence, the co-contraction of the lateral and medial muscles would render them less susceptible to the signal driving the CN. Some CN patients exhibit a vertical or torsional head posture and there is very little in the literature concerning management strategies. A recent survey sent to members of the American Association for Pediatric Ophthalmology and Strabismus found that when surgery is indicated, a graded bilateral vertical rectus recession or combined vertical rectus recession-resection procedures are usually done.[54] Since most respondents saw no cases of torsional head postures, no procedure was advocated.

Biofeedback has been advocated as a possible treatment in CN. Mezawa et al. studied the changes in CN waveform associated with biofeedback.[55] They found that their subjects were able to voluntarily damp the CN (intensity decreased by 50%) and prolong the foveation time (increased by 180%). However, after completion of the training, no clear improvement in acuity was seen, although all subjects reported a subjective improvement in their vision when suppressing their nystagmus. A key to the effectiveness of this training appears to be in the answer to the question, can they suppress while attempting an acuity test? If suppression is only possible under certain conditions and these preclude real-life situations, biofeedback, although interesting, may not prove to be a practical therapy. The value of electroretinography (ERG) in the evaluation of children with early onset nystagmus was recently examined.[56] The incidence of congenital achromatopsia in a group of otherwise undiagnosed children was 29%, with 40% being classified as having idiopathic CN. The authors concluded that there was a need to use ERG in children when the diagnosis was uncertain.

Since the last volume, in which I reviewed a paper from a group who used bitemporal, alternating current-coupled EOG to take their data, several papers have appeared from this group using the same method.[57–60] These papers contain fairly sophisticated analyses of poorly taken data and it is very difficult to separate out what can truly be inferred from their analyses and what is artifact. Specifically, the power spectra of various CN waveforms shown in these papers are *not* the complete spectra of these waveforms but only of their overly filtered data. Thus, the large amount of power in the range from direct current to 1 Hz is missing. This is *the most important* area of the waveform since it is produced by the foveation periods that we know are intimately related to acuity and the suppression of OSOP. Some of the correct descriptions of CN found in these papers (based on the work of others) are the result of high-bandwidth, direct current-coupled measurement techniques that could not have been discovered with their method. Therefore, it is disturbing to find statements denigrating both accurate descriptive analyses of CN waveforms and neurophysiologically based models in papers whose foundations are based on that knowledge. Despite many misstatements, these papers contain information that could, if properly interpreted, be useful. Unfortunately, it takes someone familiar with both areas (CN and spectral analysis) to be able to separate the good from the bad. I would strongly urge these workers to change their methods of recording eye movements to provide good input data for any future work if they hope to make meaningful contributions.

In one of their papers,[58] they correctly concluded that the model of Optican and Zee, that produced pendular waveforms from the same basic instability that caused the jerk waveforms, was incorrect. This was already known, based on observations of many patients and the independence shown between the two waveforms in those patients that had both; we concluded years ago that the pendular and jerk waveforms were independently caused. Their reasoning for the suggestion that the pendular CN waveform differs from that found in the dual jerk waveform is not supported by the many cases where the jerk waveform is variably present but the pendular waveform remains (this is also seen with convergence). Because of the differences in methods and the inability of their recording techniques to separate CN from LMLN, their two papers on the evaluation of surgery[59, 60] are almost impossible to compare to previous work; some of their confusing findings are due, in my opinion, to their poor input data.

Much praise is given to the importance of spectral analysis in these papers, but I found nothing new or that could not be easily predicted by anyone knowledgeable about frequency-domain analysis. We have looked at the total spectra (direct current to 100 Hz) of CN waveforms in the past and they merely confirmed what we expected based on simple observation of the waveforms. All analysis methods have something to add to our understanding, but none give all the answers; the total reliance by these authors on spectral analysis is misplaced and their expectation that better models will arise from that approach rather than from models closely tied to known neurophysiology ignores the early history of bioengineering modeling.

Convergence Nystagmus

A case of convergence nystagmus associated with an Arnold-Chiari type 1 malformation was presented. The nystagmus appeared in the absence of fixation and was provoked during the Valsalva maneuver and neck flexion and extension as well as being attenuated on deep inspiration.[61] The authors postulated that this nystagmus was due to a combination of mechanical distortion and abnormal transmission of cerebrospinal fluid pressure to the aqueductal region. The figures shown in the paper were of a pendular convergence nystagmus that could be quite asymmetric between the eyes.

Convergence nystagmus at approximately 1 Hz has been described in several cases of Whipple's disease.[62] The authors suggested that the nystagmus be called "pendular vergence oscillations," but since this eye sign is convergence nystagmus by defintion, there is no compelling reason for the less specific term "oscillations." The association of this convergence nystagmus with discharge of the masticatory muscles has given rise to the vague term "oculo-masticatory myorhythmia." Perhaps the best compromise here would be, "oculo-masticatory convergence nystagmus" to identify the oscillation as a nystagmus and use the prefix to indicate a connection with masticatory discharges.

Convergence-Evoked Nystagmus

Two cases of convergence-evoked nystagmus were reported to have occurred in spasmus nutans.[63] The compressed time base of the recordings shown in the paper make it difficult to determine if the nystagmus was truly disconjugate as has been reported for spasmus nutans.[64] The case description refers to the nystagmus as pendular and conjugate which would be more indicative of CN than spasmus nutans. Despite the clinical description, the two figures appear to show disconjugate nystagmus in each case. Oliva and Rosenberg presented a review of 17 patients with acquired convergence-evoked nystagmus.[65] Cases showing both vertical and horizontal nystagmus were included. A wide variety of neurologic diagnoses and other findings were included for each patient; some of these findings were not related to the nystagmus.

Dissociated Nystagmus

A peculiar form of dissociated nystagmus (divergence nystagmus) was reported with congenital adduction palsy and synergistic divergence.[66] On attempted adduction, the affected eye moved into an abducted position causing extreme divergence and simultaneous divergence nystagmus resulted. This was a jerk nystagmus with the fast phases beating temporally in both eyes. Attempted right gaze caused the affected left eye to go further to the left and optokinetic and vestibular inputs resulted in an inverse nystagmus of the affected left eye. The authors concluded that, similar to Duane's retraction syndrome, this developmental anomaly was characterized by absence of the abducens nucleus and subsequent innervation of the lateral rectus muscle by the inferior branch of the oculomotor nerve. In addition to the nystagmus, flutter was observed during intense fixation.

A dissociated nystagmus was also reported as a common sign in patients with human immunodeficiency virus (HIV).[67] Here, it was thought that the medial longitudinal fasciculus was affected and the nystagmus was indicative of the development of internuclear ophthalmoplegia (INO). If that was the case, then these oscillations were saccadic pulse trains and not nystagmus. The tracings shown resemble the so-called abduction "nystagmus" of INO; rebound nystagmus and gaze-evoked nystagmus were also seen in these patients.

Downbeat Nystagmus

Downbeat nystagmus that appeared during eye closure was reported in two patients with dizzy spells.[68] The nystagmus only appeared when the eyeballs were depressed to the midline position during eye closure. Since there were no other remarkable neurologic findings, the nystagmus was probably related to the vestibular symptoms. Weissman et al. reported downbeat nystagmus in an infant that resolved within the first year of life.[69] The nystagmus was observed by 6 weeks of age and the patient preferred to keep her head in a chin-down position. The slow phases of the nystagmus were predominantly of constant velocity, and it was suggested that the nystagmus was caused by an immaturity of central connections associated with the vertical canal pathways. Recent reports have also linked downbeat nystagmus with dolichoectasia of the vertebrobasilar artery,[70] multiple sclerosis,[71] occult breast carcinoma,[72] and alternating skew on lateral gaze (bilateral abducting hypertropia).[73] An EOG study of downbeat nystagmus has documented some of the uncommon features that may be encountered.[74] The use of alternating current–coupled EOG confounds the slow phases, although the time constant of 10 seconds is long enough to distinguish increasing velocity exponential slow phases from linear; one case did have the former. Pursuit, optokinetic, and vestibular responses were obtained and correctly interpreted as being confounded by the presence of the spontaneous nystagmus rather than being defective and the cause of the nystagmus, as has been the misinterpretation applied to other forms of spontaneous nystagmus when tested under these conditions. Possible mechanisms responsible for downbeat nystagmus were reviewed, but no conclusion was reached because of the variable nature of the downbeat nystagmus in these patients.

Drug-Induced Nystagmus

A review article by Abel and Hertle documented the effects of psychoactive drugs on ocular motor behavior.[75] The authors grouped the drugs in seven categories based on their primary functional effects. Two papers reported downbeat nystagmus induced by ingestion of lithium.[76, 77] Williams et al. studied two patients in whom lithium was administered for psychiatric illness. Several months after stopping the lithium, one patient showed a resolution of his nystagmus but the second did not. They concluded that several months of abstinence may be necessary for improvement. Halmagyi et al. studied 12 patients in whom lithium was administered. Of the six that were able to reduce or stop taking lithium, only two showed a resolution or improvement of the downbeat nystagmus. Some patients from both studies also showed gaze-evoked horizontal nystagmus in addition to the downbeat nystagmus.

Bow tie nystagmus is a drug-induced oscillation consisting of upbeat nystagmus combined with alternating horizontal saccades that are synchronized with the vertical fast phases. The resulting two-dimensional motion traces a bow tie, hence the name. The authors who first recorded bow tie nystagmus after their subject smoked tobacco have isolated the cause to the nicotine and suggested that perhaps "nicotine" nystagmus might be a better name than their original term, "bow tie."[78] I prefer bow tie for two reasons: (1) there are many drugs that induce nystagmus and creating a new name for each would unnecessarily add to an already large collection of terms; (2) bow tie describes the nystagmus correctly without linking it to any of the many possible drugs that might produce the same nystagmus. As I have urged in these chapters, new names should be descriptive of either the oscillation or, where known, the neurophysiologic mechanism.

Epileptic Nystagmus

A combination of vertical and horizontal gaze deviation and nystagmus associated with epilepsy was reported in a comatose patient with a left hemisphere subdural hematoma.[79] The vertical eye deviation and nystagmus are unusual since seizure activity usually causes a contralateral eye deviation in nystagmus. We now have the second and third accurate recordings of the epileptic nystagmus in the literature. In one, the slow phase component was found to be linear,[80] and in the other, the slow phases were both linear and of decreasing velocity.[81] These are in contrast to the first recorded case of epileptic nystagmus where a gaze-evoked, decreasing velocity slow phase was found.

Gaze-Evoked Nystagmus

Gaze-evoked nystagmus (GEN) is a jerk nystagmus, not present in primary position, elicited by attempted maintenance of eccentric eye position. GEN may have a linear or a decreasing-velocity exponential slow phase; the latter has sometimes been referred to as gaze-paretic nystagmus but, unless it is due to a nerve (gaze-paretic) or muscle (muscle-paretic) paresis, the GEN terminology is preferred. Distinction should be made between nystagmus that is truly gaze-evoked and that which is gaze-modulated. Many types of nystagmus vary with gaze angle but are present in primary position and are not GEN. Gaze-modulated nystagmus is a jerk nystagmus, present in primary position, that is increased by lateral gaze. The slow phases may be linear, decreasing-velocity or increasing-velocity exponentials. Examples of gaze-modulated nystagmus are vestibular nystagmus (VN), LMLN, and CN. Both VN and LMLN vary in intensity with gaze angle according to Alexander's law; the nystagmus increases as gaze is directed in the direction of the fast phases. CN increases as gaze is directed away from the null and, if the null is near primary position, CN may be mistaken for GEN (especially in the absence of a patient history or in a case of head trauma seen in the emergency room). These types of nystagmus increase with lateral gaze but, since their genesis is not due to gaze off primary position, they are not types of GEN. There is overlap between GEN and gaze-modulated nystagmus. Nystagmus that is modulated according to Alexander's law may be classified type I, II, or III, depending on the field of gaze in which the nystagmus first appears. Thus, a type I nystagmus (appearing only in lateral gaze) may easily be mistaken for GEN. There are both normal and pathologic types of GEN as well as of gaze-modulated nystagmus. The normal types of GEN are physiologic (end-point) nystagmus and rebound/centripetal nystagmus; the normal type of gaze-modulated nystagmus is induced VN. The pathologic types of GEN are those due to drugs or alcohol gaze nystagmus, gaze-paretic or muscle-paretic nystagmus, rebound/centripetal nystagmus, and Brun's nystagmus; pathologic types of gaze-modulated nystagmus are alcohol position nystagmus, periodic alternating nystagmus, LMLN, and CN.

Medulloblastoma has been linked with GEN and upbeat nystagmus[82] and both horizontal and vertical GEN were found in familial paroxysmal ataxia.[83] In a study of three patients with central nervous system (CNS) lesions and markedly decreased time constants of the VOR, GEN was also found.[84]

Induced Nystagmus

Information about diurnal variations of induced nystagmus in healthy and sick subjects has now been collected.[85] The authors demonstrated circadian rhythms of vestibular responses, and in some variables, significant differences were found between healthy and sick subjects.

Latent/Manifest Latent Nystagmus

In an exhaustive study of smooth pursuit and the optokinetic response (OKR) in LMLN, Dickinson and Abadi came to the following conclusions: (1) both pursuit and OKR could be symmetric in LMLN for both binocular and monocular viewing; (2) the asymmetric patterns of response often reported in LMLN result from either shifts in the zone of minimum intensity oscillation or from nonstimulus-specific increases in the LMLN.[86] Their careful work revealed that, when properly evaluated, there is no nasal-to-temporal (N-T) asymmetry in the smooth pursuit of subjects with LMLN and therefore, the hypothesis that an N-T smooth pursuit asymmetry is the *cause* of LMLN is invalid. As with CN, conventional measures of slow-phase velocity do not reveal the true performance of either pursuit or the OKR and the apparent asymmetries recorded are, in fact, merely reflections of the spontaneous LMLN oscillation and *cannot* be causative factors in the genesis of this condition. In another study on the N-T asymmetries of pursuit in strabismic amblyopes, correction for the mean velocity of the slow phases eliminated the observed asymmetry in the nonamblyopic eyes.[87] Although the authors of this study never mentioned that their subjects had LMLN, their description of the eye movements made it clear that they did. Thus, we have two studies that yielded the same conclusions: there is no N-T asymmetry in the smooth pursuit or OKR of subjects with LMLN.

Leigh et al. found that one of four patients with monocular loss of vision exhibited LMLN.[88] In addition, upbeat nystagmus was measured; gaze-evoked nystagmus was not found in these patients. In a patient with bilateral congenital blindness, they found nystagmus with horizontal and vertical components and a wandering null point; they attributed this to an abnormal neural integrator. Steinbach et al. studied spatial localization monocularly in each eye of eight patients undergoing unilateral strabismus surgery.[89] In most cases, they found that the changes in spatial localization produced by the surgery on the operated eye paralleled those found in the other eye both in magnitude and duration. Thus, unilateral surgery was found to have central effects on egocentric localization. Since the surgery forced a recalibration of one eye's position (the operated eye), a change was forced on the calibration for localization even in the unoperated eye. From this study, we can infer that the strabismus that *always* accompanies LMLN might also cause a change in the calibration necessary for spatial localization and therefore result in a shift in central egocentric localization. This paper, as well as others I have reviewed in previous volumes, provide strong support for the hypothesis that LMLN is the direct result of a shift in egocentric localization and not of asymmetry in any of the ocular motor subsystems.

Zubcov et al. studied four patients with dissociated horizontal deviation.[90] All had amblyopia and asymmetric MLN and used convergence to reduce their nystagmus when viewing with the eye having the more severe nystagmus. They concluded that an asymmetric nystagmus blockage syndrome can be found in MLN. By comparing the clinical descriptions of each patient with the nystagmus shown in eye movement recordings, the authors also reemphasized that clinical observation alone is often inadequate and ocular motor recordings are necessary for accurate diagnosis. Their findings also confirm that it is the angle of convergence and not accommodation that is related to the amplitude of MLN (also of CN).

In a study of VEP in patients with early monocular loss of vision, jerk nystagmus in the sound eye was found in 7 of 16 patients.[91] Since no ocular motor recordings were made, LMLN could not be verified. In a retrospective review of the charts of 119 children with infantile esotropia, it was found that 14 (12%) also had high-frequency, low-amplitude torsional nystagmus.[92] Ten of the 14 were said to also have MLN superimposed on the torsional nystagmus and the relatively larger MLN masked the underlying torsional nystagmus. The occurrence of torsional nystagmus in association with LMLN is not uncommon and has been reported by several authors. A recent study of LMLN in infantile esotropia misidentified the nystagmus as "abduction nystagmus."[93] The author recognized LN upon occlusion but failed to realize that what was seen in lateral gaze was the Alexander's law increase of MLN.

The effects of both surgical and optical treatment on eight cases of LMLN have revealed that MLN may be converted to LN as a result of the treatment.[94] Five of the patients had their tropia corrected surgically, and their visual acuity improved as a result of this conversion. Of the three patients who received optical treatment, in one the MLN converted to LN with improved vision and in the other two the MLN decreased in intensity and the acuity of one of these patients improved. It thus appears that surgical or optical alignment of eyes can decrease the intensity of MLN and improve binocular visual acuity. Several of these patients had both CN and MLN. The authors concluded that there was a close relationship between the level of visual acuity and the intensity of MLN. In one case, although there was MLN, the patient appeared clinically not to have any strabismus. The authors allowed for the possibility that this patient did have a small-angle tropia that was not detected because of the high amplitude of the MLN. In previous volumes, I have discussed how small tropias can be detected by properly calibrating each eye individually (while the other eye is behind cover) so that when the cover is removed, small tropias in the non-fixating eye can be easily measured.

Simonsz reported on the effect of prolonged monocular occlusion on LN in the treatment of amblyopia.[95] Whereas before occlusion the slow-phase velocity was lower when the better eye fixated, after occlusion it was lower when the worse eye fixated. He concluded that occlusion of the better eye in children with amblyopia and LN should be prescribed in days per week not in hours per day.

Optokinetic Nystagmus

Howard and Simpson developed a procedure by which OKN gain could be measured as a function of the binocular disparity of the stimulus to test the hypothesis that a linkage exists in higher mammals between the optokinetic system and the stereoscopic system.[96] They found that the gain of OKN was inversely proportional to binocular disparity. This supported their previous hypothesis that the main reason for the evolution of a cortical component to OKN is to allow animals with foveate eyes and stereoscopic vision to deal with complex motion signals that are generated by linear motion through a three-dimensional world. Another interesting finding about OKN is that it can exhibit the same predictive behavior that is known to occur in smooth pursuit.[97] Thus, the "primitive" OKN subsystem may actually be intimately linked with the "higher" pursuit subsystem; they may even both be part of one SEM subsystem responding to different inputs. It has long been my opinion[98] that there is only one SEM control subsystem and that the subsystems exhibited in models (including my own) for smooth pursuit, OKR, or VOR merely reflect the mathematical differences in signal processing of the various inputs to this unitary motor subsystem.

In another study of OKN in monkeys, it was found that although they tried to suppress OKN movements, the monkeys exhibited slow movements of low amplitude directed oppositely to the moving OKN stimulus while they were fixing a stationary object.[99] These SEM were apparently induced by a perceived motion of the stationary target in a direction opposite to the moving OKN background. When they exhibited optokinetic after-nystagmus (OKAN), it was always determined by the actual background motion and not by the perceived target motion.

Several papers investigated direction asymmetries of OKN. Van den Berg and Collewijn found no evidence for asymmetry in the horizontal direction but a clear preference for upward stimulus motion.[100] They found the decrease in OKN gain as a function of stimulus velocity was steeper for vertical than horizontal motion, and the eyes were nearly perfectly yoked for vertical OKN but not during horizontal OKN. Tracking in the nasal direction had a higher gain (by about 4%) than in the temporal direction. This difference was attributed to motor rather than sensory origin. The finding of a vertical OKN asymmetry in man is in disagreement with past reports where it was found not to be significant but in agreement with findings of vertical OKN asymmetries in rhesus monkeys, squirrel monkeys, and cats. In squirrel monkeys, the vertical OKN asymmetry was increased after bilateral sacculectomy.[101] It was also found that the asymmetry of vertical OKAN is more dominant than of OKN.

Vestibular habituation in the squirrel monkey also affects OKN.[102] Repeated clockwise vestibular stimulations caused an increase of counterclockwise OKN responses. It had been previously thought that prolonged OKN stimulus affected VOR gain but the reverse was not true; in these experiments, OKN responses were not affected for the first 5 days but thereafter there were clear and repeatable increases. Since the OKN response was back to baseline by the time of the next day's test, the authors concluded there was either no or a short-term storage.

In a study of the characteristics of saccades, the fast phases of OKN were found to be as fast as "foveating" saccades.[103] This term, introduced to distinguish foveating from braking saccades in CN waveforms, has now been extended to normal saccades that achieve target foveation.

Periodic/Aperiodic Alternating Nystagmus

An interesting case of intermittent unidirectional nystagmus that might be related to periodic alternating nystagmus (PAN) was recently described.[104] It consisted of an intermittent jerk right nystagmus occurring every 45 to 90 minutes and lasting 20 to 40 seconds; during this nystagmus, OSOP was perceived. At other times, no nystagmus could be elicited and the patient's neurologic examination was normal. The amplitude of the nystagmus followed a sinusoidal time course. The authors speculated that the nystagmus might represent dormant PAN or another type of dormant nystagmus appearing intermittently due to episodic migrainous brain stem ischemia. One paper claimed to demonstrate an alternating nystagmus appearing with infectious mononucleosis.[105] Unfortunately, the figure shown had no identification of the zero position for either eye and the methods did not describe whether the EOG signal was alternating current- or direct current-coupled, nor was the bandwidth of the system given. The only thing evident from the figure was that there was a conjugate oscillation that had both fast and slow phases. The figure did not demonstrate which of the two phases was the initiating phase and therefore we cannot determine whether this was nystagmus or saccadic pulse trains.

The effects of baclofen on PAN in both monkey and man raises the question of whether its beneficial effect lasts while the drug is continued.[106] In a 1-year study of the effects of baclofen in a patient with PAN, it was found that, although initially the PAN was abolished, continued treatment resulted in only a partial suppression. The authors concluded that baclofen does not seem to be a real therapeutic drug for PAN. The figures in this paper suffer from the same deficiencies found in the previous paper. PAN has recently been associated with administration of primidone/phenobarbital.[107] With withdrawal and discontinuation of these medications, the cycle length, velocity, and magnitude of the PAN diminished and then disappeared. Periodic alternating (ping-pong) gaze has been reportedly induced by deliberate overdose of tranylcypromine.[108] This condition resolved spontaneously, leaving no lasting impairment. This is the first report of ping-pong gaze resulting from drug therapy or toxicity.

Physiologic Nystagmus

Eizenman et al. recently published the results of a study of the three types of physiologic (end-point) nystagmus: (1) sustained; (2) unsustained; and (3) fatigue.[109] They found that the onset of end-point point nystagmus is determined by the velocity of the slow-phase drift and investigated the factors affecting drift velocity: target eccentricity, visual feedback, and fatigue. Visual feedback served to decrease drift velocity; mean drift velocity increased during the fixation period (the increase was more pronounced for larger fixation eccentricities), and mean drift velocity increased for larger fixation eccentricities. They found that when the drift velocity was less than 0.3 degrees/sec, no end-point nystagmus occurred. For drift velocities between 0.3 and 1 degree/sec, either sustained or unsustained end-point nystagmus was observed and for drift velocities above 1 degree/sec, either sustained or fatigue end-point nystagmus was apparent. The authors included the results of their study in an integrated model of ocular motor control that included saccadic, pursuit, and optokinetic subsystems. Their model demonstrated that the reduction in drift eye movement velocity during fixation of a visual target as compared to attempted fixation in the dark was mainly due to their smooth pursuit subsystem. Since the subject is not actually pursuing a moving target, it is more appropriate to describe the subsystem responsible for this reduction in drift velocity as part of the SEM subsystem that is operating during fixation rather than the part that is operating during smooth pursuit.

Pseudospontaneous Nystagmus

Blessing and Kommerell found that the small light sources of Frenzel's glasses can induce a Purkinje's figure on the retina and that this stabilized retinal figure may elicit an artificial pseudospontaneous nystagmus.[110] Since this might be mistaken for spontaneous vestibular nystagmus, they advocated the use of glasses that cannot induce a Purkinje's figure. They found that 22 of 55 normal subjects were able to produce pseudospontaneous nystagmus when instructed on how to induce a Purkinje's figure.

Rebound Nystagmus

Shallo-Hoffmann et al. recently studied both the characteristics of physiologic end-point nystagmus and rebound nystagmus.[111] With sustained lateral gaze of 40 degrees and 50 degrees, end-point nystagmus almost always appeared immediately and was sustained for 15 to 25 seconds. In five of their subjects who exhibited end-point nystagmus, they measured rebound nystagmus whose magnitude was always less than the end-point nystagmus and decayed over a 5- to 10-second time period. An important finding of this study was that rebound nystagmus can be evoked in healthy subjects even when a fixation target, in a fully lit room, is present; it had previously been thought that darkness was necessary for rebound nystagmus.

A new syndrome has been suggested based on three members of a family with motion sickness and rebound nystagmus.[112] The patients seemed to have a type I VN, saccadic pursuit, defective OKN slow phases and failure of VOR suppression. The authors suggested the name "familial vestibulocerebellar dysfunction."

See-Saw Nystagmus

Nakada and Kwee have analyzed the role of visuo-vestibular interaction in the pathogenesis of see-saw nystagmus.[113] They reviewed all known cases of see-saw nystagmus in the literature and concluded that see-saw nystagmus is an ocular oscillation brought about by an unstable visuo-vestibular interaction control system. They postulated that it was the nonavailability of retinal error signals to the inferior olivary nucleus, due to disruption of chiasmal crossing fibers, that caused the system instability. Although a model was not presented in this paper, a mathematical and control system analysis is available as a supplement by request.

Torsional Nystagmus

Morrow and Sharpe reported on three patients with lateral medullary syndrome who exhibited torsional nystagmus.[114] The slow phases of the torsional nystagmus included increasing, decreasing, and constant velocity. In addition, torsional pulsion of saccades was observed. The authors concluded that torsional nystagmus was due to an imbalance of central projections from the anterior and posterior semicircular canals and the otolith receptors. Unlike another report on torsional nystagmus published in the same year and reviewed in the last volume,[115] these authors chose to define torsional nystagmus from the point of view of the *observer* rather than the *subject*. Since all other eye movements are defined from the point of view of the subject and since such a definition makes interpretation of OSOP due to torsional, circular, or elliptical movements easier, I would urge that all future reports and recordings of these types of nystagmus adopt the Kestenbaum convention (i.e., from the point of view of *subject*). Thus, someone with a clockwise torsional slow phase (and counterclockwise quick phase) would experience a counterclockwise OSOP and presentation of a clockwise OKN stimulus would result in clockwise slow phases (counterclockwise fast phases) of OKN.

We reported a patient with a combination of torsional, see-saw, and bow tie nystagmus.[116] The patient had brain stem anomalies that appeared to have disturbed central vestibular pathways.

Uniocular Nystagmus

Pritchard et al. studied ten patients who had long-standing visual loss and monocular vertical oscillations.[117] These oscillations varied from 3 to 50 degrees with frequencies of 0.12 to 5 Hz.

The authors were particularly interested in the waveform characteristics of the vertical oscillations. Their recordings revealed that several subjects appeared to have two waveforms superimposed on, and interfering with, one another. In these patients a low-amplitude, high-frequency waveform was superimposed on a larger amplitude, low-frequency waveform. Since these were uniocular oscillations, they were probably not due to artifact. I agree with the authors that these phenomena deserve further study and suggest that perhaps another, more accurate method of recording eye movements might be used to study the interaction between the two frequencies.

Upbeat Nystagmus

Two recent papers investigated possible mechanisms responsible for upbeat nystagmus. Ranalli and Sharpe reviewed reports of upbeat nystagmus with pathologically verified lesions and concluded that upbeat nystagmus was due to bilateral damage to the ventral tegmental pathway (an upward VOR pathway) in pontomedullary disease.[118] Harada et al. investigated upbeat nystagmus in humans and cats.[119] They presented a case with a discrete vascular lesion in the lower dorsal brain stem involving the hypoglossal nucleus and adjacent structures and, in addition, they presented the results of experiments in cats where the floor of the fourth ventricle was destroyed electrolytically. From their data, they concluded that a prepositus hypoglossal lesion could result in a tonic imbalance for eye position and eye movements of the vertical axis and thereby cause upbeat nystagmus in both humans and cats. Traccis et al. described a rare case of upbeat nystagmus due to cerebellar astrocytoma.[120] Their patient developed upbeat nystagmus with increasing velocity slow phases. Surgical removal of the tumor resulted in a virtual disappearance of the upbeat nystagmus. Another report of upbeat nystagmus accompanied a focal hemorrhagic lesion of the left brachium conjunctivum, the anterior vermis, and the anterior superior left cerebellar hemisphere.[121] This nystagmus was suppressed by a contralateral head tilt, and the authors postulated that the nystagmus was inhibited by the otolith-ocular reflex.

Vertical Nystagmus

Baloh and Yee studied the records of 106 patients with spontaneous vertical nystagmus that had been evaluated over the past 10 years.[122] They found correlations between downbeat nystagmus and lesions involving the caudal midline cerebellum and with upbeat nystagmus and lesions of the central medulla. They concluded that, since the vestibular system is the main source of tonic input to the ocular motor neurons and since both the up and down VOR pathways separate beginning at the level of the vestibular nuclei, asymmetric involvement of these pathways could explain spontaneous vertical nystagmus. Thus, both upbeat and downbeat spontaneous nystagmus would, by their analysis, be types of central vestibular nystagmus resulting from an imbalance in central VOR pathways. They did not offer explanations for the changes in these types of nystagmus with lateral gaze or convergence.

Vestibular Nystagmus

An interesting study examined the effects of temperature on the magnitude of fixation suppression of the VOR.[123] Using both warm and cold caloric vestibular stimulation, the authors found that the warm media elicited more nystagmus and significantly less fixation suppression than the cool media. This effect worsened as a function of subject age. The authors concluded that separate normal upper limits for fixation and suppression need to be determined for different temperature caloric testing and age should be factored into these norms. A related study was of the test-retest repeatability of caloric responses.[124] Twenty-nine subjects were evaluated over a 6-month period and it was found that for any given subject, there was a reasonably reliable repeatability over time for testing of young and old subjects. Intersubject variability was greater in older subjects. In a study of the effects of linear acceleration, it was found that the induced L-nystagmus was modifiable.[125] Similar to the VN produced by rotation, L-nystagmus could be suppressed or augmented by appropriate visual or imaginary stimuli.

Brandt wrote an extensive review article on positional and positioning vertigo and nystagmus.[126] The review contains both theoretical mechanisms and clinical signs as well as management of many different types of positional and positioning nystagmus. It is well worth reading for the clinician who sees patients with vestibular symptoms. Positional vertigo is usually treated with various exercises meant to repeatedly elicit the vertigo.[127] Various maneuvers can be used to elicit vertigo, and this study found that since the specific maneuvers differed from patient to patient, prior testing of each patient is necessary before prescribing adequate exercises.

A recent paper reported vestibular symptoms arising from vascular compression of the eighth cranial nerve.[128] Magnetic resonance imaging documented a tortuous basilar artery compressing the eighth cranial nerve on the involved side. In another study, a review of 84 patients with vertigo resulted in a conclusion that the vestibular labyrinth is selectively vulnerable to ischemia within the vertebrobasilar system.[129] Positional vertigo also resulted from surgical trauma.[130] This patient developed vertigo due to trauma to the labyrinth during surgery for partial excision of the upper jaw for squamous carcinoma. Asymmetry in vestibular nystagmus was documented in congenital ocular motor apraxia.[131] Along with the asymmetry of VN was an asymmetric OKN. The neural and anatomical reasons for these asymmetries are not presently well understood. Head-shaking nystagmus was noted in 37 of 108 patients referred for caloric testing.[132] However, these authors found that head-shaking nystagmus and canal paresis were insensitive predictors of either hearing loss or of each other; they concluded that head-shaking nystagmus is not as powerful a test as canal paresis in detecting lesions of the eighth nerve.

Unilateral labyrinthectomy in six rhesus monkeys resulted in spontaneous VN where the slow phases could be increasing then decreasing in velocity.[133] The authors of this study concluded that peripheral vestibular lesions can alter the function of the ocular motor neural integrator. Labyrinthectomy also impaired the velocity-storage component of the OKN system. The initial reduction in the time constant of velocity storage only partially recovered. A model with bilateral central vestibular connections, including an inhibitory vestibular commisure, suggested that changes in commisural gains either played no role at all or at most only a secondary role in the restoration of static vestibular balance. In a related study,[134] the influence of visual experience on vestibular compensation was investigated. The authors found that visual experience after labyrinthectomy was essential for recovery of VOR gain but not for the resolution of spontaneous VN.

A study of 70 patients with acoustic neurinomas found a highly significant linear relationship between the tumor size and the caloric side difference.[135] For tumors larger than 20 mm, disturbed pursuit movements or GEN were frequently found. Vestibular nerve section, which is used in the management of Meniere's disease, creates a state of dysequilibrium which usually resolves. However, 6 patients have been reported who had persistent spontaneous VN after this procedure.[136] Torsional (rotatory) recovery nystagmus has been identified as an important localizing sign in endolymphatic hydrops.[137] The descriptions of torsional nystagmus in the paper were based on the observer's point of view rather than the subject's.

For those interested in epidemiology, studies on benign paroxysmal positional vertigo and Meniere's disease in Japan are available.[138, 139]

SACCADIC INTRUSIONS AND OSCILLATIONS

Nonnystagmic ocular motor oscillations and intrusions represent solely saccadic or saccadically initiated instabilities. Table 2 shows 16 varieties of saccadic oscillations and intrusions that have been characterized in the literature by the other terms shown, including 10 which erroneously contain the term "nystagmus." This section contains discussions of recent studies of saccadic oscillations and intrusions; they are in alphabetical order. For detailed discussions of these and other types of saccadic intrusions and oscillations, see previous volumes on the subject.[1-5]

Flutter

Low-amplitude flutter has been described in two cases and given the designation "microflutter."[140, 141] In one, cerebellar degeneration was the diagnosis. Ashe et al. studied five cases with microflutter and hypothesized that microflutter was not merely a case of low-amplitude flutter but a mechanistically different oscillation.[142] Their suggestion that the term, "microsaccadic flutter" is more "specific" than microflutter confuses specificity with redundancy; all flutter is, by definition, saccadic and this attempt to drive home that point is overkill. More difficult to resolve is the question of mechanism. The authors used a modification of their original model for flutter that included the local, resettable neural integrator first proposed by Abel et al.[143] to support the suggestion that different mechanisms were involved. They demonstrated that flutter might be caused by an increased delay of the feedback signal from the local integrator plus a lowered tone signal in the pause cells and that microflutter might be due to a lowered tone signal alone. They did not use the model to show that both could not be caused by some other single deficit. Since both of these are speculative mechanisms based on a putative model of the saccadic pulse generator itself and since these specific, subtle changes are more easily made on a model than in that small area of the brain stem where these cells and their connections reside, it is premature to conclude that the mechanism for microflutter is significantly different from that of flutter. The former may merely be the precursor of the latter or reflect a smaller disruption to that area of the brain stem. In keeping with the guidelines at the beginning of this chapter, microflutter is included as a subtype of flutter in Table 2.

Opsoclonus

Opsoclonus was first described in 1913[144] and again in 1927.[145] In addition to the many disorders that have since been associated with opsoclonus, we can now add organophosphate poisoning,[146] thymic carcinoma,[147] Epstein-Barr virus infection,[148] hyperosmolar stupor,[149] and hypertension.[150, 151] Also, a case of opsoclonus-myoclonus ("dancing eyes, dancing feet") was reported secondary to cocaine usage.[152] The episode was self-limited over 4 weeks and had not reappeared after 1 year.

Saccadic Lateropulsion

Two cases with leftward saccadic pulsion during vertical saccades were studied with EOG.[153] The patient with Wallenberg's syndrome exhibited lateropulsion, whereas the patient with the proximal type of the superior cerebellar syndrome had contrapulsion.

Saccadic Pulses/Pulse Trains

Gamlin et al. studied the effects (in rhesus monkeys) on convergence and conjugate eye movements of lidocaine-induced unilateral INO.[154] While a through discussion of the many findings of this study are beyond the scope of this chapter, relevant findings were: (1) uniocular vertical nystagmus with unyoked fast phases inferred independent operation of the individual saccade generators; and (2) abduction "nystagmus" was actually caused by adaptive saccadic behavior. This latter finding is yet another supporting the classification of this sign as a saccadic oscillation. A report of INO in tuberculous meningitis failed to appreciate this distinction.[155]

Square-Wave Jerks/Oscillations

Shallo-Hoffmann et al. studied the occurrence of square-wave jerks (SWJ) in healthy subjects under different conditions.[156] They concluded that SWJ were normal with the eyes closed, in darkness while looking straight ahead, and while fixating a target in a lighted room. More than 16 SWJ per minute while fixating or 20/min under the other conditions should be considered abnormal according to these authors. A difference between this and a previous report[157] on the number of

SWJ occurring in darkness was attributed to the specific instruction, "hold the eyes still" given in the other study. In a related study, Shallo-Hoffmann et al. reported the characteristics of SWJ over a broad age range.[158] Their results showed no relationship between SWJ frequency and age.

The occurrence of both SWJ and square-wave oscillations SWO has been documented in two patients with acquired immunodeficiency syndrome.[159] The SWO had a frequency of up to 5 Hz.

Square-Wave Pulses (Bursts/Single)

When "macro square-wave jerks (MSWJ)" were first recorded and named, they were of greater amplitude than SWJ and were recognized as being caused by a different mechanism since their pulse width was not the saccadic interval (200 ms) characteristic of SWJ.[160] Nevertheless, the name "macro square-wave jerks" was chosen. This name had its origin in "pendular macro-oscillations," which had been used to describe these eye movements at the bedside. Eye movement recordings showed that they were saccadic and not pendular, so MSWJ was chosen despite the mechanistic difference from SWJ. Since that time, despite several papers restating the differences,[161, 162] this doubly erroneous name (they are *not* always large and they are *not* SWJ) has continued to mislead both the scientific reader and investigator. As one of those responsible for this name, I am herein proposing that we drop "macro square-wave jerks" from the literature and use the more correct description "square-wave pulses (SWP)" for this low–pulse-width saccadic intrusion (less than the 200 ms intersaccadic latency). When bursts of these SWP appear on a strip chart recording made at normal paper speeds, the oscillation looks like narrow square pulses separated by the saccadic latency; at fast paper speeds, no saccades appear "square" but despite this, the term is well known and gives an immediate and correct picture in the mind of the reader. An example of how the term "MSWJ" may have caused confusion is in the inclusion of two patients (numbers 2 and 3) in the category of SWJ in a 1982 paper on SWJ.[163] The authors recognized that the short latency between the initiating and return saccades differed from SWJ but because of the implications of the term "macro," the low amplitude of the intrusions may have kept them from considering MSWJ; these patients' intrusions are defined by their timing not their amplitude and should be classified as SWP (at the time, MSWJ). The characteristics of SWP and other similar oscillations are summarized in Table 3.

Superior Oblique Myokymia

Morrow et al. recorded superior oblique myokymia (SOMY) in an idiopathic case and in a case of an astrocytoma involving the midbrain tectum.[164] Monocular

TABLE 3.
Characteristics of Square-Wave Instabilities*

Characteristic	SWJ	SWO	SWP	MSO
Amplitude (degrees)	0.5–5†	0.5–5†	4–30	1–30
	Constant	Constant	Variable	Increasing then decreasing
Time course	Sporadic/bursts	Bursts	Bursts/sporadic	Bursts
Latency (ms)	200	200	50–150	200
Foveation	Yes	Yes	Yes	No
Presence in darkness	Yes	Yes	Yes	No

*SWJ = square-wave jerks; SWO = square-wave oscillations; SWP = square-wave pulses; MSO = macro saccadic oscillations.
†Amplitudes occasionally may reach 10 degrees.

bursts of tonic and phasic intorsion and depression and miniature oscillations were found. In both patients, the torsional and vertical movements were synchronous with similar waveforms, but the torsional movements were about twice as large as the vertical. The waveforms of SOMY consisted of either a slow sustained tonic intorsion and depression or a phasic intorsion; each was followed by a decreasing velocity return. Occasionally there were small torsional-vertical oscillations superimposed on the tonic deviations. The tonic amplitudes were 2 to 3 degrees of intorsion and 1 to 1.5 degrees of depression. The phasic amplitudes were 0.5 to 1 degree and the small oscillations were less than 0.5 degree at up to 20 Hz. Thus, in the torsional plane, SOMY consists of either an intorsional saccade followed after some time by a decreasing velocity return (tonic) or an intorsional saccadic pulse (phasic). In addition, bursts of small pendular oscillations can be superimposed on the tonic intorsions. These movements are also seen in the vertical plane. The symptoms stopped in the second patient after tumor resection. An EOG recording of the pendular horizontal and vertical components of SOMY in a patient's right eye also appeared.[165] They looked to be in phase, resulting in a diagonal movement; the torsional component was said to be clockwise (presumably from the observer's point of view).

Ruttum and Harris reported on the results of surgery in superior oblique myokymia.[166] They found that when superior oblique tenotomy or tenectomy were used, OSOP recurs in approximately 50% of the patients; incomplete transection of the tendon, residual attachments, or postoperative adhesions were given as possible reasons for the failures. Repeat surgery with a superior oblique myectomy and trochlectomy via an anterior orbital approach was successful in one such patient.

OSCILLOPSIA

Since the identification in the early 1970s of the foveation periods in CN waveforms, their importance in visual acuity was obvious. All therapies for CN have stressed reduction of the nystagmus waveform intensity with the hoped-for result that the foveation-period durations would be increased. What was less appreciated was the importance of stable, on a beat-to-beat basis, foveation periods in the suppression of OSOP in subjects with CN. This was partially due to the early hypothesis that OSOP was suppressed in CN by efferent copy of the CN waveform.[167] Based on the premise that the best way to study OSOP in healthy subjects is to understand its suppression in those with CN, we have begun to study this phenomenon. Inherent in this premise is the hypothesis that the mechanisms used by subjects with CN to suppress OSOP do *not* represent specially developed abilities but rather result from the application of the normal capabilities present in the ocular motor system. If this hypothesis is true, the subject with CN becomes an excellent model for the study of healthy subjects who acquire OSOP due to neurologic deficits in later life and, once the mechanism used by subjects with CN is understood, we should be able to therapeutically apply this knowledge to subjects with acquired OSOP.

We studied the waveform changes in a subject with hereditary CN who experienced intermittent OSOP after an episode of loss of consciousness.[168] Using the same type of phase-plane analysis employed to study foveation periods in CN, we found that his normal CN fell into a foveation window defined by 0 ± 0.5 degrees and 0 ± 4 degrees/sec limits on eye position and velocity, respectively. However, when he complained of OSOP, he exhibited a different waveform that *never* entered this foveation window. Thus, when the foveation periods fell within this foveation window on a beat-to-beat basis, he was able to suppress OSOP and when his waveform did not allow foveation periods to fall within the window, he could not suppress OSOP. We performed the same analysis during retinal image stabilization (RIS) and the results did not change. We concluded from this that RIS by itself was insufficient to suppress OSOP and further that the mechanism that prevents OSOP in subjects with CN requires the ocular motor stability provided by the CN foveation periods; without it, OSOP is not suppressed even during RIS. Thus, we infer that all one needs to suppress OSOP is a short period of time during which the subject can foveate a target of interest with a low retinal slip velocity on a repeatable basis. In subjects with acquired oscillations, ways must now be found to alter the oscillations in such a way to achieve these periods of stable target foveation.

In a study of human horizontal VOR, it was found that high-acceleration stimuli resulted in OSOP.[169] The gaze disturbance that resulted in OSOP was attributed to the latency of the VOR, which was found to be 6 to 15 ms. The instability of gaze during locomotion has also been studied.[170] Two patients with bilaterally deficient vestibular function complained of OSOP during walking. It was found that during sitting and standing their gaze was as stable as in healthy subjects, but during walking in place the gaze velocity was double that of healthy subjects. Their VOR compensated well during active head motions but not during locomotion; this was attributed to the predictable nature of active head movements. The authors concluded that testing of such patients should include perturbations similar to those that occur during locomotion. Anticonvulsant therapy also affects the VOR and can cause OSOP.[171] In a study of eight patients with epilepsy receiving anticonvulsants who had recurrent visual disturbances (diplopia and OSOP) in both the horizontal and vertical planes, it was found that both the vergence and version mechanisms (smooth pursuit and gaze-holding) were affected. Spontaneous vertical nystagmus and up-down asymmetry of the VOR were found; the former caused OSOP with a stationary head and the latter during vertical head motion. OSOP has also been reported in a case of otolith Tullio phenomenon.[172] This sound-induced OSOP results from paroxysms of the ocular tilt reaction. When the Valsalva maneuver was performed, both the tonic eye movements and OSOP induced were opposite in direction to those produced by the sound, reflecting the push-pull nature of the otoliths. Sound stimulation elicited a paroxysmal ocular tilt reaction with both phasic and tonic components. Initially there was rapid phasic clockwise (reported as counterclockwise with respect to the observer) rotary-upward deviation that was followed by a similar tonic effect as long as the sound stimulation lasted. Switching the sound off produced a rapid return of the eye to primary position.

A first-person account of OSOP secondary to Wallenberg's syndrome by an experienced observer is worth reading.[173] The accompanying paper describes the eye movements associated with the OSOP.[174] Clear examples of dysmetria and SWO were recorded in this patient. An up-to-date chapter on the management of OSOP is available.[175] In it are descriptions of new optical treatments to alleviate OSOP. Acquired nystagmus causing OSOP has also been treated with botulinum.[176] Two patients were treated and OSOP diminished with an increase in acuity that lasted for 3 to 18 weeks.

ACKNOWLEDGMENTS

The editorial assistance of Lorna Murph is gratefully acknowledged.

REFERENCES

1. Dell'Osso LF: Nystagmus and other ocular motor oscillations, in Lessell S, Van Dalen JTW (eds): *Neuro-Ophthalmology-1980*, vol I. Amsterdam, Excerpta Medica, 1980, pp 146–177.

2. Dell'Osso LF: Nystagmus and other ocular motor oscillations, in Lessell S, Van Dalen JTW (eds): *Neuro-Ophthalmology-1982*, vol II. Amsterdam, Excerpta Medica, 1982, pp 148–171.

3. Dell'Osso LF: Nystagmus and other ocular motor oscillations and intrusions, in Lessell S, Van Dalen JTW (eds): *Neuro-Ophthalmology-1984*, vol III. Amsterdam, Excerpta Medica, 1984, pp 157–204.

4. Dell'Osso LF: Nystagmus and other ocular motor oscillations and intrusions, in Lessell S, Van Dalen JTW (eds): *Current Neuro-Ophthalmology*, vol 1. Chicago, Year Book Medical Publishers, 1987, pp 139–172.

5. Dell'Osso LF: Nystagmus, saccadic oscillations/intrusions and oscillopsia, in Lessell S, Van

Dalen JTW (eds): *Current Neuro-Ophthalmology,* vol 2. Chicago, Year Book Medical Publishers, 1989, pp 147–182.

6. Stevens GT: *Motor Apparatus of the Eyes.* Philadelphia, FA Davis Co, 1906, p 436.

7. Juhola M, Pyykkö I: Effects of sampling frequencies on the velocity of slow and fast phases of nystagmus. *Int J Bio-Med Comp* 1987; 20:253–263.

8. Becker W, Fuchs AF: Prediction in the oculomotor system: Smooth pursuit during transient disappearance of a visual target. *Exp Brain Res* 1985; 57:562–575.

9. Traccis S, Rosati G, Monaco MF, et al: Successful treatment of acquired pendular elliptical nystagmus in multiple sclerosis with isoniazid and base-out prisms. *Neurology* 1990; 40:492–494.

10. Dell'Osso LF, Van der Steen J, Collewijn H, et al: Foveation dynamics in congenital nystagmus. *Invest Ophthalmol Vis Sci (ARVO Suppl)* 1988; 29:166.

11. Abadi RV, Pascal E, Whittle J, et al: Retinal fixation behavior in human albinos. *Optom Vis Sci* 1989; 66:276–280.

12. Mezawa M, Ukai K, Yamada T, et al: Quantitative indices of congenital nystagmus: Characteristics and their relations. *Acta Soc Ophthalmol Jpn* 1987; 91:1008–1014.

13. Bedell HE, White JM, Abplanalp PL: Variability of foveations in congenital nystagmus. *Clin Vision Sci* 1989; 4:247–252.

14. Abadi RV, Worfolk R: Retinal slip velocities in congenital nystagmus. *Vision Res* 1989; 29:195–205.

15. Guo S, Reinecke RD, Goldstein HP: Visual acuity determinants in infantile nystagmus. *Invest Ophthalmol Vis Sci (ARVO Suppl)* 1990; 31:83.

16. Bedell HE, Loshin DS: Interrelations between measures of visual acuity and parameters of eye movement in congenital nystagmus. *Invest Ophthalmol Vis Sci,* 1991; 32:416–421.

17. Demer JL, Porter FI, Goldberg J, et al: Predictors of functional success in telescopic spectacle use by low vision patients. *Invest Ophthalmol Vis Sci* 1989; 30:1652–1665.

18. Dell'Osso LF, Van der Steen J, Collewijn H, et al: Pursuit and VOR dynamics in congenital nystagmus. *Invest Ophthalmol Vis Sci (ARVO Suppl)* 1989; 30:50.

19. Kurzan R, Büttner U: Smooth pursuit mechanisms in congenital nystagmus. *Neuroophthalmol* 1989; 9:313–325.

20. Lueck CJ, Tanyeri S, Mossman S, et al: Unilateral reversal of smooth pursuit and optokinetic nystagmus. *Rev Neurol (Paris)* 1989; 145:656–660.

21. Kelly BJ, Rosenberg ML, Zee DS, et al: Unilateral pursuit-induced congenital nystagmus. *Neurology* 1989; 39:414–416.

22. Takahashi H: An analysis of congenital nystagmus, velocity characteristics of the slow eye movements of pursuit stimulation in four families. *Acta Soc Ophthalmol Jpn* 1986; 90:839–847.

23. Tusa RJ, Repka MX: Early visual deprivation in monkeys results in persistent strabismus and nystagmus. *Invest Ophthalmol Vis Sci (ARVO Suppl)* 1990; 31:120.

24. Reinecke RD, Suqin G, Goldstein HP: Waveform evolution in infantile nystagmus: An electro-oculo-graphic study of 35 cases. *Binocular Vision* 1988; 3:191–202.

25. Parks MM: Congenital esotropia vs infantile esotropia. *Graefe's Arch Clin Exp Ophthalmol* 1988; 226:106–107.

26. Gresty MA, Bronstein AM, Page NG, et al: Congenital-type nystagmus emerging in later life. *Neurology,* 1991; 44:653–656.

27. Weiss AH, Biersdorf WR: Visual sensory disorders in congenital nystagmus. *Ophthalmology* 1989; 96:517–523.

28. Lambert SR, Taylor D, Kriss A: The infant with nystagmus, normal appearing fundi, but an abnormal ERG. *Surv Ophthalmol* 1989; 34:173–186.

29. Gelbert SS, Hoyt CS: Congenital nystagmus: A clinical perspective in infancy. *Graefe's Arch Clin Exp Ophthalmol* 1988; 226:178–180.

30. Shallo-Hoffmann J, Watermeier D, Peterson J, et al: Fast-phase instabilities in normally sighted relatives of congenital nystagmus patients-autosomal dominant and x-chromosome recessive modes of inheritance. *Neurosurg Rev* 1988; 11:151–158.

31. Funahashi K, Kuwata T, Yabumoto M, et al: Congenital vertical pendular nystagmus in sisters. *Ophthalmologica* 1988; 196:137–142.

32. Price MJ, Judisch GF, Thompson HS: X-linked congenital stationary night blindness with myopia and nystagmus without clinical complaints of nyctalopia. *J Pediatr Ophthalmol Strabismus* 1988; 25:33–36.

33. Pearce WG, Reedyk M, Coupland SG: Variable expressivity in X-linked congenital stationary night blindness. *Can J Ophthalmol* 1990; 25:3–10.

34. Goldstein DJ, Ward RE, Moore E, et al: Overgrowth, congenital hypotonia, nystagmus, strabismus, and mental retardation: Varient of dominantly inherited Sotos sequence? *Am J Med Genet* 1988; 29:783–792.

35. Williams CA, Cantú ES, Friás JL: Brief clinical report: Metaphyseal dysostosis and congenital nystagmus in a male infant with the fragile X syndrome. *Am J Med Genet* 1986; 23:207–211.

36. Lowry RB, Wood BJ, Cox TA, et al: Epiphyseal dysplasia, microcephaly, nystagmus and retinitis pigmentosa. *Am J Med Genet* 1989; 33:341–345.

37. Grossman SA, Peyman GA: Long-term visual results after pars plicata lensectomy-vitrectomy for congenital cataracts. *Br J Ophthalmol* 1988; 72:601–606.

38. Oliver MD, Dotan SA, Chemke J, et al: Isolated foveal hypoplasia. *Br J Ophthalmol* 1987; 71:926–930.

39. Kruis JA, Houtman WA, Van Weerden TW: Congenital absence of conjugate horizontal eye movements. *Doc Ophthalmol* 1987; 67:13–18.

40. Apkarian P, Spekreijse H, Collewijn H: Oculomotor behavior in human albinos, in Kolder HEJW (ed): *Documenta Ophthalmologica Proceedings Series,* vol 37. The Hague, Dr W Junk, 1983, pp 361–372.

41. Apkarian P, Reits D, Spekreijse H, et al: A decisive electrophysiological test for human albinism. *EEG Clin Neurophysiol* 1983; 55:513–531.

42. Apkarian P, Spekreijse H: The VEP and misrouted pathways in human albinism, in Cracco RQ, Bodis-Wollner I (eds): *Evoked Potentials.* New York, AR Liss, 1986, pp 211–226.

43. Apkarian P, Reits D: Global stereopsis in human albinos. *Vision Res* 1989; 29:1359–1370.

44. Guo S, Reinecke RD, Fendick M, et al: Visual pathway abnormalities in albinism and infantile nystagmus: VECPs and stereoacuity measurements. *J Pediatr Ophthalmol Strabismus* 1989; 26:97–104.

45. Russell-Eggitt I, Kriss A, Taylor DSI: Albinism in childhood: A flash VEP and ERG study. *Br J Ophthalmol* 1990; 74:136–140.

46. Abplanalp P, Bedell HE: Visual improvement in an albinotic patient with an alteration of congenital nystagmus. *Am J Optom Physiol Optics* 1987; 64:944–951.

47. Dell'Osso LF, Traccis S, Abel LA, et al: Contact lenses and congenital nystagmus. *Clin Vision Sci* 1988; 3:229–232.

48. Dell'Osso LF, Leigh RJ, Daroff RB: Suppression of congenital nystagmus by cutaneous stimulation. *Neuro-ophthalmol,* in press.

49. Hatayama R, Kawai K, Matsuzaki H: A study of prismatic treatment of congenital nystagmus by the electro-oculogram-fixation, pursuit eye movement and optokinetic nystagmus. *Acta Soc Ophthalmol Jpn* 1986; 90:263–271.

50. Young JDH: Head posture measurement. *J Pediatr Ophthalmol Strabismus* 1988; 25:86–89.

51. Castanera AM: Length-tension diagrams of medial rectus muscles after Cüppers' fadenoperation. *Ophthalmologica* 1989; 198:46–52.

52. Sendler S, Shallo-Hoffmann J, Mühlendyck H: Die Artifizielle-Divergenz-Operation beim kongenitalen Nystagmus. *Fortschr Ophthalmol* 1990; 87:85–89.

53. Gamlin PDR, Gnadt JW, Mays LE: Abducens internuclear neurons carry an inappropriate signal for ocular convergence. *J Neurophysiol* 1989; 62:70–81.

54. Sigal MB, Diamond GR: Survey of management strategies for nystagmus patients with vertical or torsional head posture. *Ann Ophthalmol* 1990; 22:134–138.

55. Mezawa M, Ishikawa S, Ukai K: Changes in waveform of congenital nystagmus associated with biofeedback treatment. *B J Opthalmol* 1990; 74:472–476.

56. Good PA, Searle AET, Campbell S, et al: Value of the ERG in congenital nystagmus. *Br J Ophthalmol* 1989; 73:512–515.

57. Reccia R, Roberti G, Russo P: Computer analysis of ENG spectral features from patients with congenital nystagmus. *J Biomed Eng* 1990; 12:39–45.

58. Reccia R, Roberti G, Russo P: Spectral analysis of pendular waveforms in congenital nystagmus. *Ophthalmic Res* 1989; 21:83–92.

59. D'Exposito M, Reccia R, Roberti G, et al: Amount of surgery in congenital nystagmus. *Ophthalmologica* 1989; 198:145–151.

60. Bosone G, Reccia R, Roberti G, et al: On the variations of the time constant of the slow-phase eye movements produced by surgical therapy of congenital nystagmus: A preliminary report. *Ophthalmic Res* 1989; 21:345–351.

61. Mossman SS, Bronstein AM, Gresty MA, et al: Convergence nystagmus associated with Arnold-Chiari malformation. *Arch Neurol* 1990; 47:357–359.

62. Selhorst JB, Schwartz MA, Ochs AL, et al: Pendular vergence oscillations, in Ishikawa S (ed): *Highlights in Neuro-Ophthalmology. Proceedings of the Sixth Meeting of the International Neuro-Ophthalmology Society.* Amsterdam, Aeolus Press, 1987, pp 153–162.

63. Chrousos GA, Matsuo V, Ballen AE, et al: Near-evoked nystagmus in spasmus nutans. *J Pediatr Ophthalmol Strabismus* 1986; 23:141–143.

64. Weissman BM, Dell'Osso LF, Abel LA, et al: Spasmus nutans: A quantitative prospective study. *Arch Ophthalmol* 1987; 105:525–528.

65. Oliva A, Rosenberg MI: Convergence-evoked nystagmus. *Neurology* 1990; 40:161–162.

66. Cruysberg JRM, Mtanda AT, Duinkerke-Eerola KU, et al: Congenital adduction palsy and synergistic divergence: A clinical and electro-oculographic study. *Br J Ophthalmol* 1989; 73:68–75.

67. Pfister HW, Einhäupl KM, Büttner U, et al: Dissociated nystagmus as a common sign of ocular motor disorders in HIV-infected patients. *Eur Neurol* 1989; 29:277–280.

68. Kitamura K: Downbeat nystagmus during eye closure. *J Laryngol Otol* 1987; 101:1075–1078.

69. Weissman BM, Dell'Osso LF, Discenna A: Downbeat nystagmus in an infant. Spontaneous resolution during infancy. *Neuro-ophthalmol* 1988; 8:317–319.

70. Jacobson DM, Corbett JJ: Downbeat nystagmus with dolichoectasia of the vertebrobasilar artery. *Arch Neurol* 1989; 46:1005–1008.

71. Masucci EF, Kurtzke JF: Downbeat nystagmus secondary to multiple sclerosis. *Ann Ophthalmol* 1988; 20:347–348.

72. Guy JR, Schatz NJ: Paraneoplastic downbeating nystagmus. A sign of occult malignancy. *J Clin Neuro-ophthalmol* 1988; 8:269–272.

73. Moster ML, Schatz NJ, Savino PJ, et al: Alternating skew on lateral gaze (bilateral abducting hypertropia). *Ann Neurol* 1988; 23:190–192.

74. Crevits L, Reynaert C: Downbeat nystagmus. An electro-oculographic study. *Neuro-ophthalmol* 1989; 9:43–48.

75. Abel LA, Hertle RW: Effects of psychoactive drugs on ocular motor behavior, in Johnston CW, Pirozzolo FJ (eds): *Neuropsychology of Eye Movements.* Hillsdale, Lawrence Erlbaum Associates, 1988, pp 83–114.

76. Williams DP, Troost BT, Rogers J: Lithium-induced downbeat nystagmus. *Arch Neurol* 1988; 45:1022–1023.

77. Halmagyi GM, Lessell I, Curthoys IS, et al: Lithium-induced downbeat nystagmus. *Am J Ophthalmol* 1989; 107:664–670.

78. Sibony PA, Evinger C, Manning K, et al: Nicotine and tobacco-induced nystagmus. *Ann Neurol* 1990; 28:198.

79. Kaplan PW, Lesser RP: Vertical and horizontal epileptic gaze deviation and nystagmus. *Neurology* 1989; 39:1391–1393.

80. Furman JMR, Crumrine PK, Reinmuth OM: Epileptic nystagmus. *Ann Neurol* 1990; 27:686–688.

81. Tusa RJ, Kaplan PW, Hain TC, et al: Ipsiversive eye deviation and epileptic nystagmus. *Neurology* 1989; 40:662–665.

82. Elliott AJ, Simpson EM, Oakhill A, et al: Nystagmus after medulloblastoma. *Dev Med Child Neurol* 1989; 31:43–46.

83. Vighetto A, Froment JC, Trillet M, et al: Magnetic resonance imaging in familial paroxysmal ataxia. *Arch Neurol* 1988; 45:547–549.

84. Baloh RW, Beykirch K, Tauchi P, et al: Ultralow vestibuloocular reflex time constants. *Ann Neurol* 1988; 23:32–37.

85. Wolf M, Ashkenazi IE, Leventon G: Circadian variation of nystagmus in healthy and sick subjects. *Arch Otolaryngol Head Neck Surg* 1990; 116:221–223.

86. Dickinson CM, Abadi RV: Pursuit and optokinetic responses in latent/manifest latent nystagmus. *Invest Ophthalmol Vis Sci* 1990; 31:1649–1652.

87. Bedell HE, Yap YL, Flom MC: Fixational drift and nasal-temporal pursuit asymmetries in strabismic amblyopes. *Invest Ophthalmol Vis Sci* 1990; 31:968–976.

88. Leigh RJ, Thurston SE, Tomsak RL, et al: Effect of monocular visual loss upon stability of gaze. *Invest Ophthalmol Vis Sci* 1989; 30:288–292.

89. Steinbach MJ, Smith D, Crawford JS: Egocentric localization changes following unilateral strabismus surgery. *J Pediatr Ophthalmol Strabismus* 1988; 25:115–118.

90. Zubcov AA, Reinecke RD, Calhoun JH: Asymmetric horizontal tropias, DVD, and manifest latent nystagmus: An explanation of dissociated horizontal deviation. *J Pediatr Ophthalmol Strabismus* 1990; 27:59–64.

91. Ciancia AO: Oculomotor disturbances and VER findings in patients with early monocular loss of vision. *Graefe's Arch Clin Exp Ophthalmol* 1988; 226:108–110.

92. Clarke WN, Nöel LP, Blaylock JF: Rotatory nystagmus in infantile esotropia. *Can J Ophthalmol* 1988; 23:270–272.

93. Ciancia AO: Infantile esotropia with abduction nystagmus. *Int Ophthalmol Clin* 1989; 29:24–29.

94. Zubcov AA, Reinecke RD, Gottlob I, et al: Treatment of manifest latent nystagmus. *Am J Ophthalmol* 1990; 110:160–167.

95. Simonsz HJ: The effect of prolonged monocular occlusion on latent nystagmus in the treatment of amblyopia. *Doc Ophthalmol* 1989; 72:375–384.

96. Howard LP, Simpson WA: Human optokinetic nystagmus is linked to the stereoscopic system. *Exp Brain Res* 1989; 78:309–314.

97. Wyatt HJ, Pola J: Predictive behavior of optokinetic eye movements. *Exp Brain Res* 1988; 73:615–626.

98. Dell'Osso LF, Daroff RB: Functional organization of the ocular motor system. *Aerosp Med* 1974; 45:873–875.

99. Waespe W, Schwarz U: Slow eye movements induced by apparent target motion in monkey. *Exp Brain Res* 1987; 67:433–435.

100. Van den Berg AV, Collewijn H: Directional asymmetries of human optokinetic nystagmus. *Exp Brain Res* 1988; 70:597–604.

101. Igarashi M, Himi T: Asymmetry of vertical optokinetic nystagmus and afternystagmus. *ORL* 1988; 50:219–224.

102. Usami S-I, Igarashi M, Ishii M, et al: Unidirectional vestibular habituation in the squirrel monkey. *Acta Otolaryngol (Stockh)* 1988; 106:124–129.

103. Whittaker SG, Cummings RW: Foveating saccades. *Vision Res* 1990; 30:1363–1366.

104. Nazarian SM, Jay WM: Intermittent unidirectional nystagmus. *Ann Ophthalmol* 1990; 22:177–178.

105. Reis J, Eber A-M, Warter J-M, et al: Alternating nystagmus and infectious mononucleosis. *Neuro-ophthalmol* 1989; 9:289–292.

106. Uemura T, Inoue H, Hirano T: The effects of baclofen on periodic alternating nystagmus and experimentally induced nystagmus. *Adv Oto-Rhino-Laryngol* 1988; 42:254–259.

107. Schwankhaus JD, Kattah JC, Lux WE, et al: Primidone/phenobarbital-induced periodic alternating nystagmus. *Ann Ophthalmol* 1989; 21:230–232.

108. Watkins HC, Ellis CJK: Ping pong gaze in reversible coma due to overdose of monoamine oxidase inhibitor. *J Neurol Neurosurg Psychiatry* 1989; 52:539.

109. Eizeman M, Cheng P, Sharpe JA, et al: End-point nystagmus and ocular drift: An experimental and theoretical study. *Vision Res* 1990; 6:863–877.

110. Blessing R, Kommerell G: Pseudo-Spontannystagmus unter der Frenzel-Brille. *Laryngol Rhinol Otol* 1988; 67:453–456.

111. Shallo-Hoffmann J, Schwarze H, Simonsz HJ, et al: A reexamination of end-point and rebound nystagmus in normals. *Invest Ophthalmol Vis Sci* 1990; 31:388–392.

112. Theunissen EJJM, Huygen PLM, Verhagen WIM: Familial vestibulocerebellar dysfunction: A new syndrome? *J Neurol Sci* 1989; 89:149–155.

113. Nakada T, Kwee IL: Seesaw nystagmus. Role of visuovestibular interaction in its pathogenesis. *J Clin Neuro-ophthalmol* 1988; 8:171–177.

114. Morrow MJ, Sharpe JA: Torsional nystagmus in the lateral medullary syndrome. *Ann Neurol* 1988; 24:390–398.

115. Noseworthy JH, Ebers GC, Leigh RJ, et al: Torsional nystagmus: Quantitative features and possible pathogenesis. *Neurology* 1988; 38:992–994.

116. Weissman JD, Seidman SH, Dell'Osso LF, et al: Torsional, see-saw, "bow-tie" nystagmus in association with brain stem anomalies. *Neuro-ophthalmology*, in press.

117. Pritchard C, Flynn JT, Smith JL: Wave form characteristics of vertical oscillations in longstanding vision loss. *J Pediatr Ophthalmol Strabismus* 1988; 25:233–236.

118. Ranalli PJ, Sharpe JA: Upbeat nystagmus and the ventral tegmental pathway of the upward vestibulo-ocular reflex. *Neurology* 1988; 38:1329–1330.

119. Harada K, Kato I, Koike Y, et al: Primary position upbeat nystagmus in man and cats. *Adv Oto-Rhino-Laryngol* 1988; 42:190–194.

120. Traccis S, Rosati G, Aiello I, et al: Upbeat nystagmus as an early sign of cerebellar astrocytoma. *J Neurol* 1989; 236:359–360.

121. Kattah JC, Dagi TF: Compensatory head tilt in upbeating nystagmus. *J Clin Neuro-ophthalmol* 1990; 10:27–31.

122. Baloh RW, Yee RD: Spontaneous vertical nystagmus. *Rev Neurol* 1989; 145:527–532.

123. Jacobson GP, Henry KG: Effect of temperature on fixation suppression ability in normal subjects: The need for temperature and age-dependent normal values. *Ann Otol Rhinol Laryngol* 1989; 98:369–372.

124. Davidson J, Wright G, McIlmoyl L, et al: The reproducibility of caloric tests of vestibular function in young and old subjects. *Acta Otolaryngol (Stockh)* 1988; 106:264–268.

125. Baloh RW, Beykirch K, Honrubia V, et al: Eye movements induced by linear acceleration on a parallel swing. *J Neurophysiol* 1988; 60:2000–2013.

126. Brandt T: Positional and positioning vertigo and nystagmus. *J Neurol Sci* 1990; 95:3–28.

127. Norre ME, Beckers AM: Vestibular habituation training. *Arch Otolaryngol Head Neck Surg* 1988; 114:883–886.

128. Benecke JE, Hitselberger WE: Vertigo caused by basilar artery compression of the eighth nerve. *Laryngoscope* 1988; 98:807–809.

129. Grad A, Baloh RW: Vertigo of vascular origin: clinical and electronystagmographic features in 84 cases. *Arch Neurol* 1989; 46:281–284.

130. Nigam A, Moffat DA, Varley EWB: Benign paroxysmal positional vertigo resulting from surgical trauma. *J Laryngol Otol* 1989; 103:203–204.

131. Catalano RA, Calhoun JH, Reinecke RD, et al: Asymmetry in congenital ocular motor apraxia. *Can J Ophthalmol* 1988; 23:318–321.

132. Wei D, Hain TC, Proctor LR: Head-shaking nystagmus: Associations with canal paresis and hearing loss. *Acta Otolaryngol (Stockh)* 1989; 108:362–367.

133. Fetter M, Zee DS: Recovery from unilateral labyrinthectomy in rhesus monkey. *J Neurophysiol* 1988; 59:370–393.

134. Fetter M, Zee DS, Proctor LR: Effect of lack of vision and of occipital lobectomy upon recovery from unilateral labyrinthectomy in rhesus monkey. *J Neurophysiol* 1988; 59:394–407.

135. Bergenius J, Magnusson M: The relationship between caloric response, oculomotor dysfunction and size of cerebello-pontine angle tumours. *Acta Otolaryngol (Stockh)* 1988; 106:361–367.

136. Shotton JC, Ludman H, Davies R: Persisting nystagmus following vestibular nerve section for Menière's disease. *J Laryngol Otol* 1989; 103:263–268.

137. Parnes LS, McClure JA: Rotatory recovery nystagmus: An important localizing sign in endolymphatic hydrops. *J Otolaryngol* 1990; 19:96–99.

138. Mizukoshi K, Ino H, Ishikawa K, et al: Epidemiological survey of definite cases of Meniere's disease collected by the seventeen members of the Meniere's disease research committee of Japan in 1975–1976. *Adv Oto-Rhino-Laryngol* 1979; 25:106–111.

139. Mizukoshi K, Watanabe Y, Shojaku H, et al: Epidemiological studies on benign paroxysmal positional vertigo in Japan. *Acta Otolaryngol (Stockh)* 1988; 447:67–72.

140. Carlow TJ: Medical treatment of nystagmus and other ocular motor disorders. *Int Ophthalmol Clin* 1986; 26:251–263.

141. Sharpe JA, Fletcher WA: Disorders of visual fixation, in Smith JL (ed): *Neuroophthalmology Now.* Chicago, Year Book Medical Publishers, 1986, pp 267–284.

142. Ashe J, Hain TC, Zee DS, et al: Microsaccadic flutter. *Brain,* 1991; 114:461–472.

143. Abel LA, Dell'Osso LF, Daroff RB: Analog model for gaze-evoked nystagmus. *IEEE Trans Biomed Eng* 1978; BME-25:71–75.

144. Orzechowski K, Walichiewicz T: Przypadek operowanej torbieli śródpajęczy móżdżka (operated cyst of the cerebellum). *Lwowski Tygodnik Lekarski* 1913; 18:219–227.

145. Orzechowski K: De l'ataxie dysmetrique des yeux: remarques sur l'ataxie des yeux dite myoclonique (opsoclonie, opsochorie). *J Psychiatry Neurol* 1927; 35:1–18.

146. Pullicino P, Aquilina J: Opsoclonus in organophosphate poisoning. *Arch Neurol* 1989; 46:704–705.

147. Schwartz M, Sharf B, Zidan J: Opsoclonus as a presenting symptom in thymic carcinoma. *J Neurol Neurosurg Psychiatry* 1990; 53:534.

148. Delreux V, Kevers L, Callewaert A, et al: Opsoclonus secondary to an Epstein-Barr virus infection. *Arch Neurol* 1989; 46:480–481.

149. Weissman BM, Devereaux M, Chandar K: Opsoclonus and hyperosmolar stupor. *Neurology* 1989; 39:1401–1402.

150. Tychsen L, Engelken EJ, Austin EJ: Periodic saccadic oscillations and tinnitus. *Neurology* 1990; 40:549–551.

151. Wolpow ER, Davis KR, Kamitsuka PF, et al: Case records of the Massachusetts General Hospital. Case 9–1988. *N Engl J Med* 1988; 318:563–570.

152. Scharf D: Opsoclonus-myoclonus following the intranasal usage of cocaine. *J Neurol Neurosurg Psychiatry* 1989; 52:1447–1448.

153. Uno A, Mukuno K, Sekiya H, et al: Lateropulsion in Wallenberg's syndrome and contrapulsion in the proximal type of the superior cerebellar artery syndrome. *Neuro-ophthalmol* 1989; 9:75–80.

154. Gamlin PDR, Gnadt JW, Mays LE: Lidocaine-induced unilateral internuclear ophthalmoplegia: Effects on convergence and conjugate eye movements. *J Neurophysiol* 1989; 62:82–95.

155. Teoh R, Humphries MJ, Chan JCN, et al: Internuclear ophthalmoplegia in tuberculous meningitis. *Tubercle* 1989; 70:61–64.

156. Shallo-Hoffmann J, Petersen J, Mühlendyck H: How normal are "normal" square wave jerks? *Invest Ophthalmol Vis Sci* 1989; 30:1009–1011.

157. Herishanu YO, Sharpe JA: Normal square wave jerks. *Invest Ophthalmol Vis Sci* 1981; 20:268–272.

158. Shallo-Hoffmann J, Sendler B, Mühlendyck H: Normal square wave jerks in differing age groups. *Invest Ophthalmol Vis Sci* 1990; 31:1649–1652.

159. Friedman DI, Feldon SE: Eye movements in acquired immunodeficiency syndrome. *Arch Neurol* 1989; 46:841.

160. Dell'Osso LF, Troost BT, Daroff RB: Macro square wave jerks. *Neurology* 1975; 25:975–979.

161. Dell'Osso LF, Abel LA, Daroff RB: "Inverse latent" macro square wave jerks and macro saccadic oscillations. *Ann Neurol* 1977; 2:57–60.

162. Abel LA, Traccis S, Dell'Osso LF, et al: Square wave oscillation. The relationship of saccadic intrusions and oscillations. *Neuro-ophthalmol* 1984; 4:21–25.

163. Sharpe JA, Herishanu YO, White OB: Cerebral square wave jerks. *Neurology (NY)* 1982; 32:57–62.

164. Morrow MJ, Sharpe JA, Ranalli PJ: Superior oblique myokymia associated with a posterior fossa tumor: Oculographic correlation with an idiopathic case. *Neurology* 1990; 40:367–370.

165. Nai-chuan Z, Cong W, Hou-ren W: Superior oblique myokymia. *Chin Med J* 1988; 101:815–817.

166. Ruttum MS, Harris GJ: Superior oblique myectomy and trochlectomy in recurrent superior oblique myokymia. *Graefe's Arch Clin Exp Ophthalmol* 1988; 226:145–147.

167. Dell'Osso LF: *A Dual-Mode Model for the Normal Eye Tracking System and the System with Nystagmus* (unpublished thesis). Laramie, University of Wyoming, January 1968.

168. Dell'Osso LF, Leigh RJ: Foveation periods and oscillopsia in congenital nystagmus. *Invest Ophthalmol Vis Sci (ARVO Suppl)* 1990; 31:122.

169. Maas EF, Huebner WP, Seidman SH, et al: Behavior of human horizontal vestibulo-ocular reflex in response to high-acceleration stimuli. *Brain Res* 1989; 499:153–156.

170. Grossman GE, Leigh RJ: Instability of gaze during locomotion in patients with deficient vestibular function. *Ann Neurol* 1990; 27:528–532.

171. Remler BF, Leigh RJ, Osorio I, et al: The characteristics and mechanisms of visual disturbance associated with anticonvulsant therapy. *Neurology* 1990; 40:791–796.

172. Dieterich M, Brandt T, Fries W: Otolith function in man. Results from a case of otolith Tullio phenomenon. *Brain* 1989; 112:1377–1392.

173. Werner DL, Ciuffreda KJ, Tannen B: Wallenberg's syndrome: A first-person account. *J Am Optom Assoc* 1989; 60:745–747.

174. Tannen B, Ciuffreda KJ, Werner DL: A case of Wallenberg's syndrome: Ocular motor abnormalities. *J Am Optom Assoc* 1989; 60:748–752.

175. Leigh RJ: Management of oscillopsia, in Barber HO, Sharpe JA (eds): *Vestibular Disorders.* Chicago, Year Book Medical Publishers, 1988, pp 201–211.

176. Helveston EM, Pogrebniak AE: Treatment of acquired nystagmus with botulinum A toxin. *Am J Ophthalmol* 1988; 106:584–586.

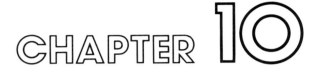

CHAPTER 10

Supranuclear and Nuclear Disorders of Eye Movement

Ekkehard Mehdorn, M.D.

Marienhospital Aachen, Aachen, Federal Republic of Germany

OBSERVATIONS OF TOPOLOGICAL AND PATHOPHYSIOLOGIC IMPORTANCE

Paramedian Pontine Reticular Formation and Other Pontine Structures

The essential features of the brain stem circuitry subserving the generation of rapid eye movements are well understood,[1] and patients exhibiting the classic picture of gaze palsy are recognized easily.[2] Unfortunately, the clinical neuroophthalmologist is confronted often with complex eye movement abnormalities that do not fit into the well-defined descriptions from neurophysiologic experiments.

Neuroimaging techniques, which are becoming more refined, narrow the gap between basic neurophysiologic research and clinical observation and may help define the lesions underlying more complex eye movement disorders. A promising clinical approach to the topographic analysis of gaze disturbances was presented in a comparative study of eye movement recordings and magnetic resonance imaging (MRI) in 51 patients with abnormalities of horizontal gaze.[3, 4] The lesions responsible for isolated abducens paralysis, conjugate paralysis, and different types of internuclear ophthalmoplegia were determined by overlapping individual MRI scans at comparable brain stem levels of patients exhibiting the same type of eye movement disorder. A statistical procedure was developed to exclude the possibility that the areas of overlap occurred by chance. The study confirmed that isolated lateral rectus muscle weakness is correlated with lesions of the posterior part of the abducens fasciculus, but never with lesions of the abducens nucleus. Unilateral gaze paralysis was observed with lesions in the paramedian area of the pons, including the abducens nucleus, the lateral part of the nucleus reticularis pontis caudalis and the nucleus reticularis pontis oralis. Lesions responsible for bilateral gaze paralysis involved the raphe pontis, which contains the omnipause neurons. This finding suggests that damage to omnipause neurons produces slowing of saccades rather than opsoclonus. Lesions with internuclear ophthalmoplegia (INO) were frequently not confined to the medial longitudinal fasciculus (MLF). In fact, this may explain the various eye movement abnormalities that are often associated with INO.

MRI is clearly superior to computed tomography (CT) in the demonstration of subtle brain stem lesions and should be the neuroophthalmologist's first choice in a patient with an eye movement disorder probably originating in the brain stem.[5] Lateral gaze paralysis is usually related to intrinsic brain stem lesions, but compression of the brain stem due to a giant aneurysm of the posterior fossa has been reported.[6]

Recently, smooth pursuit deficits caused by brain stem lesions have gained more attention. The case of a pontine tuberculoma has been reported in which a unilateral paramedian pontine reticular formation (PPRF) lesion (confirmed with MRI) was associated not only with a saccadic paralysis but also with an abolition of ipsilateral smooth pursuit.[7] Smooth pursuit recovered during treatment whereas the saccadic paralysis remained unchanged. Three similar cases with abolished saccades and preserved pursuit were reported.[8] These observations, along with earlier clinical reports,[7, 8] let us assume tonic neurons in the lower pons near the PPRF. Indeed, there is recent neurophysiologic evidence that several pontine nuclei, especially the dorsolaterral pontine nucleus, serve as a smooth pursuit interface between the cerebral hemispheres and the cerebellar vermis.[9, 10]

Internuclear Ophthalmoplegia and One-and-a-Half Syndrome

Vertical smooth eye movements were quantified with magnetic search coil oculography in seven patients with INO and compared to those in age-matched control subjects.[11] The upward and downward vestibulo-ocular reflex (VOR) had reduced gain and abnormal phase lag in both unilateral and bilateral INO during active head motion. Vertical smooth pursuit was only mildly affected. Cancellation of the vertical VOR was more impaired than smooth pursuit. The results indicate that the MLF or neighboring tegmental tracts convey bidirectional signals for vertical pursuit, cancellation of the VOR, and vestibular smooth eye movements in man. Some of the deficits that were recorded in this study[11] may be related to interruption of the ascending vestibulo-oculomotor three-neuron arc.

Forty percent of 53 patients with probable brain stem multiple sclerosis had subclinical abnormalities of saccadic eye movement, mainly long saccadic latencies and INO.[12] The detection rate of abnormalities with saccadic eye movement recordings was equal to that of visual evoked responses, but more than that of brain stem auditory evoked responses. Saccadic abnormalities in multiple sclerosis were also compared to findings with MRI: both methods were equally sensitive.[13]

There is now anatomic and neurophysiologic evidence that the MLF contains not only ascending fibers but descending fibers, which relay burst-tonic information of both vertical and horizontal saccades and eye position to the flocculus via a cell group that is called "cell group of the paramedian tracts" or "paramedian continuum."[14] This paramedian continuum is interspersed between the fascicles of the MLF and the paramedian tracts in the caudal pons and medulla, and also constitutes the rostral part of the classic abducens nucleus.[14] Damage to the descending MLF pathway should lead to a disturbance of gaze-holding in the horizontal and vertical plane, a disturbance that has been observed in primates and patients with MLF lesions.[14]

As mentioned previously, INO may be caused by almost everything. As rare causes of bilateral INO, a fourth ventricular dermoid tumor[15] and acute cervical hyperextension have been reported.[16] The clinical picture of a complete bilateral INO was simulated in a patient with botulinum intoxication.[17] Another cause of increasing importance that has to be included in the differential diagnosis of INO is human immunodeficiency virus (HIV) encephalitis.[18, 19]

Two cases with a one-and-a-half syndrome were reported, again illustrating the utility of MRI for the detection of small brain stem lesions.[20, 21] Myasthenic pseudo one-and-a-half syndrome now has joined myasthenic pseudo-INO.[22]

Disturbances of Vertical Gaze

The clinical picture of eye movement disorders resulting from midbrain lesions was reviewed by Bogousslavsky.[23] Keane has presented an extensive analysis of 206 patients with the pretectal syndrome he examined over an 18-year period.[24] He stresses the possible misinterpretation of peripheral eye movement abnormalities (e.g., myasthenia, thyroid eye disease, Miller-Fisher disease) or bilateral tonic pupils as a pretectal syndrome. Hydrocephalus, stroke, and tumor were the three most common causes of the pretectal syndrome. A case report of a fascicular third nerve paralysis with decreased vertical saccade velocity of the contralateral eye illustrates the diagnostic problem of distinguishing supranuclear from third cranial nerve nuclear disorders in patients with lesions including not only the third cranial nerve nucleus but spreading into neighboring supranuclear structures.[25] A clinicopathologic correlation study demonstrated that a vertical gaze paralysis can be produced by selective involvement of the rostral interstitial nucleus of the medial longitudinal fasciculus (riMLF).[26] The authors speculate whether the unilateral riMLF lesion may have disrupted bilateral upgaze excitatory and inhibitory inputs and unilateral downgaze excitatory inputs.

Lid movements are intimately coordinated with vertical eye movements. In vertical supranuclear gaze paralysis, marked lid retraction usually appears on attempted upgaze. A careful clinico-pathologic analysis of the opposite condition; i.e., a ptosis accompanying a supranuclear downgaze paralysis, was presented by Büttner-Ennever et al.[27] The patient had bilateral ptosis unaffected by any eye movement, a downgaze paralysis with absent saccades and smooth pursuit but intact VOR. Postmortem examination showed an astrocytoma invading the oculomotor nucleus including the central caudal nucleus, which probably caused the ptosis. The additional destruction of the supraoculomotor nucleus, which takes part in the supranuclear control of lid movements, may have aggravated the ptosis.

Lid-eye coordination during vertical gaze changes was examined with the magnetic search coil technique in man and monkey.[28] It was shown that the lid followed the eye almost as a shadow, and that the burst-tonic lid innervation is a copy of the oculomotor neuron activity associated with the concomitant vertical saccades. An enigma remains: how can the upper lid execute downward saccades in the absence of any electromyography activity?

Another mystery is the so-called double elevator paralysis, which now has been observed on the same side in identical twins.[29] Interestingly, Bell's phenomenon was preserved in the affected eye, which excludes a muscular or infranuclear defect and favors a supranuclear origin.

Hemispheric Control of Saccades and Pursuit

For a brief review of the hemispheric control of saccades, the reader is referred to reference 30. As this review shows, there is growing experimental and clinical evidence that the frontal lobe may participate in the generation of voluntary saccades, whereas the superior colliculus may be involved in reflexive saccades. This concept was supported by a detailed analysis of different saccadic tasks in a patient with a unilateral frontal lobe deficit.[31] Another problem represents the hemispheric lateralization of gaze mechanisms. By means of intracarotid sodium amylobarbitone injections hemispheric specialization was tested in 90 patients.[32] The results are consistent with right cerebral dominance for attentional intentional mechanisms directed at external space. The cerebral asymmetry for gaze may be considered a consequence of the evolutionary loss of attentional intentional gaze mechanisms by the left hemisphere as language function developed. Manual reaction time and reaction time to initiate a saccade to a predicted or unpredicted target were measured in patients with right and left frontal lobe and right parietal lobe lesions.[33] Men with right parietal lobe lesions and women with right frontal lobe lesions showed an overall elevation of manual but not of saccadic reaction time. This indicates that the cortical areas studied apparently were not necessary for directing visual attention with a saccadic task. However, patients with right frontal lobe lesions executed smaller saccades than healthy subjects if the target appeared in the direction previously indicated, and larger saccades if the target appeared opposite to the direction previously indicated. The effect was opposite following damage to the right parietal lobe. Although the processes of saccadic eye movements and attention and the phenomena of neglect and horizontal gaze paralysis are closely related, the underlying mechanisms and the causative lesions are separable as evidenced by a comparison of CT analysis and clinical observation in 48 patients with acute stroke syndrome.[34]

A negative presaccadic scalp potential most prominent at the vertex and a widespread positive presaccadic potential over the posterior scalp were recorded in healthy volunteers before self-initiated saccades.[35] The authors assume that these potentials reflect an activation of the supplementary eye field in the mesial frontal cortex and a presaccadic activation of the parietal occipital lobe even in the absence of visual targets. Cortical stimulation of the frontal lobes via chronically implanted subdural electrodes in fully alert patients always elicited contralateral saccades, either purely horizontal or oblique upward.[36] This finding is in good agreement with Foville's first description of conjugate gaze deviation after stroke.[37] An analogous observation of periods of rightward eye deviation and right-beating nystagmus, which alternated with upward eye deviation and upbeating nystagmus during epileptic seizures, was made in a comatose patient with a subdural hematoma in the left temporal region.[38] These two studies make it difficult to understand how the intact frontal lobe can take over the generation of ipsilateral saccades after a lesion to the contralateral frontal lobe.[39]

Horizontal smooth pursuit was recorded in 28 patients with discrete unilateral cerebral hemispheric lesions.[40] Gain was reduced in both directions in most patients. Of ten patients who had a lower gain for tracking toward the lesioned side, two had frontal lobe lesions and the other eight provided evidence for a pursuit pathway that originates from Brodmann areas 19 and 39 and descends to the brain stem through the posterior limb of the internal capsule. In another analysis of hemispheric tracking deficits that used step-ramp paradigms to control the retinal location of the visual stimulus, it has been possible to identify two distinct deficits of horizontal visual tracking that occur with unilateral cerebral lesions.[41] The first is a bidirectional deficit that affects both saccades and pursuit to stimuli moving in the visual hemifield contralateral to the side of the lesion and may be permanent. It is probably related to the temporal-occipital-parietal pit. The second tracking deficit is a unidirectional impairment of smooth pursuit for targets moving toward the side of the lesion and occurs in both hemifields. A short case report contains observations that may fit these basic studies. It presents conjugate eye deviation and nystagmus slow phases directed toward the side of temporo-occipital seizure activity.[42] The authors postulate epileptic activation of smooth pursuit pathways originating from temporo-occipital cortex.

It is still not clear how the cerebral hemispheres project to the motor nuclei of the brain stem and spinal cord. A recent clinico-pathologic study did not present any corticofugal projections to the ocular motor nuclei of the third and sixth cranial nerves.[43]

Diseases of the Nervous System Causing Disorders of Eye Movement

Fisher's Syndrome

The interest in Fisher's syndrome has faded in the past few years after some passionate debates. Three cases with repeatedly normal MRI images were reported to support a peripheral origin of the syndrome.[44] Contrast-enhanced CT scans and MRI images were also normal in a patient with uremia who developed Fisher's syndrome acutely after dialysis.[45] A supranuclear affection was postulated to explain the bilateral lid lag observed in three patients with Guillain-Barré syndrome.[46] Guillain-Barré syndrome with peripheral cranial nerve involvement may accompany the early stages of acquired immunodeficiency syndrome (AIDS).[47]

Acquired Immunodeficiency Syndrome

Recent reports suggest that early HIV infection of the central nervous system may directly affect ocular motility. Perhaps eye movement recordings may serve as a predictor of central nervous system involvement, especially in the AIDS-dementia complex[48] and help monitor responsiveness to therapy. Peak saccadic velocity was significantly lower and saccadic duration longer in patients with AIDS than in a control group.[49] Saccadic intrusions, hypometria, hypermetria, wrong-way saccades opposite to the target direction, and longer latencies were reported by others.[50] Further disorders were conjugate gaze paralysis with ipsilateral facial paresis, bilateral abducens paralysis, gaze paresis, internuclear ophthalmoplegia, and abducens nerve paresis.[18, 19, 51] Brain stem involvement and cortical lesions may give rise to oculomotor disturbances in patients with AIDS as illustrated by a case of acquired ocular motor apraxia related to bilateral frontoparietal lesions.[52] Effects on peripheral cranial nerves in patients with AIDS has been mentioned.[47] It is evident from these few reports that HIV infection has to be included in the differential diagnosis of oculomotor disorders of cortical, brain stem, or peripheral origin, especially in younger patients.

Neurodegenerative Diseases

The basal ganglia are thought to play an important role in the control of eye movements. The basal ganglia, pars reticularis, and caudate nucleus contribute to the suppression and initiation of saccadic eye movements by imposing or removing a tonic inhibition on the superior colliculus.[53] The major involvement of the basal ganglia appears to be the generation of voluntary saccades and the suppression of reflex saccades.[54] The observed saccadic abnormalities in Huntington disease and Parkinson's disease conform well to known disease pathologic progression and recent neurophysiologic data, whereas the disease process in progressive supranuclear palsy (PSP) and Wilson's disease is more widespread, making it difficult to assess the role of the basal ganglia in these diseases.[54] Neuropathologic findings in patients with PSP included extensive neuronal loss in deep subcortical gray matter such as globus pallidus, subthalamic nuclei, substantia nigra, red nucleus, dentate nucleus, and inferior olivary nucleus; neurofibrillary tangles were noted in the thalamus, hypothalamus, corpus striatum, nucleus basalis, locus coeruleus, pontine nuclei, midbrain pontine, and medullary reticular formation as well as in various cranial nerve nuclei.[55, 56] The role of the basal ganglia in the generation of smooth pursuit is not well understood.

In a group of 40 patients with PSP, many had longer or shorter saccadic latencies than those in healthy subjects when asked to refixate a peripheral target after removal of a central fixation mark (gap task).[57] Patients with short latencies made more mistakes when asked to saccade away from a peripheral target (antisaccade task), a behavior that may be related to frontal dysfunction. There was also a correlation between latency and frontal dysfunction as evaluated with neuropsychologic tests. The study suggests a severe impairment of the frontal inhibitory system involved in saccade initiation.

Saccade latency, amplitude and peak velocity, smooth pursuit peak velocity, optokinetic nystagmus maximal and mean velocities, and vestibulo-ocular reflex suppression were significantly altered in 45 patients with Parkinson's disease.[58] Saccade amplitude improved 90 minutes after a single oral dose of L-dopa, which suggests a possible dopaminergic control of some ocular movements. Saccades to a novel peripheral target were unimpaired in seven patients with Parkinson's disease in contrast to saccades to a remembered target location, which were dysmetric with a characteristic multistepping pattern.[59] These results support the assumption that there is a neural pathway for visually elicited saccades that can be distinguished from a pathway for non-visual saccades, which includes the basal ganglia and may be selectively impaired in Parkinson's disease. Antisaccadic tasks were not impaired in mild-to-moderate Parkinson's disease as opposed to saccades toward remembered target location.[60] Saccadic latency, gain, duration, or peak velocity of vertical saccades were not significantly different from normal in mild-to-moderate Parkinson's disease.[61] Supranuclear disturbances of ocular motility in Lytico-Bodig (amyotrophic lateral sclerosis/parkinsonism-dementia complex of Guam) were universal and sometimes very prominent as opposed to earlier reports in the literature.[62]

Eye movement recordings in 20 patients with mild cases of Huntington disease demonstrated lower saccadic peak velocities in the younger onset group and longer latencies in the older onset group, whereas the ability to maintain steady fixation in the face of a distracting visual stimulus was decreased to the same degree in both groups.[63] Saccadic latency and velocity-amplitude relationship were examined over 6 years in a patient with Huntington disease and in a patient with Alzheimer's disease.[64] The patient with Huntington disease showed some fluctuation of ocular motility dysfunction but no correlation with the clinical deterioration as opposed to the patient with Alzheimer's disease who suddenly showed prolonged latencies 1 year prior to the progression of the dementia. Both patients showed a significant correlation between latency and peak velocity, longer latencies being correlated to lower peak velocities, suggesting a common source within the frontal eyefields for both saccadic initiation and motor programming. A failure to inhibit anticipatory saccades was a prominent feature in patients with Alzheimer's disease.[65] Patients with Alzheimer's disease exhibited longer latencies and hypometria without an obvious correlation to the degree of the dementia. This is in contrast to patients with Huntington disease or PSP.

Ocular Motor Apraxia

The clinical expression of congenital ocular motor apraxia is variable and the spectrum of associated neuroradiologic abnormalities wide, allowing no definite correlation between cerebral defect and oculomotor deficit.[66] Hypoplasia of the corpus callosum and the cerebellum have been found to be associated malformations.[66] Another case of purely vertical ocular motor apraxia with normal horizontal saccades in a 4-year-old boy has been reported.[67] MRI demonstrated bilateral lesions at the mesencephalic-diencephalic junction.

A syndrome mimicking ataxia-telangiectasia is characterized by slowly progressive ataxia, choreoathetosis, and ocular motor apraxia in both the horizontal and the vertical planes.[68]

REFERENCES

1. Henn V, Hepp K, Vilis T: Rapid eye movement generation in the primate. Physiology, pathophysiology, and clinical implications. *Rev Neurol* 1989; 145:540–545.
2. Tan E, Kansu T: Bilateral horizontal gaze palsy in multiple sclerosis. *J Clin Neuro-ophthalmol* 1990; 10:124–127.
3. Bronstein AM, Morris J, DuBoulay G, et al: Abnormalities of horizontal gaze. Clinical, oculographic and magnetic resonance imaging findings. I. Abducens palsy. *J Neurol Neurosurg Psychiatry* 1990; 53:194–199.
4. Bronstein AM, Rudge P, DuBoulay G, et al: Abnormalities of horizontal gaze. Clinical, oculographic and magnetic resonance imaging findings. II. Gaze palsy and internuclear ophthalmoplegia. *J Neurol Neurosurg Psychiatry* 1990; 53:200–207.
5. Hommel M, Besson G, Tarel V, et al: L'imagerie par resonance magnétique dans les parlysies de l'oculomotricité horizontale par infarctus. *Rev Neurol* 1989; 144:18–24.
6. Masson C, Prier S, Masson M, et al: Paralysie unilatérale des saccades due à un tuberculome du pont. *Rev Neurol* 1989; 145:652–655.
7. Morgan DW, Honan W: Lateral gaze palsy due to a giant aneurysm of the posterior fossa. *J Neurol Neurosurg Psychiatry* 1988; 52:883–886.
8. Pierrot-Desilligny C, Rivaud S, Samson Y, et al: Some instructive cases concerning the circuitry of ocular smooth pursuit in the brainstem. *Neuro-ophthalmology* 1989; 9:31–42.
9. Mustari MJ, Fuchs A, Wallman J: Response properties of dorsolateral pontine units during smooth pursuit in the rhesus monkey. *J Neurophysiol* 1988; 60:664–686.
10. Suzuki DA, May JG, Keller EL, et al: Visual motion response properties of neurons in dorsolateral pontine nucleus of the alert monkey. *J Neurophysiol* 1990; 63:37–59.
11. Ranalli PJ, Sharpe JA: Vertical vestibulo-ocular reflex, smooth pursuit and eye-head tracking dysfunction in internuclear ophthalmoplegia. *Brain* 1988; 111:1299–1317.

12. Pitt MC, Rawles JM: The value of measuring saccadic eye movement in the investigation of non-compressive myelopathy. *J Neurol Neurosurg Psychiatry* 1989; 52:1157–1161.

13. Tedeschi G, Alloca S, Di Costanzo A, et al: Role of saccadic analysis in the diagnosis of multiple sclerosis in the era of magnetic resonance imaging. *J Neurol Neurosurg Psychiatry* 1989; 52:967–969.

14. Büttner-Ennever JA, Horn AKE, Schmidtke K: Cell group of the medial longitudinal fasciculus and paramedian tracts. *Rev Neurol* 1989; 145:533–539.

15. Tekkok IH, Ayberk G, Kansu T, et al: Bilateral internuclear ophthalmoplegia associated with fourth ventricular dermoid tumor. *J Clin Neuro-ophthalmol* 1989; 9:254–257.

16. Jammes JL: Bilateral internuclear ophthalmoplegia due to acute hyperextension without head trauma. *J Clin Neuro-ophthalmol* 1989; 9:112–115.

17. Ehrenreich H, Garner CG, Witt TN: Complete bilateral internal ophthalmoplegia as sole clinical sign of botulism: Confirmation of diagnosis by single fibre electromyography. *J Neurol* 1989; 236:243–245.

18. Fuller GN, Guiloff RJ, Scaravilli F, et al: Combined HIV-CMV encephalitis presenting with brainstem signs. *J Neurol Neurosurg Psychiatry* 1989; 52:957–979.

19. Pfister HW, Einhäupl KM, Büttner U, et al: Dissociated nystagmus as a common sign of ocular motor disorders in HIV-infected patients. *Eur Neurol* 1989; 29:277–280.

20. Hitchings L, Crum A, Troost BT: Isolated one-and-a-half syndrome from focal brainstem hypertensive hemorrhage: Precise localization with MRI. *Neurology* 1988; 38:1501–1502.

21. Martyn CN, Kean D: The one-and-a-half syndrome. Clinical correlation with a pontine lesion demonstrated by nuclear magnetic resonance imaging in a case of multiple sclerosis. *Br J Ophthalmol* 1988; 72:515–517.

22. Davis TL, Lavin PJM: Pseudo one-and-a-half syndrome with ocular myasthenia. *Neurology* 1989; 39:1553.

23. Bogousslavsky J: Syndromes oculomoteurs résultant de lésions mésencéphaliques chez l'homme. *Rev Neurol* 1989; 145:546–559.

24. Keane JR: The pretectal syndrome: 206 patients. *Neurology* 1990; 40:684–690.

25. Ferbert A, Mülliges W, Binopiek R: Fascicular third nerve palsy with decreased vertical saccade velocity of the contralateral eye. *Neuro-ophthalmology* 1989; 10:33–38.

26. Bogousslavsky J, Miklossy J, Regli F, et al: Vertical gaze palsy and selective unilateral infarction of the rostral interstitial nucleus of the medial longitudinal fasciculus (riMLF). *J Neurol Neurosurg Psychiatry* 1990; 53:67–71.

27. Büttner-Ennever JA, Acheson JF, Büttner U, et al: Ptosis and supranuclear downgaze paralysis. *Neurology* 1989; 39:385–389.

28. Becker W, Fuchs AF: Lid-eye coordination during vertical gaze changes in man and monkey. *J Neurophysiol* 1988; 60:1227–1252.

29. Bell JA, Fielder AR, Viney S: Congenital double elevator palsy in identical twins. *J Clin Neuro-ophthalmol* 1990; 10:32–34.

30. Pierrot-Deseilligny Ch: Contrôle cortical des saccades. *Rev Neurol* 1989; 145:596–604.

31. Moser A, Kömpf D: Unilateral visual exploration deficit in a frontal lobe lesion. *Neuro-ophthalmol* 1990; 10:39–44.

32. Meador KJ, Loring DW, Lee GP, et al: Hemispheric asymmetry for eye gaze mechanisms. *Brain* 1989; 112:103–111.

33. Nagel-Leiby S, Buchtel HA, Welch KMA: Cerebral control of directed visual attention and orienting saccades. *Brain* 1990; 113:237–276.

34. Kömpf D, Gmeiner H-J: Gaze palsy and visual hemineglect in acute hemisphere lesions. *Neuro-ophthalmology* 1989; 9:49–53.

35. Moster ML, Goldberg G: Topography of scalp potentials preceding self-initiated saccades. *Neurology* 1990; 40:644–648.

36. Godoy J, Lüders H, Dinner DS, et al: Versive eye movements elicited by cortical stimulation of the human brain. *Neurology* 1990; 40:296–299.

37. Foville AL: Note sur une paralysie peu connue de certains muscles de l'oeil et sa liaison avec quelques points d'anatomie et la physiologie de la protubérance annulaire. *Bull Soc Anat* 1858; 33:373–405.

38. Kaplan PW, Lesser RP: Vertical and horizontal epileptic gaze deviation and nystagmus. *Neurology* 1989; 39:1391–1393.

39. Steiner I, Melamed E: Conjugate eye deviation after acute hemispheric stroke. *Ann Neurol* 1984; 16:509–511.

40. Morrow MJ, Sharpe JA: Cerebral hemispheric localization of smooth pursuit asymmetry. *Neurology* 1990; 40:284–292.

41. Leigh RJ: Cortical control of ocular pursuit movements. *Rev Neurol* 1989; 145:605–612.

42. Tusa RJ, Kaplan PW, Hain TC, et al: Ipsiversive eye deviation and epileptic nystagmus. *Neurology* 1990; 40:662–665.

43. Iwatsubo T, Kuzura S, Kanemitsu A, et al: Corticofugal projections to the motor nuclei of the brainstem and spinal cord in humans. *Neurology* 1990; 40:309–312.

44. Ropper AH: Three patients with Fisher's syndrome and normal MRI. *Neurology* 1988; 38:1630–1631.

45. Galassi G, Cappelli G, Trevisan C: Acute Fisher's syndrome during the course of chronic uremia: Is the hemodialysis implicated in onset and relapse? *Eur Neurol* 1990; 30:84–86.

46. Tan E, Kansu T, Kirkali P, et al: Lid lag and the Guillain-Barré syndrome. *J Clin Neuroophthalmol* 1990; 10:121–123.

47. Bélec L, Gherardi R, Georges AJ, et al: Peripheral facial nerve paralysis and HIV infection: Report of four african cases and review of the literature. *J Neurol* 1989; 236:411–414.

48. Currie J, Benson E, Ramsden B, et al: Eye movement abnormalities as a predictor of the acquired immunodeficiency syndrome dementia complex. *Arch Neurol* 1988; 45:949–953.

49. Nguyen N, Rimmer S, Katz B: Slowed saccades in acquired immunodeficiency syndrome. *Am J Ophthalmol* 1989; 107:356–360.

50. Friedman DI, Feldon SE: Eye movements in acquired immunodeficiency syndrome. *Arch Neurol* 1989; 46:841.

51. Hamed LM, Schatz NJ, Galetta SL: Brainstem ocular motility defects and AIDS. *Am J Ophthalmol* 1988; 106:437–442.

52. Brekelmans GFJ, Tijssen CC: Acquired ocular motor apraxia in an AIDS patient with bilateral fronto-parietal lesions. *Neuro-ophthalmology* 1990; 10:53–56.

53. Hikosaka O: Role of basal ganglia in saccades. *Rev Neurol* 1989; 145:580–586.

54. Kennard C, Lueck CJ: Oculomotor abnormalities in diseases of the basal ganglia. *Rev Neurol* 1989; 145:587–595.

55. Kida M, Koo H, Grossniklaus HE, et al: Neuropathologic findings in progressive supranuclear palsy. *J Clin Neuro-ophthalmol* 1988; 8:161–170.

56. Destee A, Gray F, Parent M, et al: Comportement compulsif d'allure obsessionnelle et paralysie supranucléaire progressive. *Rev Neurol* 1990; 146:12–18.

57. Pierrot-Deseilligny C, Rivaud S, Pillon B, et al: Lateral visually guided saccades in progressive supranuclear palsy. *Brain* 1989; 112:471–487.

58. Rascol O, Clanet M, Montastruc JL, et al: Abnormal ocular movements in Parkinson's disease. Evidence for involvement of dopaminergic systems. *Brain* 1989; 112:1193–1214.

59. Crawford TJ, Henderson L, Kennard C: Abnormalities of nonvisually-guided eye movements in Parkinson's disease. *Brain* 1989; 112:1573–1586.

60. Lueck CJ, Tanyeri S, Crawford TJ, et al: Antisaccades and remembered saccades in Parkinson's disease. *J Neurol Neurosurg Psychiatry* 1990; 53:284–288.

61. Tanyeri S, Lueck CJ, Crawford TJ, et al: Vertical and horizontal saccadic eye movements in Parkinson's disease. *Neuro-ophthalmology* 1989; 9:165–177.

62. Lepore FE, Steele JC, Cox TA, et al: Supranuclear disturbances of ocular motility in Lytico-Bodig. *Neurology* 1988; 38:1849–1853.

63. Lasker AG, Zee DS, Hain TC, et al: Saccades in Huntington's disease: Slowing and dysmetria. *Neurology* 1988; 38:427–431.

64. Abel LA, DellÓsso LF, Rustad LC: Longitudinal saccadic changes in Huntington's disease and Alzheimer's disease. *Neuro-ophthalmology* 1988; 8:307–315.

65. Hotson JR, Steinke GW: Vertical and horizontal saccades in aging and dementia. Failure to inhibit anticipatory saccades. *Neuro-ophthalmology* 1988; 8:267–273.

66. Steinlin M, Martin E, Largo R, et al: Congenital ocular motor apraxia: A neurodevelopmental and neuroradiological study. *Neuro-ophthalmology* 1990; 10:27–32.

67. Ebner R, Lopez L, Ochoa S, et al: Vertical ocular motor apraxia. *Neurology* 1990; 40:712–713.

68. Aicardi J, Barbosa C, Andermann E, et al: Ataxia-ocular motor apraxia: A syndrome mimicking ataxia-telangiectasia. *Ann Neurol* 1988; 24:497–502.

CHAPTER 11

Nonmyasthenic Ophthalmoplegia

John W. Gittinger, Jr., M.D.

Professor of Surgery and Neurology, University of Massachusetts Medical School, Worcester, Massachusetts

ACQUIRED NEUROMUSCULAR OPHTHALMOPLEGIA

New evidence concerning the relationship of chronic progressive external ophthalmoplegia to mitochondrial metabolism has emerged. Although there are still unanswered questions, most cases of chronic progressive external ophthalmoplegia (CPEO) appear to be caused by deletions in mitochondrial DNA (mtDNA). The properties of mtDNA explain many of the clinical features of this syndrome.

Both mitochondria and nuclei contain DNA, but human mtDNA—a circular, double-stranded 16.5 kilobase molecule—encodes only 37 genes: a large and small ribosomal RNA (rRNA), 22 transfer RNAs (tRNA), and 13 structural peptides.[1] All 13 peptides are components of the multipeptide enzymes in the five mitochondrial respiratory chain complexes that perform oxidative phosphorylation to generate adenosine triphosphate, the carrier of the high-energy phosphate bond that is the energy currency of the cell.[2] MtDNA contains only about 1/200,000th of the genetic information present in the nuclear chromosomes,[3] and the remaining genes necessary to produce mitochondrial enzymes and other components of the organelle are nuclear. Each mitochondrion is thus the joint genetic product of nuclear and mitochondrial DNA.

Since mitochondria are thought to be descendants of aerobic bacteria that colonized primitive glycolytic eukaryotic cells, this implies a transfer of genetic information from the mitochondria to the nucleus over evolutionary time. The movement of genes to nuclear chromosomes may have stopped when the genetic code used by mtDNA diverged slightly from that used by all other living organisms.[1]

There are multiple copies (two to ten) of its DNA in each mitochondrion, and hundreds of mitochondria in each cell. As cells divide, the mitochondria randomly distribute among the daughter cells, allowing genetic diversity among daughter cell lines and the potential for selection in growing cell populations. MtDNA mutates at least five times as often as nuclear DNA, but the effects of a mutation may only appear when the number of copies of mtDNA containing this mutation reach a critical level. Cells containing a mixture of wild-type mtDNA and mutant mtDNA are termed heteroplasmic; those with pure wild or mutant mtDNA, homoplasmic. Tissues vary in their dependence on mitochondrial energy: the central nervous system most, followed by skeletal muscle, heart muscle, kidney, and liver.[2]

The presence of deletions in mtDNA is detected with an enzyme that cuts the circle at one point. The resulting linear DNA is electrophoresed: if there is a deletion in some of the DNA, two lines representing the two subpopulations, one migrating faster than normal, appear on the gel. Depending on the relative size of the two bands, the proportion of mtDNA with deletions can be estimated.

In early 1988, Holt and coworkers described deletions in 9 of 25 patients with mitochondrial myopathies, but did not further characterize the clinical features.[4] Lestienne and Ponsot then reported deletions in a patient with Kearns-Sayre syndrome,[5] prompting Holt and coworkers to summarize the clinical features of patients in their series, which had grown to 44 cases.[6] All 16 patients with deletions had CPEO, including 4 with Kearns-Sayre syndrome.

Subsequently, Zeviani and coworkers found deletions of mtDNA in all 7 cases of Kearns-Sayre syndrome studied, but no deletions in 3 patients with isolated ophthalmoplegia with ragged red fibers or in 6 patients with other mitochondrial encephalomyopathies.[7] Each of these 7 patients had at least 45% deleted mtDNA, and the deletions were not always the same.

This series was also expanded and, of 123 patients studied by Moraes and associates,[8] mtDNA deletions were present in 11 of 14 patients with typical Kearns-Sayre syndrome, 4 of 4 patients with probable Kearns-Sayre syndrome, and 17 of 36 patients with "ocular myopathy" alone. No deletions were encountered in a variety of other mitochondrial myopathies or encephalomyopathies, and the relative proportion of affected genomes varied from 27% to 85%. In total, they detected deletions in 32 of 123 patients; all 32 had CPEO. In 1 of the cases, a deletion was present in leukocyte mtDNA, but the proportion was lower than in muscle. Johns and coworkers had found an identical deletion in blood and muscle, also with a lower proportion in the blood.[9]

In a third and more extensive paper, Holt and coworkers detected deletions in 30 of 72 cases studied.[10] All 30 patients with deletions had CPEO, as did 12 of 42 patients without detectable deletions. In this series, deletions were found in muscle, but not blood, mitochondria.

Thus it appears that detectable deletions of mtDNA are characteristic of chronic progressive external ophthalmoplegia, but not of the mitochondrial encephalomyopathies in general. A patient with Kearns-Sayre syndrome is more likely to have a detectable deletion than a patient with isolated CPEO. A possible genetic justification for the separation of Kearns-Sayre syndrome from isolated CPEO as a distinct entity is the suggestion by Shanske and coworkers that patients with CPEO have deletions only in skeletal muscle, while those with Kearns-Sayre syndrome have more generalized abnormalities.[11] Their autopsy results of a 22-year-old woman with Kearns-Sayre syndrome found deletions in 50% to 60% of skeletal muscle mtDNA, 40% to 50% of brain mtDNA, and 14% to 19% of liver mtDNA, which were all the tissues examined. Southern blot analyses of five patients with isolated CPEO and two with Kearns-Sayre syndrome appear to support this hypothesis: heteroplasmic mtDNA was detectable only in muscle in isolated CPEO, but in all organs investigated in Kearns-Sayre.[12]

The explanation for the occurrence of Kearns-Sayre syndrome without detectable mtDNA deletions is uncertain. Two hypotheses are the limitations of current methods of detection—point or small mutations at critical sites would be missed—or the existence of two different diseases with the same manifestations, the second perhaps the result of a nuclear mutation. Genetic studies imply that nuclear genes are involved in some cases of mitochondrial myopathy.[13] Full sequencing of portions of the mtDNA in such patients may be necessary to answer this question. The genetic picture is further complicated by the existence of cases in which the mtDNA is duplicated, not deleted.[14]

Deletions of mtDNA have been traced to a portion of the genome coding for parts of the respiratory chain complex, which would explain the partial decrease in cytochrome c oxidase activity observed biochemically and histochemically[15] and the severe deficiency of cytochrome aa_3.[16] The deletions are not the same size in each case, but are consistent in samples taken from one individual and appear preferentially to affect "hot spots" on the mitochondrial genome. At least one of these hotspots lies between two 13 base-pair repeats, suggesting either what is called "a homologous recombination event," something that had only been previously recognized in lower eucaryotes and plants,[17] or "slip-replication" during transcription.[18] Deleted mtDNA genomes are transcribed but not translated, because of the lack of indispensable mtDNA-encoded tRNAs, resulting in the failure of synthesis of respiratory-chain polypeptides.[19]

In one study, treatment with coenzyme Q10 improved neurologic function but had no effect on the ophthalmoplegia or the electrocardiogram.[20] The treatment of another patient with succinate and coenzyme Q10 led to improvement of vital capacity, with respiratory failure when the drugs were discontinued.[18]

The reason why external ophthalmoplegia is such an important manifestation of mtDNA deletion disorders is unknown. One hypothesis is that small muscles, such as ocular muscles, are derived from relatively few embryonic cells. The proportion of mitochondria with deletions could be higher than that in a large muscle and the metabolic demands greater.[10] Also, the mitochondrial volume fraction of extraocular muscles is higher than in limb muscles.[8]

Another unique feature of mtDNA is its exclusive maternal transmission. This has demonstrated relevance in Leber's hereditary optic neuropathy, the other major neuro-ophthalmic disorder related to mtDNA.[21] Most cases of mitochondrial myopathy appear to be caused by mutations in the oocyte or zygote, rather than by direct inheritance from the mother.[8, 12] Similar but not identical deletions, however, have been demonstrated in one mother and daughter with CPEO.[22] Rowland and coworkers discuss the genetic implications of Kearns-Sayre syndrome in Polish twins in the same issue of *Neurology* in which deletions are reported.[23]

Endomyocardial biopsy specimens of nine patients with Kearns-Sayre syndrome revealed abnormal mitochondria.[24] The criteria for pacemaker implantation are discussed in two patients,[25] and dilated cardiomyopathy developed years after pacemaker placement in another man, suggesting eventual exhaustion of cardiac mitochondrial function.[26] Lesions resembling demyelination may be detected on cerebral magnetic resonance imaging (MRI) in Kearns-Sayre syndrome.[27]

Wilson and associates review a more prosaic form of acquired neuromuscular ophthalmoplegia that they prefer to call Brown's syndrome rather than Brown's superior oblique tendon sheath syndrome.[28] Their well-argued thesis is that both congenital and acquired Brown's syndrome are part of a continuum of dysfunction at the trochlear/tendon complex. Superior oblique tenotomy with or without inferior oblique recession is the recommended procedure of choice in congenital Brown's syndrome, and injection of steroids in the region of the trochlea may be useful in acquired inflammatory syndromes. Many acquired and some congenital cases of Brown's syndrome improve spontaneously, indicating a conservative approach unless the deficit is severe (i.e., produces abnormal head posture) and persistent. Two siblings with bilateral Brown's syndrome are described,[29] as are another set of monozygotic twins with mirror-image Brown's syndrome,[30] confirming a genetic factor. Causes of acquired Brown's syndrome include peribulbar anesthesia,[31] blepharoplasty,[32] frontal sinus osteoma,[33] and pansinusitis.[34] Surgery in the region of the trochlea may also cause isolated superior oblique dysfunction.[35]

Diffuse infiltration of the extraocular muscles in primary systemic amyloidosis produced ophthalmoplegia.[36] Although pathologic confirmation has been obtained only in secondary amyloidosis, it seems reasonable to add primary systemic amyloidosis to the long list of processes other than Grave's orbitopathy that enlarge the extraocular muscles.[37]

CONGENITAL NEUROMUSCULAR OPHTHALMOPLEGIA

Congenital bilateral superior oblique palsy is a common feature of Apert's syndrome (craniosynostosis with syndactyly of the toes and fingers).[38] At surgery, the superior oblique tendon was often absent or rudimentary. Neuro-imaging studies have also demonstrated the congenital absence or hypoplasia of extraocular muscles in congenital superior oblique palsy[39] and in congenital fibrosis of the inferior rectus muscles with blepharoptosis.[40]

MRI of a child with congenital bilateral third nerve palsies, however, demonstrated hypoplasia of the ventral midbrain.[41] Only computed tomography (CT) was performed in a woman with arthrogryposis multiplex congenita and bilateral ophthalmoplegia.[42] This and other studies failed to elucidate the mechanism for the congenital ophthalmoplegia.

Arthrogryposis multiplex congenita is most often associated with Möbius' syndrome, but an affected individual who also had synergistic divergence was studied by Cruysberg and coworkers.[43] On the basis of this case and another and a review of the literature, these authors concur that synergistic divergence is a variant of Duane's syndrome. Brodsky and coworkers provide a cogent discussion of a truly remarkable child with the combination of congenital fibrosis, synergistic divergence, Marcus Gunn jaw winking, and oculocutaneous albinism.[44] The neural misconnections in this little boy boggle the mind.

The basis for the diagnosis of cat-eye syndrome in a child with Duane's syndrome and multiple congenital anomalies is obscure, since neither anal atresia nor iris colobomas are described.[45] The third example of discordance for Duane's syndrome in identical twins has been reported.[46] (An instance of twins concordant for congenital double elevator palsy is described.[47]) Dissociated vertical deviation was present in an 18-year-old woman with bilateral Duane's syndrome.[48] Seven of 44 patients with Duane's syndrome who were screened had hearing impairment.[49]

The spectrum of limb deformities associated with Möbius' syndrome is exhaustively reviewed by Miller and coworkers.[50] A native American child had Möbius' syndrome, transposition of the great vessels, and absence of the left hand.[51] Harbord and coworkers explain the association of Möbius' syndrome and unilateral cerebellar hypoplasia by a vascular disruption in the basilar artery circulation early in development.[52] Lipson and coworkers review the evidence in rats and humans that Möbius' syndrome is the consequence of a transient ischemic/hypoxic insult to the fetus,[53] and Möbius' is the "Syndrome of the Month" in the *Journal of Medical Genetics*.[54]

ACQUIRED LESIONS OF THE OCULAR MOTOR NERVES

Third Cranial Nerve Palsies

Neuro-ophthalmologists should not share the contempt many academics have for case reports, since much of what we know is the cumulative experience contained in many single cases. Even though thousands of patients with isolated ocular motor cranial nerve palsies have been reported, new insights from individual cases still are possible. In brief papers whose titles could serve as their abstracts, Lustbader and Miller[55] describe a third cranial nerve palsy complete except for the pupil, and Good[56] reports isolated ptosis, both caused by aneurysms. Those who like to cling to clinical maxims will note that the pupil-sparing third cranial nerve palsy was painless, and the ptosis was accompanied by headache. In another case with headache, ptosis was found initially, a partial third cranial nerve palsy evolved and then resolved, but angiography revealed a posterior communicating aneurysm.[57]

The age limits for aneurysmal third cranial nerve palsies have also been stretched. A case in a 14-year-old girl occasions a reassessment of the evidence, with the conclusion that angiography is unnecessary under age 10 if a neuro-imaging study is normal.[58] An accompanying editorial by a neuro-radiologist points out that MRI is not yet a substitute for angiography in the demonstration of small aneurysms.[59] Two other cases of aneurysms in 6- and 15-year-old patients had abnormalities on contrast-enhanced CT scans.[60, 61]

Do these observations mean that all patients with third cranial nerve palsies should undergo angiography? Trobe again wrestles with this issue and concludes that even though, with careful clinical criteria, some aneurysmal third cranial nerve palsies will be missed unless angiography is performed, his answer is still no.[62] The decision to perform a test depends on several variables: the prevalence of the disease in the population that the patient represents (aneurysmal third cranial nerve palsies must be pretty uncommon in children if the reported cases can be counted on the fingers of one hand), the risk of the test (angiography in a child includes the risk of general anesthesia), the likelihood that intervention will be successful (attempts at occluding the basilar aneurysm in Lustbader and Miller's case were not), and the sensitivity and specificity of the test (how much more sensitive is angiography than MRI in demonstrating aneurysms?).

These factors are difficult but not impossible to quantify and can be analyzed formally. A perusal of the considerable literature on clinical decision-making may not change the way you think, but certainly expands your vocabulary. For an introduction to Bayesean statistics, interested readers may want to consult Sox's brief review.[63]

My own tentative conclusion is that neuro-imaging studies are warranted in almost all cases of third cranial nerve dysfunction, with MRI preferable in adults or older children in whom sedation is not required to perform the study and there are no contraindications (pacemaker, other metallic foreign bodies) to MRI. I would still not image a truly isolated ptosis; i.e. not accompanied by headache or other findings.

Although ptosis was the presenting complaint in three patients with pituitary adenoma encountered by Yen and coworkers,[64] all three had other abnormalities on careful neuro-ophthalmic examination. Recurrent ptosis with headache led to the diagnosis of pituitary adenoma in an 11-year-old girl.[65]

MRI has also forced revision of the localization of isolated, partial third cranial nerve palsies. While some clinical observations suggested a mesencephalic site,[66] most cases studied pathologically had peripheral lesions. Imaging studies now commonly localize vascular (and demyelinating[67]) partial third cranial nerve palsies to the brain stem.[68-70] Selective involvement of superior division functions does not reliably localize the lesion to the anatomic superior division.[71]

The site of the lesion in a 29-year-old woman with a partial third cranial nerve palsy that responded to time or steroids and led to the diagnosis of systemic lupus erythematosus was not identified.[72] Likewise, a transient superior division palsy in a 13-year-old girl is attributed to ophthalmoplegic migraine because of a history of three episodes of transient ptosis without diplopia and an otherwise negative workup including angiography but not MRI.[73] A patient with bilateral, almost complete ophthalmoplegia is said to have ophthalmoplegic migraine, but had increased cerebrospinal fluid protein and may have had the Fisher variant of Guillain-Barré syndrome.[74]

A painful third cranial nerve palsy may be the only manifestation of posteriorly draining dural-cavernous sinus shunts, which do not necessarily initially manifest the tortuous episcleral veins typical of anteriorly draining shunts.[75] Repeat imaging of children with chronic third cranial nerve palsies may eventually demonstrate tumors presumed to be schwannomas.[76] From the endocrinologic literature comes the interesting but unsurprising observation that pupil-sparing diabetic third cranial nerve palsies recover more rapidly (about 6 weeks) than those involving the pupil (about 14 weeks).[77] What is thought to be the seventh family with recurrent facial and ocular motor palsies beginning after age 30 years is reported from Denmark.[78] Animal studies indicate that the CO_2 milliwatt laser may be useful in surgical repair of severed ocular motor nerves.[79]

The multiple functions subserved by the third cranial nerve lead to some interesting phenomena. A child with periodic movements of the lid and pupil probably had partial ocular motor palsy with cyclic spasms.[80] Ephaptic transmission is resurrected to explain transient oculomotor synkinesis.[81] Guy and coworkers make a valiant effort to provide a mechanism for contralateral synkinesis when movements typical of oculomotor synkinesis appear in the fellow eye of a patient with traumatic third cranial nerve palsy.[82] Jordan and coworkers attribute widening of the palpebral fissure on abduction in a 26-year-old man with bilateral aberrant regeneration of the third cranial nerve to connections between injured third and sixth cranial nerves in the superior orbital fissure.[83] Rhythmic pupillary contractions in a post-traumatic third cranial nerve palsy are a mystery.[84]

Fourth Cranial Nerve Palsies

Caudal mesencephalic lesions that cause fourth cranial nerve palsies are also being imaged.[85] In two cases, bilateral fourth cranial nerve palsies were one sign of a spontaneous brain stem hemorrhage.[86, 87] Inpatient evaluation of an isolated right fourth cranial nerve palsy led to demonstration by MRI of a vascular malformation replacing a portion of the right inferior colliculus and projecting into the quadrigeminal cistern.[88] A fourth cranial nerve palsy and headache following subconcussive head trauma were attributed to a tentorial vascular malformation when the imaged lesion, initially thought to represent a meningioma, spontaneously resolved.[89] Guy and coworkers confirm that the combination of fourth cranial nerve palsy on one side and Horner's syndrome on the other points to a lesion in the mesencephalon on the side of the Horner's syndrome.[90]

With regard to specific causes of fourth cranial nerve palsies, a small intracavernous aneurysm was detected but not surgically treated, and the isolated palsy resolved with time and management of hypertension.[91] The reasoning that led to angiography is not apparent. An orbital apex mass was imaged in a woman with Waldenström's macroglobulinemia and a fourth cranial nerve palsy; the mass and the palsy resolved with corticosteroid and radiation therapy.[92] Bilateral fourth cranial nerve palsy and papilledema were the presentation of a cerebellar hemangioblastoma,[93] and bilateral superior oblique palsies were part of the clinical syndrome in three cases of hydrocephalus.[94] In two of the patients with hydrocephalus, improvement ensued after shunting.

Of 50 consecutive cases of superior oblique palsy seen at Montreal Children's Hospital, 22 were congenital, 9 post-traumatic, and 19 idiopathic.[95] In a series from Israel, 75% of 24 post-traumatic fourth cranial nerve palsies resolved spontaneously in an average of 9.2 months.[96] Complicating the interpretation of this statistic is the inclusion of 11 patients who recalled minor trauma only after direct questioning. Imaging in a chronic fourth cranial nerve palsy may only demonstrate atrophy of the superior oblique muscle.[97]

Entering the neuro-ophthalmologic twilight zone, consider the case of a 38-year-old man with neurofibromatosis whose surgery for a cerebellopontine angle tumor led to the incidental discovery of a meningotheliomatous meningioma of the trochlear nerve. This was removed, along with the nerve itself, but ocular motility remained normal.[98] Similarly, a schwannoma of the fourth cranial nerve caused weakness and clumsiness of the right arm and leg and slurring of speech with normal ocular motility.[99] Or perhaps you prefer to contemplate a patient with rheumatoid arthritis, a chronic fourth cranial nerve palsy, and an episode of transient oscillopsia and downbeating nystagmus with normal MRI, who developed limitation of abduction thought to be caused by infiltration of the medial rectus muscle by a rheumatoid nodule.[100]

Sixth Cranial Nerve Palsy

Anyone surprised to learn that intrapontine lesions causing isolated sixth cranial nerve palsies are being imaged with increasing frequency should re-read the sections on third and fourth cranial nerve palsies.[101, 102] An elegant analysis of MRI points to the posterior half of the abducens fasciculus as the critical lesion site when the palsy is associated with other findings.[103] Even with modern neuro-imaging studies, however, the etiology of chronic sixth cranial nerve palsies may be elusive. Galletta and Smith offer a 25-year perspective that supports the proposition that slow-growing tumors—brain stem gliomas, chordomas, chondrosarcomas, and meningiomas—should be suspected.[104] In two patients with trigeminal schwannomas, the presentation was an isolated sixth cranial nerve palsy without fifth cranial nerve dysfunction, and CT was initially normal.[105]

A solitary intracranial plasmacytoma represents a potentially treatable cause of chronic sixth cranial nerve palsy.[106] The discovery of an intracavernous aneurysm in a young woman with isolated sixth cranial nerve palsy does not justify the conclusion that angiography should be performed in all such cases, but instead argues for MRI.[107] Pain was prominent in a 56-year-old man whose sixth cranial nerve palsy was initially attributed to temporal arteritis.[108] Serendipitous treatment with corticosteroids produced improvement in what was eventually proven by biopsy to be idiopathic inflammation of the orbit and cavernous sinus—the Tolosa-Hunt syndrome. MRI may be superior to CT in imaging the cavernous sinus abnormalities seen in Tolosa-Hunt syndrome.[109] A report of 165 isolated sixth cranial nerve palsies from Germany confirms the causes found in previous series, although a surprisingly large number (11 cases) are attributed to multiple sclerosis.[110]

Two almost identical cases of trigemino-abducens synkinesis following severe head trauma indicate that the motor fibers of the fifth cranial nerve can reconnect via aberrant regeneration to the ipsilateral sixth cranial nerve.[111, 112] The eye abducts on jaw movement.

Since transient sixth cranial nerve palsies are well-known complications of lumbar punctures, the explanation that iopamidol used in myelography is potentially neurotoxic seems superfluous.[113] A transient sixth cranial nerve palsy complicated acute psittacosis in a 49-year-old English woman.[114]

A temporal artery biopsy in a 79-year-old man with slowly progressive bilateral sixth cranial nerve palsies led to the diagnosis—despite lack of visceral involvement—of polyarteritis nodosa.[115] Since the pathologic findings were only apparent in a branch artery segment, the authors suggest that an attempt be made to include such branches in biopsy specimens. Bilateral sixth cranial nerve palsy with unilateral Horner's syndrome resulted from a pontine hemorrhage.[116]

ACQUIRED MULTIPLE CRANIAL NEUROPATHY

The report from Turkey in the *Journal of Clinical Neuro-ophthalmology* of a papillary carcinoma and abscess of the sphenoid sinus could use some editing.[117] For one thing, the patient has an orbital apex syndrome, not a cavernous sinus syndrome. A cavernous sinus syndrome was the presentation of a malignant lymphoma.[118] The diagnosis was made at craniotomy. Craniotomy and biopsy of the clivus and posterior orbital apex failed to demonstrate the tumor in a 44-year-old man with third, fourth, and fifth cranial nerve palsies.[119] Given the unimpressive CT scans, this is not surprising. At postmortem, a primary central nervous system melanoma infiltrating the leptomeninges was found. Lentigo malignant melanoma of the forehead extended neurotropically into the cavernous sinus to produce painful ophthalmoplegia, underwent neurosarcomatous degeneration, and then invaded the orbit.[120] This type of tumor must be identified with immunocytochemical staining.

A 74-year-old man sagely refused to return to his neurologist for further workup when his ophthalmoplegia and facial and corneal sensory changes spontaneously resolved.[121] The clinical significance of the beautiful MRI studies demonstrating dolichoectasia in this case is thus unclear. Sixth cranial nerve and contralateral seventh cranial nerve palsy were the focal signs of a brain stem hemorrhage in a 23-year-old pregnant woman.[122] A cavernous hemangioma was identified and successfully removed. Embolic infarction was the presumed cause of partial right third and left fourth cranial nerve palsies following percutaneous transluminal coronary angioplasty, although the lesion was not imaged.[123] The authors of this report struggle to localize the responsible lesion, discarding a brain stem site because of unilateral ptosis. Intrafascicular central lesions would, however, explain their findings.

Wilson and coworkers attribute transient ophthalmoparesis ipsilateral to carotid occlusion to ischemia in the nutrient circulation of the ocular motor nerves.[124] All three cases had blindness from central retinal artery occlusion, and the possibility of an ischemic myopathy is not considered. Low intraocular pressures would have supported acute orbital ischemia, but the results of tonometry are not mentioned. Another small series confirms that many post-zoster ophthalmoplegias recover spontaneously.[125]

Facial palsy followed by transient ipsilateral complete external ophthalmoplegia sparing the pupil is attributed to cavernous sinus ischemia.[126] The discussion does not address the fact that the facial nerve passes nowhere near the cavernous sinus.

REFERENCES

1. Zeviani M, Bonilla E, DeVivo DC, et al: Mitochondrial diseases. *Neurol Clin* 1989; 7:123–156.
2. Wallace DC: Mitochondrial DNA mutations and neuromuscular disease. *Trends Genet* 1989; 5:9–13.
3. Morris MA: Mitochondrial mutations in neuro-ophthalmological diseases: A review. *J Clin Neuro Ophthalmol* 1990; 10:159–166.
4. Holt IJ, Harding AE, Morgan-Hughes JA: Deletions of muscle mitochondrial DNA in patients with mitochondrial myopathies. *Nature* 1988; 331:717–719.
5. Lestienne P, Ponsot G: Kearns-Sayre syndrome with muscle mitochondrial DNA deletion. *Lancet* 1988; 1:885.
6. Holt IJ, Cooper JM, Morgan-Hughes JA, et al: Deletions of muscle mitochondrial DNA. *Lancet* 1988; 1:1462.
7. Zeviani M, Moraes CT, DiMauro S, et al: Deletions of mitochondrial DNA in Kearns-Sayre syndrome. *Neurology* 1988; 38:1339–1346.
8. Moraes CT, DiMauro S, Zevani M, et al: Mitochondrial DNA deletions in progressive external ophthalmoplegia and Kearns-Sayre syndrome. *N Engl J Med* 1989; 320:1293–1299.
9. Johns DR, Drachman DB, Hurko O: Identical mitochondrial DNA deletion in blood and muscle. *Lancet* 1989; 1:393–394.
10. Holt IJ, Harding AE, Cooper JM, et al: Mitochondrial myopathies: Clinical and biochemical features of 30 patients with major deletions of muscle mitochondrial DNA. *Ann Neurol* 1989; 26:699–708.

11. Shanske S, Moraes CT, Lombes A, et al: Widespread tissue distribution of mitochondrial DNA deletions in Kearns-Sayre syndrome. *Neurology* 1990; 40:24–28.

12. Zeviani M, Gellera C, Pannacci M, et al: Tissue distribution and transmission of mitochondrial DNA deletions in mitochondrial myopathies. *Ann Neurol* 1990; 28:94–97.

13. Harding AE, Petty RKH, Morgan-Hughes JA: Mitochondrial myopathy: A genetic study of 71 cases. *J Med Genet* 1988; 25:528–535.

14. Poulton J, Deadman ME, Gardiner RM: Duplications of mitochondrial DNA in mitochondrial myopathy. *Lancet* 1989; 1:236–240.

15. Romero NB, Lestienne P, Marsac C, et al: Immunocytological and histochemical correlation in Kearns-Sayre syndrome with mtDNA deletion and partial cytochrome c oxidase deficiency in skeletal muscle. *J Neurol Sci* 1989; 93:297–309.

16. Martens ME, Peterson PL, Lee CP: Kearns-Sayre syndrome: Biochemical studies of mitochondrial metabolism. *Ann Neurol* 1988; 24:630–637.

17. Schon EA, Rizzuto R, Moraes CT, et al: A direct repeat is a hotspot for large-scale deletion of human mitochondrial DNA. *Science* 1989; 244:346–349.

18. Shoffner JM, Lott MT, Voljavec AS, et al: Spontaneous Kearns-Sayre/chronic external ophthalmoplegia plus syndrome associated with a mitochondrial DNA deletion: A slip-replication model and metabolic therapy. *Proc Natl Acad Sci USA* 1989; 86:7952–7956.

19. Nakase H, Moraes CT, Rizzuto R, et al: Transcription and translation of deleted mitochondrial genomes in Kearns-Sayre syndrome: Implications for pathogenesis. *Am J Hum Genet* 1990; 46:418–427.

20. Bresolin N, Bet L, Binda A, et al: Clinical and biochemical correlations in mitochondrial myopathies treated with coenzyme Q10. *Neurology* 1988; 38:892–899.

21. Harding AE: The mitochondrial genome—breaking the magic circle. *N Engl J Med* 1989; 320:1341–1343.

22. Ozawa T, Yoneda M, Tanaka M, et al: Maternal inheritance of deleted mitochondrial DNA in a family with mitochondrial myopathy. *Biochem Biophys Res Commun* 1988; 154:1240–1247.

23. Rowland LP, Hausmanowa-Petrusewicz I, Bardurska B, et al: Kearns-Sayre syndrome in twins: Lethal dominant mutation or acquired disease? *Neurology* 1988; 38:1399–1402.

24. Schwartzkopff B, Frenzel H, Breithardt G, et al: Ultrastructural findings in endomyocardial biopsy of patients with Kearns-Sayre syndrome. *J Am Coll Cardiol* 1988; 12:1522–1528.

25. Polak PE, Zijlstra F, Roelandt RTC: Indications for pacemaker implantation in the Kearns-Sayre syndrome. *Eur Heart J* 1989; 10:281–282.

26. Tveskov C, Angelo-Nielsen K: Kearns-Sayre syndrome and dilated cardiomyopathy. *Neurology* 1990; 40:553–554.

27. Elsas T, Rinck PA, Isaksen C, et al: Cerebral nuclear magnetic resonance in Kearns syndrome. *Acta Ophthalmol* 1988; 66:469–473.

28. Wilson ME, Eustis HS Jr, Parks MM: Brown's syndrome. *Surv Ophthalmol* 1989; 34:153–172.

29. Moore AT, Walker J, Taylor D: Familial Brown's syndrome. *J Pediatr Ophthalmol Strabismus* 1988; 25:202–204.

30. Wortham EV, Crawford JS: Brown's syndrome in twins. *Am J Ophthalmol* 1988; 105:562–563.

31. Erie JC: Acquired Brown's syndrome after peribulbar anesthesia. *Am J Ophthalmol* 1990; 109:349–350.

32. Neely KA, Ernest JT, Mottier M: Combined superior oblique paresis and Brown's syndrome after blepharoplasty. *Am J Ophthalmol* 1990; 109:347–349.

33. Biedner B, Monos T, Frilling F, et al: Acquired Brown's syndrome caused by frontal sinus osteoma. *J Pediatr Ophthalmol Strabismus* 1988; 25:226–229.

34. Saunders RA, Stratas BA, Gordon RA, et al: Acute-onset Brown's syndrome associated with pansinusitis. *Arch Ophthalmol* 1990; 108:58–60.

35. Couch JM, Somers ME, Gonzalez C: Superior oblique muscle dysfunction following anterior ethmoidal artery ligation for epistaxis. *Arch Ophthalmol* 1990; 108:1110–1113.

36. Katz B, Leja S, Melles RB, et al: Amyloid ophthalmoplegia; Ophthalmoparesis secondary to primary systemic amyloidosis. *J Clin Neuro Ophthalmol* 1989; 9:39–42.

37. Patrinely JR, Osborn AG, Anderson RL, et al: Computed tomographic features of nonthyroid extraocular muscle enlargement. *Ophthalmology* 1989; 96:1038–1047.

38. Pollard ZF: Bilateral superior oblique muscle palsy associated with Apert's syndrome. *Am J Ophthalmol* 1988; 106:337–340.

39. Matsuo T, Ohtsuki H, Sogabe Y, et al: Vertical abnormal retinal correspondence in three patients with congenital absence of the superior oblique muscle. *Am J Ophthalmol* 1988; 106:341–345.

40. Hupp SL, Williams JP, Curran JE: Computerized tomography in the diagnosis of congenital fibrosis syndrome. *J Clin Neuro Ophthalmol* 1990; 10:135–139.

41. Flanders M, Watters G, Draper J, et al: Bilateral congenital third cranial nerve palsy. *Can J Ophthalmol* 1989; 24:28–30.

42. Zeiter JH, Boniuk M: Ophthalmologic findings associated with arthrogryposis multiplex congenita: Case report and review of the literature. *J Pediatr Ophthalmol Strabismus* 1989; 26:204–207.

43. Cruysberg JRM, Mtanda AT, Duinkerke-Eerola KU, et al: Congenital adduction palsy and synergistic divergence: A clinical and electro-oculography study. *Br J Ophthalmol* 1989; 73:68–75.

44. Brodsky MC, Pollock SC, Buckley EG: Neural misdirection in congenital ocular fibrosis syndrome: Implications and pathogenesis. *J Pediatr Ophthalmol Strabismus* 1989; 26:159–161.

45. Kalpakian B, Choy AE, Sparkes RS, et al: Duane syndrome associated with features of the cat-eye syndrome and mosaicism for a supernumerary chromosome probably derived from number 22. *J Pediatr Ophthalmol Strabismus* 1988; 25:293–297.

46. Kaufman LW, Folk ER, Miller MT: Monozygotic twins discordant for Duane's retraction syndrome. *Arch Ophthalmol* 1989; 107:324–325.

47. Bell JA, Fielder AR, Viney S: Congenital double elevator palsy in identical twins. *J Clin Neuro Ophthalmol* 1990; 10:32–34.

48. Rimmer S, Katz B: Dissociated vertical deviation in a patient with Duane's retraction syndrome. *J Clin Neuro Ophthalmol* 1990; 10:38–40.

49. Ro A, Chernoff G, MacRae D, et al: Auditory function in Duane's retraction syndrome. *Am J Ophthalmol* 1990; 109:75–78.

50. Miller MT, Ray V, Owens P, et al: Möbius and Möbius-like syndromes (TTV-OFM, OMLH). *J Pediatr Ophthalmol Strabismus* 1989; 26:176–188.

51. Raroque HG Jr, Hershewe GL, Snyder RD: Möbius syndrome and transposition of the great vessels. *Neurology* 1988; 38:1894–1895.

52. Harbord MG, Finn JP, Hall-Craggs MA, et al: Moebius' syndrome with unilateral cerebellar hypoplasia. *J Med Genet* 1989; 26:579–582.

53. Lipson AH, Webster WS, Brown-Woodman PDC, et al: Moebius syndrome: Animal model—human correlations and evidence for a brainstem vascular etiology. *Teratology* 1989; 40:339–350.

54. Kumar D: Moebius syndrome. *J Med Genet* 1990; 27:122–126.

55. Lustbader JM, Miller NR: Painless, pupil-sparing but otherwise complete oculomotor nerve paresis caused by basilar artery aneurysm. *Arch Ophthalmol* 1988; 106:583–584.

56. Good EF: Ptosis as the sole manifestation of compression of the oculomotor nerve by an aneurysm of the posterior communicating artery. *J Clin Neuro Ophthalmol* 1990; 10:59–61.

57. Greenspan BN, Reeves AG: Transient partial oculomotor nerve paresis with posterior communicating artery aneurysm; A case report. *J Clin Neuro Ophthalmol* 1990; 10:56–58.

58. Gabianelli EB, Klingele TG, Burde RM: Acute oculomotor nerve palsy in childhood; Is angiography necessary? *J Clin Neuro Ophthalmol* 1989; 9:33–36.

59. Fox AJ: Angiography for third nerve palsy in children. *J Clin Neuro Ophthalmol* 1989; 9:37–38.

60. Ebner R: Angiography for IIIrd nerve palsy in children. *J Clin Neuro Ophthalmol* 1990; 10:154–155.

61. Pollard ZF: Aneurysm causing third nerve palsy in a 15-year-old boy. *Arch Ophthalmol* 1988; 106:1647–1648.

62. Trobe JD: Third nerve palsy and the pupil: Footnotes to the rule. *Arch Ophthalmol* 1988; 106:601–602.

63. Sox HC Jr: Probability theory in the use of diagnostic tests; An introduction to critical study of the literature. *Ann Intern Med* 1986; 104:60–66.

64. Yen MY, Liu JH, Jaw SJ: Ptosis as the early manifestation of pituitary tumour. *Br J Ophthalmol* 1990; 74:188–191.

65. Small KW, Buckley EG: Recurrent blepharoptosis secondary to a pituitary tumor. *Am J Ophthalmol* 1988; 106:760–761.

66. Hopf HC, Gutmann L: Diabetic 3rd nerve palsy: Evidence for a mesencephalic lesion. *Neurology* 1990; 40:1041–1045.

67. Newman NJ, Lessell S: Isolated pupil-sparing third-nerve palsy as the presenting sign of multiple sclerosis. *Arch Neurol* 1990; 47:817–818.

68. Brean LA, Farris BK, Gutmann L, et al: Pupil-sparing oculomotor nerve palsy due to a midbrain infarct. *Neurology* 1989; 39:355.

69. Ksiazek SM, Repka MX, Maguire A, et al: Divisional oculomotor nerve paresis caused by intrinsic brainstem disease. *Ann Neurol* 1989; 26:714–718.

70. Castro O, Johnson LN, Mamourian AC: Isolated inferior oblique paresis from brain-stem infarction; Perspective on oculomotor fascicular organization in the ventral midbrain tegmentum. *Arch Neurol* 1990; 47:235–237.

71. Guy JR, Day AL: Intracranial aneurysms with superior division paresis of the oculomotor nerve. *Ophthalmology* 1989; 96:1071–1076.

72. Rosenstein ED, Sobelman J, Kramer N: Isolated, pupil-sparing third nerve palsy as initial manifestation of systemic lupus erythematosus. *J Clin Neuro Ophthalmol* 1989; 9: 285–288.

73. Katz B, Rimmer S: Ophthalmoplegic migraine with superior ramus oculomotor palsy. *J Clin Neuro Ophthalmol* 1989; 9:181–183.

74. Hutchinson DO, Donaldson IM: Ophthalmoplegic migraine with bilateral involvement. *J Neurol Neurosurg Psychiatry* 1989; 52:807–808.

75. Hawke SHB, Mullie MA, Hoyt WF, et al: Painful oculomotor nerve palsy due to dural-cavernous sinus shunt. *Arch Neurol* 1989; 46:1252–1255.

76. Abdul-Rahim AS, Savino PJ, Zimmerman RA, et al: Cryptogenic oculomotor nerve palsy; The need for repeated neuroimaging studies. *Arch Ophthalmol* 1989; 107:387–390.

77. Naghmi R, Subuhi R: Diabetic oculomotor mononeuropathy: Involvement of pupillomotor fibres with slow resolution. *Horm Metab Res* 1990; 22:38–40.

78. Sørensen TT: Familial recurrent cranial nerve palsies. *Acta Neurol Scand* 1988; 78:542–543.

79. Seifert V, Stolke D: Laser-assisted reconstruction of the oculomotor nerve: Experimental study on the feasibility of cranial nerve repair. *Neurosurgery* 1989; 25:579–583.

80. Friedman DI, Wright KW, Sadun AF: Oculomotor palsy with cyclic spasms. *Neurology* 1989; 39:1262–1264.

81. Johnson LN, Pack WL: Transient oculomotor nerve misdirection in a case of pituitary tumor with hemorrhage. *Arch Ophthalmol* 1988; 106:584–585.

82. Guy J, Engel HM, Lessner AM: Acquired contralateral oculomotor synkinesis. *Arch Neurol* 1989; 46:1021–1023.

83. Jordan DR, Miller DG, Anderson RL: Acquired oculomotor-abducens synkinesis. *Can J Ophthalmol* 1990; 25:148–151.

84. Keane JR: Rhythmic pupillary oscillations accompanying a complete third-nerve palsy. *J Clin Neuro Ophthalmol* 1989; 9:169–170.

85. Burgerman RS, Wolf AL, Kelman SE, et al: Traumatic trochlear nerve palsy diagnosed by magnetic resonance imaging; Case report and review of the literature. *Neurosurgery* 1989; 25:978–981.

86. Dussaux P, Plas J, Brion S: Parésie bilatérale du muscle grand oblique par hématome de la calotte mésencéphalique. *Rev Neurol (Paris)* 1990; 146:45–47.

87. Tachibana H, Mimura O, Shiomi M, et al: Bilateral trochlear nerve palsy from a brainstem hematoma. *J Clin Neuro Ophthalmol* 1990; 10:35–37.

88. Gonyea EF: Superior oblique palsy due to a midbrain vascular malformation. *Neurology* 1990; 40:554–555.

89. Jacobson DM, Warner JJ, Choucair AK, et al: Trochlear nerve palsy following minor head trauma; A sign of structural disorder. *J Clin Neuro Ophthalmol* 1988; 8:263–268.

90. Guy J, Day AL, Mickle JP, et al: Contralateral trochlear nerve paresis and ipsilateral Horner's syndrome. *Am J Ophthalmol* 1989; 107:73–76.

91. Maurice-Williams RS, Harvey PK: Isolated palsy of the fourth cranial nerve caused by an intracavernous aneurysm. *J Neurol Neurosurg Psychiatry* 1989; 52:679.

92. Moulis H, Mamus SW: Isolated trochlear nerve palsy in a patient with Waldenström's macroglobulinemia: Complete recovery with combination therapy. *Neurology* 1989; 39:1399.

93. Sawle GV, Sarkies NJC: Bilateral fourth nerve palsy due to cerebellar haemangioblastoma. *J R Soc Med* 1989; 82:111–112.

94. Guy JR, Friedman WF, Mickle JP: Bilateral trochlear nerve paresis in hydrocephalus. *J Clin Neuro Ophthalmol* 1989; 9:105–111.

95. Flanders M, Draper J: Superior oblique palsy: Diagnosis and treatment. *Can J Ophthalmol* 1990; 25:17–24.

96. Teller J, Karmon G, Savir H: Long-term follow-up of traumatic unilateral superior oblique palsy. *Ann Ophthalmol* 1988; 20:424–425.

97. Horton JC, Tsai R-K, Truwit CL, et al: Magnetic resonance imaging of superior oblique muscle atrophy in acquired trochlear palsy. *Am J Ophthalmol* 1990; 110:315–316.

98. Tada T, Shigeta H, Kobayashi H, et al: Trochlear nerve meningioma in von Recklinghausen's disease. *Neurochirurgia* 1988; 31:226–227.

99. Maurice-Williams RS: Isolated schwannoma of the fourth cranial nerve: Case report. *J Neurol Neurosurg Psychiatry* 1989; 52:1442–1443.

100. Goldmann JA, Spector RH: Diplopia due to 4th nerve palsy and enlargement of the right medial rectus muscle. *J Rheumatol* 1989; 16:1010–1011.

101. Donaldson D, Rosenberg NL: Infarction of abducens nerve fascicle as cause of isolated sixth nerve palsy related to hypertension. *Neurology* 1988; 38:1654.

102. Johnson LN, Hepler RS: Isolated abducens nerve paresis from intrapontine, fascicular abducens nerve injury. *Am J Ophthalmol* 1989; 108:459–461.

103. Bronstein AM, Morris J, Du Boulay G, et al: Abnormalities of horizontal gaze. Clinical, oculographic and magnetic resonance imaging findings. I. Abducens palsy. *J Neurol Neurosurg Psychiatry* 1990; 53:194–199.

104. Galetta SK, Smith JL: Chronic isolated sixth nerve palsies. *Arch Neurol* 1989; 46:79–82.

105. Del Priore LV, Miller NM: Trigeminal Schwannoma as a cause of chronic, isolated sixth nerve palsy. *Am J Ophthalmol* 1989; 108:726–729.

106. O'Sullivan F, Elton JS, Rossor M: Solitary intracranial plasmacytoma presenting as lateral rectus palsy. *Neuro Ophthalmol* 1990; 10:109–113.

107. Stracciari A, Ciucci G, Bianchedi G, et al: Isolated sixth nerve palsy due to intracavernous carotid aneurysm in a young woman. *Acta Neurol Belg* 1988; 88:148–151.

108. Goadsby PJ, Lance JW: Clinicopathological correlation in a case of painful ophthalmoplegia: Tolosa-Hunt syndrome. *J Neurol Neurosurg Psychiatry* 1989; 52:1290–1293.

109. Goto Y, Hosogawa S, Goto I, et al: Abnormalities in the cavernous sinus in three patients with Tolosa-Hunt syndrome: MRI and CT findings. *J Neurol Neurosurg Psychiatry* 1990; 53:231–234.

110. Berlit P, Reinhardt-Eckstein, Krause K-H: Die isolierte abduzensparese—eine retrospektive studie an 165 patienten. *Fortschr Neurol Psychiatr* 1989; 57:32–40.

111. McGovern ST, Crompton JL, Ingham PN: Trigemino-abducens synkinesis: An unusual case of aberrant regeneration. *Aust NZ J Ophthalmol* 1986; 14:275–279.

112. Nelson SK, Kline LB: Acquired trigemino-abducens synkinesis. *J Clin Neuro Ophthalmol* 1990; 10:111–114.

113. Bell JA, Dowd TC, McIlwaine GG, et al: Postmyelographic abducent nerve palsy in association with the contrast agent iopamidol. *J Clin Neuro Ophthalmol* 1990; 10:115–117.

114. Zumla A, Lipscomb G, Lewis D: Sixth cranial nerve palsy complicating psittacosis. *J Neurol Neurosurg Psychiatry* 1989; 52:1462.

115. Sedwick LA, Margo CE: Sixth nerve palsies, temporal artery biopsy, and necrotizing vasculitis. *J Clin Neuro Ophthalmol* 1989; 9:119–121.

116. Kellen RI, Burde RM, Hodges FJ III, et al: Central bilateral sixth nerve palsy associated with a unilateral preganglionic Horner's syndrome. *J Clin Neuro Ophthalmol* 1988; 8:179–184.

117. Çolak A, Benli K, Dönmez T, et al: Papillary carcinoma of the sphenoid sinus associated with sphenoid sinus abscess presenting as cavernous sinus syndrome; A case report. *J Clin Neuro Ophthalmol* 1990; 10:18–20.

118. Delpassand ES, Kirkpatrick JB: Cavernous sinus syndrome as the presentation of malignant lymphoma: Case report and review of the literature. *Neurosurgery* 1988; 23:501–504.

119. Fish LA, Friedman DI, Sadun AA: Progressive cranial polyneuropathy caused by primary central nervous system melanoma. *J Clin Neuro Ophthalmol* 1990; 10:41–44.

120. Hufnagel TJ, Savino PJ, Zimmerman RA, et al: Painful ophthalmoplegia caused by neurotropic malignant melanoma. *Can J Ophthalmol* 1990; 25:38–41.

121. Durand JR, Samples JR: Dolichoectasia and cranial nerve palsies; A case report. *J Clin Neuro Ophthalmol* 1989; 9:249–253.

122. Ondra SL, Doty JR, Mahla ME, et al: Surgical excision of a cavernous hemangioma of the rostral brain stem: Case report. *Neurosurgery* 1988; 23:490–493.

123. Drummond GT, Wuebbolt G: Bilateral ophthalmoplegia during percutaneous transluminal coronary angioplasty. *Can J Ophthalmol* 1990; 25:152–155.

124. Wilson WB, Leavengood JM, Ringel SP, et al: Transient ocular motor paresis associated with acute internal carotid occlusion. *Ann Neurol* 1989; 25:286–290.

125. Archambault P, Wise JS, Rosen J, et al: Herpes zoster ophthalmoplegia; Report of six cases. *J Clin Neuro Ophthalmol* 1988; 8:185–191.

126. Luco CF, Valenzuela RF: Diabetic complete external ophthalmoplegia. *J Clin Neuro Ophthalmol* 1990; 10:206–209.

PART THREE

THE PUPIL

CHAPTER 12

The Pupil

H. Stanley Thompson, M.D.
Professor of Ophthalmology, Director of Neuro-ophthalmology Service, University of Iowa College of Medicine, Iowa City, Iowa

Randy H. Kardon, M.D., Ph.D.
Assistant Professor of Ophthalmology, University of Iowa College of Medicine, Neuro-ophthalmology Service, Iowa City, Iowa

HORNER'S SYNDROME

Professor Horner died in 1886 and the 100th anniversary of his death was marked by some biographical sketches,[1, 2] some discussion of the naming of the syndrome,[3-5] and a symposium held in his honor.[6] But most importantly, a book was published[7] by Koelbing and Mörgeli, medical historians at the University of Zürich, that reprints Horner's autobiographical notes, freshly edited from the original manuscript, and includes an appreciation of Horner as the founder of Swiss ophthalmology. Much useful bibliographic material is included: lists of his publications, his students' dissertations, references to 254 people and sources mentioned in the autobiography, and several pages of pictures of the leading characters.

Some unusual causes of Horner's syndrome turned up this year: tuberculosis[8] rather than malignancy produced a Rowland-Payne syndrome (preganglionic Horner's syndrome, vocal cord paralysis, and phrenic nerve palsy due to involvement of lymph nodes in the neck at the C6 level).

A local anesthetic solution placed by catheter between the two layers of the pleura for relief of chest pain will, with the help of gravity, also produce a Horner's syndrome—presumably by soaking through the parietal pleura. This is a stellate ganglion block from below.[9]

Two patients with Horner's syndrome are described, who were "shot in the neck in Spain," but (perhaps for the sake of their catchy title[10]) the authors fail to mention the case of Edward Mooney, aged 24 years, who was shot in the neck at Chancellorsville on May 3, 1863, and whose case was reported in fascinating detail in 1864 by Mitchell, Moorehouse, and Keen.[4]

A patient with Horner's syndrome, presumed to be postganglionic because facial sweating was normal, had ipsilateral hemifacial pain and trigeminal nerve dysfunction. This "Raeder's syndrome" was thought, because of the clinical context and course, to be of syphilitic origin.[11] We are reminded that nasal stuffiness is often a troublesome feature of Horner's syndrome,[12] and that superior mediastinal masses can produce a Horner's syndrome; for example, a bronchogenic cyst,[13] or a schwannoma.[14]

The term "alternating Horner's syndrome" suggests that the oculosympathetic palsy alternates from side to side. That is, it is intermittent on each side, but at the moment when the left side is dysfunctional the right side is working well, and vice versa. This would indeed be hard to explain.[15, 16] Another interpretation of the phrase (and the observations) is that the sympathetic outflow remains normal on one side, while on the affected side it alternates between insufficiency (Horner's syndrome) and excess (Pourfour du Petit sign).[17, 18]

It is interesting that of 40 cases of Horner's syndrome in which the lesion was judged to be in the preganglionic neuron, 20% (8/40) were associated with malignancy, 40% were due to injury, either accidental or surgical, and in the remaining 40%, no cause was found. Four of the 8 patients with malignancy had breast cancer, 3 had lung cancer, and 1 had a mixed lymphoma. All of these tumors were advanced. Horner's syndrome is seldom an early sign of malignancy, so, if in the evaluation of a preganglionic Horner's syndrome enhanced magnetic resonsance imaging of the neck and upper chest is negative, fears of cancer may be set aside.[19]

Dr. Rosenberg has found that one can safely disregard the warning "Never Use Alcohol!" that comes with most plastic prism bars. He degreases both the bar and the forehead with an alcohol swab, allows them to dry, and finds that the back of the plastic bar slips easily over the dry skin on the side of the Horner's syndrome, but tends to stick to normally innervated skin.[20] Air conditioners and nerve regeneration will no doubt throw this test some curve balls, but it is certainly worth trying.

The Iowa group has restudied the role of cocaine eyedrops in the diagnosis of Horner's syndrome. It appears that the odds of having Horner's syndrome increase with increasing degrees of pupillary inequality measured 45 minutes after the instillation of 10% cocaine in both eyes. It is not necessary to compare before and after measurements; a post-cocaine anisocoria of 0.8 mm is taken as evidence of Horner's syndrome.[21, 22]

The same group has reviewed the value of hydroxyamphetamine eyedrops in trying to localize the lesion in Horner's syndrome.[23] The clinician would like to know where the lesion is in Horner's syndrome because that knowledge directs the radiographic workup; e.g., to the internal carotid artery rather than to the pulmonary apex. Horner's syndrome sometimes presents itself in such a characteristic setting that further efforts at localizing the lesion are not needed. This is true of patients with cluster headaches and patients with Wallenberg's syndrome. In about half of their ambulatory patients with Horner's syndrome, the location of the lesion was satisfactorily identified by the nature and location of the injury or disease. The other half of the patients with Horner's syndrome offered no clues as to the location of the damage, and a pharmacologic localization of the lesion in these patients would have been most helpful.

The authors tried to apply what could be learned about hydroxyamphetamine mydriasis in the first half of the patients (the ones with a known location of the lesion) to the second half of the patients. It turns out that postganglionic lesions (along the carotid artery) can be separated from the nonpostganglionic lesions (in the brain stem, spinal cord, upper lung, and lower neck) with a degree of certainty that varies with the amount of anisocoria induced when the drops are put in both eyes. The difference in the dilation of the two pupils was measured (change in normal pupil minus change in Horner's pupil, 45 minutes after two drops of 1% hydroxyamphetamine). If the anisocoria increased by at least 0.8 mm (because the normal pupil dilated more than the Horner's pupil) then the lesion could be considered postganglionic with reasonable certainty. Conversely, if the Horner's pupil dilated more than the normal pupil so that it became the larger one, then the lesion was probably in the preganglionic neuron and the final neuron was intact.

The mydriatic Paredrine (bottled and sold by SmithKline Beecham) has been unavailable for the past 2 years. It was the clinician's only supply of a 1% hydroxyamphetamine HBr solution, so neuro-ophthalmologists have been conserving their last few drops. It now appears that Allergan Pharmaceuticals is going to take over the manufacture of the drop even though they expect to lose money at it.[24] Paredrine's mydriatic effect may vary quite a lot from one individual to the next, but it dilates the right and left pupils of a single healthy subject about the same amount.[25-27]

Dr. Mindel has come up with a possible substitute for cocaine eye drops for the diagnosis of Horner's syndrome.[28] The substance is a metabolite of nortriptyline that has far less anticholinergic side effects than nortriptyline but still retains nortriptyline's ability to block the re-uptake of norepinephrine at the adrenergic nerve ending. It seems that it doesn't bother the corneal epithelium any more than cocaine does, and it has zero street value.

Cocaine, when used as a test for Horner's syndrome, produces no psychoactive effect, but the urine will test positive for cocaine metabolites in 100% of the patients at 24 hours and in 50% at 36 hours.[29] Patients should be warned about this.

AFFERENT PUPILLARY DEFECTS

The clinician trying to make careful, accurate measurements of the relative afferent pupillary defect keeps running into potential sources of error that have to be taken into account. For example, the eye under a patch becomes dark adapted and, with only one eye patched, a significant difference in retinal sensitivity between the two eyes can develop that may last for several minutes after the patch has been removed.[30, 31] Interestingly, a unilateral cataract, even though it blocks a lot of light, does not produce a relative afferent pupillary defect in the cataractous eye. In fact, a dense unilateral cataract will produce a clearly visible relative afferent pupillary defect (0.4 log) in the other eye.[32] Lam suggested that despite the obvious reflection and absorption of the stimulus light by the cataract, the light that enters the cataractous lens is probably sufficiently scattered around within the eye to enhance the pupillary response. Sadun, agreeing that photochemical dark adaptation must play a role, was reluctant to believe that scatter was a sufficiently potent factor to explain the effect. He pointed out that transmission photometry of extracted cataracts has shown that the percentage of light blocked by the lens in a 60 year old rises from about 88% (0.9 log) to about 97% (1.5 log) as increasing density of cataract drops the acuity from 20/20 to 20/400 or worse.[33] Sadun postulated the existence of another mechanism for controlling retinal sensitivity, a sustained neuronal adaptive process, presumably intraretinal, that is much slower to kick in.[34] It may be that the relative afferent pupillary defect in the eye without the cataract is clinically visible because all three mechanisms are at work and potentiating each other. Is the Stiles-Crawford effect demonstrably affected by a dense cataract? Would a good trans-scleral bleach of both retinas bring out a relative afferent pupillary defect in the eye with the cataract?

Another case of a pretectal afferent defect has been reported.[35] This time the authors include a recording of both pupils during two separate light reactions. When the right eye was stimulated, both pupils had a response of similar amplitude, but when the left eye was stimulated the direct response (OS) was much stronger than the consensual response (OD). This pupillographic scrap brings up the possibility that a pretectal lesion may unbalance the midbrain decussation of the light reflex path and thus uncover a contraction anisocoria that was previously hidden to full field stimulation.

An alternative technique for estimating the size of an asymmetry of pupillomotor input has received some fresh attention.[36, 37] Kestenbaum, in 1946, suggested that the strength of the direct light reaction of each eye could be estimated by simply measuring the size of each pupil while the other eye was in darkness. This can be done with a pupil gauge and a hand light and, provided there is nothing wrong with the innervation of any of the iris muscles in either eye, the difference in the diameter of the two pupils (measured in millimeters with the other eye in darkness) comes very close to the relative afferent pupillary defect (measured in log units of neutral density filter required to balance the reactions in the two eyes).

This measurement of Kestenbaum's number may seem a little rough, but there are situations in which a rough measure is better than no measure at all.

Relative afferent pupillary defects were simulated in healthy subjects by holding a neutral density filter over one eye and alternating the light from one eye to the other.[38] The responses were recorded pupillographically so that various features of the pupil response could be studied. It was found that the contraction amplitude was the best indicator of small differences in pupillomotor input between the two eyes.

It has been confirmed by Firth that a substantial number of amblyopic eyes (32.3% in this study) show a relative afferent pupillary defect.[39] Afferent defects were more common in anisometropic amblyopia than in pure strabismic amblyopia. The possibility was discussed that this asymmetry of pupillary input might be an expression of a retinal ganglion abnormality, which in turn might be a contributing factor in the genesis of the amblyopia. It seems to us that this matter will not be settled until careful two-channel pupillometry is performed with some kind of synoptophore-like device with absolute control of fixation. The fixing eye will have to be elegantly alternated by some means that is independent of the light stimulus before we can be sure that the 32.3% of patients with amblyopia and a clinically visible afferent defect are not just the ones who would rather not take up fixation with their bad eye.

ADIE'S TONIC PUPIL

Damage to the innervation of the iris sphincter, resembling Adie's syndrome, was reported in association with temporal arteritis,[40] with systemic lupus erythematosus,[41] with botulism,[42] with a hypereosinophilic syndrome,[43] and with an epidemic nephropathy/iritis syndrome due to the Puumala virus.[44]

On hearing that the cornea in Adie's syndrome might have a decreased sensitivity to touch, Dr. Utsumi[45] wondered if topical pilocarpine might penetrate the cornea more readily in an eye with Adie's syndrome, and if so, whether this might account for the apparent supersensitivity of the iris sphincter to pilocarpine in the affected eye. To answer this question, he studied six patients with Adie's syndrome and seven age-matched control subjects with a fluorophotometer and showed that the amount of fluorescein reaching into the corneal stroma and into the anterior chamber was the same in both groups. There was no correlation in individual cases between the amount of miosis produced by the weak topical pilocarpine and the fluorescein concentration in the anterior chamber. From this, Dr. Utsumi concluded that the supersensitivity of the iris sphincter in Adie's syndrome is real and not just an artifact of increased corneal permeability.

Ukai and Ishikawa[46] have used a two-channel continuously recording infrared accommodometer to study two patients with Adie's syndrome. The affected eye had a normal range of accommodative power but two obvious abnormalities were noted:

1. All the high frequency instability of accommodation seen in healthy subjects and in the unaffected eye was gone in the affected eye. This matches the behavior of the pupil: an Adie's tonic pupil shows no hippus.
2. There is a very odd overshoot of accommodation in the affected eye with a near effort; apparently enough to produce a brief anisometropic aniseikonic blur. Does cholinergic supersensitivity have a hand in this? The same authors have studied healthy subjects with the same equipment during a vigorous near effort.[47] Interestingly, in some subjects, the pupils tend to stay small for several minutes after the accommodative effort has stopped and accommodation has returned to normal.

The whole matter of using weak pilocarpine drops for relief of symptoms in Adie's syndrome has been reviewed.[48] Some patients are happy with slightly stronger bifocals than their age would indicate, because when they don't accommodate they don't get a new cylinder or a cramp of accommodation. These authors suggest that during the workup of a patient with Adie's syndrome, the Randot Stereoacuity test be performed before and after the application of 0.1% pilocarpine. If the stereoacuity improves with weak pilocarpine, then the patient deserves a trial of these drops.

A patient with Ross's syndrome is described[49] in whom the segmental anhidrosis is not progressive and does not produce heat stroke with exercise.

A careful series of experiments in monkeys[50] showed that taking out the ciliary ganglion resulted in supersensitivity to pilocarpine, and a lack of response to eserine and to electrical stimulation of the Edinger-Westphal nuclei, Six months later, a good recovery had occurred, complete with evidence for a synapse in the pathway serving accommodation—as there had been before the surgery.

A special effort was made to study the effect of cataract extraction on pupillary function.[51] Four patients were studied before and after surgery and none showed a significant change in the amplitude or velocity of the light reaction, or in the pupil size. Nor did any of them develop a segmental palsy of the sphincter or a dilation lag. The same group studied the effect of touching the cornea on the effectiveness of a mydriatic solution.[52] The cornea of one eye was touched lightly, either by the applanation tonometer or at the inferior limbus by a cotton-tipped applicator. The other eye served as a control. It was found that the corneal touch enhanced the mydriasis six times more in darkly pigmented subjects than it did in lightly pigmented subjects.

For some reason, the size and reactivity of the pupils of the premature baby are at center stage this year. It is not enough that the newborn finds itself plunged into a world of light against which it keeps its lids and pupils tightly closed,[53] but now it must contend with waves of well-meaning doctors and nurses each with a light in hand. The observations Isenberg has been making seem important, however.[54,55]

When a premature baby is awakened and examined in dim light, the pupil size is 3.6 mm (0.9 mm). There is gerorally no light reaction until the baby has reached 31 weeks of gestational age, but the response to light then increases steadily until it is almost 2 mm reaction at term. This is thought to be due to the advancing maturity of the innervation of the iris sphincter.

Only 9% of Isenberg's premature infants were seen to have an anisocoria of 0.5 mm or more in dim light. A higher frequency of anisocoria was noted in full-term infants.[56] Robinson and Fielder[57] also noted that preterm infants do not have any light reaction until 30 weeks of gestational age, so it is important not to misinterpret 4 mm, unreactive pupils in premature infants as a sign of neurologic disease or blindness—at least not until after 32 weeks of gestational age.[55]

THE DUAL INNERVATION OF THE INTRAOCULAR MUSCLES

Remember when you thought the parasympathetic innervation to the iris sphincter and the sympathetic supply to to the dilator were simple and easy to understand? Well, hold on to your α and β receptors: it's not as straightforward as the textbooks say.

Does a Horner's pupil dilate slowly in darkness *only* because there is no tone in the dilator muscle? Could it be that the sphincter is also reluctant to let go—because this letting go is something that is normally facilitated by sympathetic innervation? These questions are not easily answered. With a psychosensory stimulus like a sudden noise, there is sympathetic outflow to the dilator muscle and at the same time there is central inhibition of the Edinger-Westphal nucleus that shuts down the iris sphincter muscle. Both of these actions serve to dilate the pupil.

This seems complicated enough without invoking a *peripheral* cross-inhibition between the sympathetic and parasympathetic systems. Yet studies of isolated iris muscles suspended on hooks in a supportive bath have shown some interesting adrenergic effects on the iris sphincter, and cholinergic effects on the dilator. Several species have been used, including humans.

Convincing evidence has been provided that the iris sphincter and dilator muscles receive functional, double reciprocal innervation by both cholinergic and adrenergic systems.[58] In other words, cholinergic excitatory nerves to the sphincter cause it to contract, but at the same time cholinergic *inhibitory* nerves to the dilator cause it to relax, thus enhancing the miosis. On the other hand, mydriasis consists of direct adrenergic excitatory input to the dilator, causing it to contract. At the same time, not only is the central, cholinergic output to the sphincter inhibited, but it appears that adrenergic *inhibitory* input to the sphincter helps it to let go—the result is a brisk pupil dilation.

The cholinergic inhibitory system to the dilator has been demonstrated in the cat,[59,60] dog,[58] rat,[61] ox,[62] and human.[63] Most of these studies involve testing of isolated strips of iris muscle in an organ bath hooked up to a mechanical transducer to measure contraction and relaxation in response to electrical stimulation in the presence of various pharmacologic agents. The preparations appear very reproducible and convincing. The physiologic studies have also been complemented by histochemical studies. In cynomolgus monkeys, 75% of the nerve terminals to the dilator were found to be adrenergic, whereas 25% were cholinergic.[64]

On the adrenergic side, inhibition of the sphincter has also been demonstrated. In the dog iris, activation of the α-2 receptors (blocked by yohimbine) and the β-1 receptors (blocked by timolol or atenolol) cause the sphincter to relax.[58] Conversely, activation of α-1 adrenergic receptors seems to potentiate sphincter contraction, which is blocked by the α-1 blocker prazocin. See Table 1 for a summary.

One clinical correlate of the adrenergic inhibition of the sphincter may lie with the Horner's pupil that dilates very slowly. In some cases, interruption of the sympathetic nerves may not only cause a deficit in dilator activation, but also a deficit of sphincter inhibition. It's also interesting that the effects of topical timolol (0.5%) were studied in humans pupillographically by Johnson et al.,[65] who found no clinically significant effect except for a statistically significant decrease in the amplitude of pupil redilation after a light stimulus, which the authors could not fully explain. Is it possible that the timolol effect may have resulted in β blockade of the inhibitory fibers to the sphincter? This would have kept the sphincter from relaxing properly, thus slowing dilation.

Perhaps with thoughtful selection of receptor-specific agonists and antagonists and continuous recording of the behavior of both pupils, the pharmacology of the human iris can be carefully picked apart and better understood. In the meantime, we can bear in mind that every time we use a dilating drop we are probably stimulating one of the iris muscles and also inhibiting its antagonist. The wiring for the central nervous system orchestration of each set of reciprocal excitatory/inhibitory pathways to the sphincter and dilator isn't fully understood as yet, but a number of the pieces are starting to fall into place, and may be discussed in the next volume of this book.

Finally, it's well known to every cataract surgeon that mechanical and chemical irritation of the eye can cause a strong miotic response that is noncholinergic and fails to reverse with autonomically acting drugs. In rabbits and cats, the response

TABLE–1.

Iris Sphincter and Dilator Responses

Input	Sphincter		Dilator	
	Action	Result*	Action	Result
Cholinergic	Excites	Miosis	Inhibits	Miosis
Adrenergic α1	Excites	Miosis	?	?
Adrenergic α2	Inhibits	Mydriasis	Excites	Mydriasis
Adrenergic β1	Inhibits	Mydriasis	Inhibits	?

*Some of these actions may not cause any significant effect on static pupil size, but may influence the rate of pupil constriction or dilation.

seems to be due to the release of substance P or closely related peptides from the sensory nerve endings, but in monkeys and humans, substance P has little or no miotic effect. At the 1990 Association for Research in Vision and Ophthalmology (ARVO) meeting, Almegard et al.[66] reported that cholecystokinin (in nanomolar amounts) caused contraction of isolated iris sphincter from monkeys and humans. Intracameral injections in monkeys caused miosis that was not prevented by tetrodotoxin or indomethacin, indicating that the miosis was not caused by stimulation of nerve endings or release of prostaglandins, but by direct action on sphincter receptors. Interestingly, the cholecystokinin antagonist lorglumide caused competitive inhibition of the response. Next time you have a Big Mac attack and put your gall bladder sphincter into spasm, look in the mirror—your pupils may be up to something!

REFERENCES

1. Thompson HS: Johann Friedrich Horner (1831–1886). *Am J Ophthalmol* 1986; 102:792–795.

2. Breathnach CS: Horner. *Ir Med J* 1986; 79:362.

3. Loewenfeld IE: Horner's syndrome; What's in a name?, in Huber A (ed): *Sympathicus und Auge*. Stuttgart, Ferdinand Enke, 1990, pp 43–78.

4. Trautman JC: An early American's contribution to Horner's syndrome: S. Weir Mitchell, MD, in Huber A (ed): *Sympathicus und Auge*. Stuttgart, Ferdinand Enke, 1990, pp 105–114.

5. Almaric P: Le Syndrome de Claude Bernard-Horner, in Huber A (ed): *Sympathicus und Auge*. Stuttgart, Ferdinand Enke, 1990, pp 231–233.

6. Huber A: *Sympathicus und Auge*. Stuttgart, Ferdinand Enke, 1990, pp 257.

7. Koelbing HM, Mörgeli C: *Johann Friedrich Horner (1831–1886). Der Begründer der Schweizer Augenheilkunde in seiner Autobiographie*. Zürich, Hans Rohr, 1986, p 113.

8. Ismail M, Hodkinson H, Tuling B: Horner's syndrome and tuberculosis. *S Afr Med J* 1988; 74:586–587.

9. Parkinson SMJ, Rich T, Little W: Unilateral Horner's syndrome associated with interpleural catheter injection of local anesthetic. *Anesth Analg* 1989; 68:61–62.

10. Singh P, Green S, Craig G, et al: Shot in the neck in Spain (a rare cause of an isolated Horner's syndrome). *Injury* 1987; 18:407–408.

11. Watanabe K, Tanahashi N, Nara M: Neurosyphilis presenting with Raeder's syndrome. *Ann Neurol* 1989; 25:418.

12. Whittet HB, Fisher EW: Nasal obstruction after cervical sympathectomy: Horner's syndrome revisited. *Otorhinolaryngology* 1988; 50:246–250.

13. Matsuda S, Tsutsui H, Shimase J, et al: A case of bronchogenic cyst in the superior mediastinum with Horner's syndrome. *Nippon Naika Gakkai Zasshi* 1988; 77:1229–1232.

14. Mathew B, Jones R, Campbell M: Horner's syndrome due to superior-mediastinal schwannoma (letter). *J Neurol Neurosurg Psychiatry* 1988; 51:1460–1461.

15. Tan E, Kansu T, Saygi S, et al: Alternating Horner's syndrome. A case report and review of the literature. *Neuro-ophthalmology* 1989; 10:19–22.

16. Thompson HS: The pupil, in Dalen SLaJTWV (ed): *Neuro-ophthalmology 1982*. Amsterdam, Excerpta Medica, 1982, pp 226–240.

17. Byrne P, Clough C: A case of Pourfour du Petit syndrome following parotidectomy. *J Neurol Neurosurg Psychiatry* 1990; 53:1014.

18. Schnapp M, Mays KS: Contralateral spread of anaesthetic solutions. *Can Anaesthetist's Soc J* 1987; 34:828–829.

19. Thompson HS, Maxner CE, Corbett JJ: Horner's syndrome due to damage to the preganglionic neuron of the oculosympathetic pathway, in Huber A (ed): *Sympathicus und Auge.* Stuttgart, Ferdinand Enke Verlag, 1990, pp 99–104.

20. Rosenberg M: The friction sweat test as a new method for detecting facial anhidrosis in patient with Horner's syndrome. *Am J Ophthalmol* 1989; 108:443–447.

21. Kardon RH, Denison CE, Brown CK, et al: Critical evaluation of the cocaine test in the diagnosis of Horner's syndrome. *Arch Ophthalmol* 1990; 108:384–387.

22. Moster ML: The cocaine test and Horner's syndrome (letter and reply by Kardon, Denison, Brown, et al). *Arch Ophthalmol* 1990; 108:1667–1668.

23. Cremer SA, Thompson HS, Digre KB, et al: Hydroxyamphetamine mydriasis in Horner's syndrome. *Am J Ophthalmol* 1990; 110:71–76.

24. Burde RM, Thompson HS: Hydroxyamphetamine. A good drug lost? (editorial). *Am J Ophthalmol* 1991; 111:100–102.

25. Cremer SA, Thompson HS, Digre KB, et al: Hydroxyamphetamine mydriasis in normal subjects. *Am J Ophthalmol* 1990; 110:66–70.

26. Heitman K, Bode DD: The paredrine test in normal eyes. A controlled study. *J Clin Neuro Ophthalmol* 1986; 6:228–231.

27. Semes LP, Bartlett JD: Mydriatic effectiveness of hydroxyamphetamine. *J Am Optom Assoc* 1982; 53:899–904.

28. Mindel JS, Rubin MA, Kharlamb AB: The pupil response to E-10-hydroxynortriptyline in rabbits with ocular sympathetic paresis. *J Auton Nerv Syst* 1990; 30:175–177.

29. Bralliar BB, Skarf B, Owens JB: Ophthalmic use of cocaine and the urine test for benzoylecgonine. *N Engl J Med* 1989; 320:1757–1758.

30. Lam BL, Thompson HS: Relative afferent pupillary defect induced by patching (the other eye). *Am J Ophthalmol* 1989; 107:305–306.

31. DuBois LG, Sadun AA: Occlusion-induced contralateral afferent pupillary defect. *Am J Ophthalmol* 1989; 107:306–307.

32. Lam BL, Thompson HS: A unilateral cataract produces a relative afferent pupil defect in the contralateral eye. *Ophthalmology* 1989; 97:334–337.

33. Sadun AA, Libondi T: Transmission of light through cataracts. *Am J Ophthalmol* 1990; 110:710–712.

34. Sadun AA, Bassi CJ, Lessell S: Why cataracts do not produce afferent pupillary defects. *Am J Ophthalmol* 1990; 10:712–714.

35. Forman S, Behrens MM, Odel JG, et al: Relative afferent pupillary defect with normal visual function. *Arch Ophthalmol* 1990; 108:1074–1075.

36. Gruber H, Lessel M: Modifikation des Swinging Flashlight Tests. *Klin Monatsbl Augenheilkd* 1982; 181:402–403.

37. Jiang M-Q, Thompson HS, Lam BL: Kestenbaum's number as an indicator of pupillomotor input asymmetry. *Am J Ophthalmol* 1989; 107:528–530.

38. Cox T: Pupillographic charateristics of simulated relative afferent pupillary defects. *Invest Ophthalmol Vis Sci* 1989; 30:1127–1131.

39. Firth AY: Pupillary responses in amblyopia. *Br J Ophthalmol* 1990; 74:676–680.

40. Rabinowich L, Mehler MF: Parasympathetic pupillary involvement in biopsy-proven temporal arteritis. *Ann Ophthalmol* 1988; 20:400–402.

41. Herson D, Krivitzky A, Douche C, et al: Familial lupus and Adie's tonic pupil (letter). *Ann Med Intern (Paris)* 1989; 140:56–57.

42. Friedman DI, Fortanasce VN, Sadun AA: Tonic pupils as a result of botulism. *Am J Ophthalmol* 1990; 109:236–237.

43. Catalano L, Scala A, Rotoli B: Adie's syndrome (benign pupillotonia) and hypereosinophilic syndrome. *Haematologica (Pavia)* 1988; 73:549.

44. Pärssinen O, Kuronen J: Tonic pupillary reaction after epidemic nephropathy and transient myopia. *Am J Ophthalmol* 1989; 108:201–202.

45. Utsumi T: Corneal permeability in patients with tonic pupil. *J Clin Neuro Ophthalmol* 1990; 10:52–55.

46. Ukai K, Ishikawa S: Accomodative fluctuations in Adie's syndrome. *Ophthalmic Physiol Opt* 1989; 9:76–78.

47. Tsuchiya K, Ukai K, Ishikawa S: A quasistatic study of pupil and accommodation after-effects following near vision. *Ophthalmic Physiol Opt* 1989; 9:385–391.

48. Flach AJ, Dolan BJ: The therapy of Adie's syndrome with dilute pilocarpine hydrochloride solutions. *J Ocular Pharmacol* 1985; 1:353–362.

49. Tzeng S-S, Liu W-C: Adie's syndrome with segmental anhidrosis. Report of one case. *Chin Med J* 1987; 40:331–334.

50. Erickson-Lamy KA, Kaufman PL: Reinnervation of primate ciliary muscle following ciliary ganglionectomy: *Invest Ophthalmol Vis Sci* 1987; 28:927–933.

51. Peters DR, Tychsen L: Recovery of pupillomotor function after cataract surgery. *Aviat Space Environ Med* 1989; 1:586–588.

52. Carlson DW, Tychsen L: Touching the cornea enhances pharmacologic dilation of the pupil, mainly in the dark iris. *Aviat Space Environ Med* 1989; 60:994–995.

53. Peyresblanques J: The photomotor reflex at birth. *Bull Soc Ophthalmol France* 1989; 89:1319–1323.

54. Isenberg SJ, Dang Y, Jotterand V: The pupils of term and preterm infants. *Am J Ophthalmol* 1989; 108:75–79.

55. Isenberg SJ, Molarte A, Vazquez M: The fixed and dilated pupils of premature neonates. *Am J Ophthalmol* 1990; 110:168–171.

56. Roarty JD, Keltner JL: Normal pupil size and anisocoria in newborn infants. *Arch Ophthalmol* 1990; 108:94–95.

57. Robinson J, Fielder AR: Pupillary diameter and reaction to light in preterm neonates. *Arch Disease Child* 1990; 65:35–38.

58. Yoshitomi T, Ito Y: Double reciprocal innervations in the dog iris sphincter and dilator muscles. *Invest Ophthalmol Vis Sci* 1986; 27:83–91.

59. Schaeppi U, Koelle WP: Adrenergic innervation of the cat iris sphincter. *Am J Physiol* 1964; 207:273–278.

60. Ehinger B, Falck B, Persson H: Function of cholinergic nerve fibers in the cat iris dilator. *Acta Physiol Scand* 1968; 72:139–147.

61. Narita S, Watanabe M: Response of isolated rat iris dilator to adrenergic and cholinergic agents and electrical stimulation. *Life Sci* 1982; 30:1211–1218.

62. Suzuki R, Oso T, Kobayashi S: Cholinergic inhibitory response in the bovine iris dilator. *Invest Ophthalmol Vis Sci* 1983; 24:760–765.

63. Yoshitomi T, Ito Y, Inomata H: Adrenergic excitatory and cholinergic inhibitory innervations in the human iris dilator. *Exp Eye Res* 1985; 40:453–459.

64. Nomura T, Smelser GK: The identification of adrenergic and cholinergic nerve endings in the trabecular meshwork. *Invest Ophthalmol* 1974; 13:525–532.

65. Johnson S, Brubaker R, Trautman J: Absence of an effect of timolol on the pupil. *Invest Ophthalmol* 1978; 17:924–926.

66. Almegård B, Andersson S, Stjernschantz J, et al: Cholecystokinin causes contraction of the iridial sphincter muscle in monkey and man. *Invest Ophthalmol Vis Sci* 1990; 31:167.

PART FOUR

THE RETINA

CHAPTER 13

The Retina

Joseph F. Rizzo III, M.D.

Assistant Professor of Ophthalmology, Department of Ophthalmology, Harvard Medical School, Massachusetts Eye and Ear Infirmary, Boston, Massachusetts

VARIABILITY IN NEURONAL POPULATIONS OF THE RETINA

The ability to see must, to a great extent, be determined by the anatomy of the visual system. Primates are known to have the capacity for well-developed central acuity, and the large number of retinal cells devoted to the central retina subserve that function. What would it mean if an individual had considerably fewer cells in the central retina?

Marked variability in retinal cell number between individuals has been recognized for photoreceptors, amacrine cells, ganglion cells, and optic nerve axons.[1-6] Substantial variability has been shown to exist even for animals that are thought to be genetically identical, with variations of up to 30%. In species that are outbred, with a more diverse genetic pool, the variation is even greater.[2]

The fact that commensurate degrees of variability in visual function have not been recognized in humans may simply reflect the fact that the current battery of psychophysical tests is not especially sensitive at the high end of the performance spectrum. The clinical value of these observations relates to the fact that some people may be able to better withstand a disease process because they have a larger number of nerves. For instance, it has been long recognized that some patients with elevated intraocular pressure do not develop visual defects as readily as others. This apparent resilience may be related to a larger initial population of optic nerve fibers, among other factors.

RETINAL VASCULAR DISEASE

The most unassuming report that I reviewed is one that describes the use of nitroglycerin for treatment of embolic central retinal artery occlusion.[7] Two patients showed a dramatic recovery of vision shortly after a single 0.4 mg dose of sublingual nitroglycerin—they had also received the more standard forms of therapy.

In one instance, a thrombus was observed to move distally minutes after the medication was given. Nitroglycerin nonspecifically dilates all smooth muscle irrespective of its innervation, and the side effects associated with controlled administration are not forbidding. Its use in a case of otherwise devastating visual loss seems reasonable, at least until its tract record can be assessed further. It would be prudent to initially give a low dose of nitroglycerin (0.15 mg or 1/600 g), with the patient supine. Blood pressure should be taken 1 to 2 minutes later and, if acceptable, a 0.4 mg (1/150 g) dose could be given, followed by another check of blood pressure.

Transient Monocular Blindness

Recognition of the relationship between carotid artery disease and stroke was provided by C. Miller Fisher with his 1951 landmark article. What better person to now admonish that substitution of the term amaurosis fugax for transient monocular blindness is fraught with imprecision.[8] In his historical review of these terms, Fisher points out that amaurosis fugax was formerly used to describe transient monocular or bilateral visual loss, whether of central or peripheral origin: "Transient monocular blindness speaks for itself."

Not persuaded, the Amaurosis Fugax Study Group published their consensus on a wide range of topics related to transient monocular visual loss.[9] A thorough presentation of the rationale for their conclusions is not presented in this abridged form; this is accomplished to a greater degree in the original publication of the report in book form, which I reviewed in the last volume on *Current Neuro-Ophthalmology*.[2] Even the more complete publication was somewhat disappointing in its failure to comprehensively review some controversial topics. Eugene Bernstein, editor of the book, subsequently published an interesting article that proposes a new classification for clinical episodes related to stroke.[10] This CHAT system is a shorthand method of signifying those *C*linical, *H*istorical, *A*rterial (indicating the site and pathologic process of arterial disease), and *T*arget (demonstrated site of brain pathologic conditions) features that relate to the occurrence of a stroke. Amaurosis fugax is given a specific notation in this system. Using this classification in a retrospective review of 480 consecutive carotid endarterectomies performed at the Scripps Clinic, a life-table analysis of the probability of stroke-free survival after surgery demonstrated a significantly better prognosis for patients who experienced amaurosis fugax vs. cortical ischemia related to carotid artery disease.

The value of surgical treatment for patients who experience attacks of retinal ischemia is reported to be of minor importance as a preventative measure against subsequent cerebral infarction, at least for persons living in the Northern Jutland of Denmark.[11] This study is of interest because it was community-based and prospective in nature, having solicited the referral of every new case of amaurosis fugax over a 3-year period. Such community-based data are unique. Given that there were no exclusion factors, it is curious that there were so few young patients. Transient visual loss related to migraine is highly prevalent and often a confounding issue when attempting to sort out the results of earlier studies.[2] For whatever reason, the small number of young patients was fortuitous since this effectively resulted in a more selective study of the subgroup of patients with transient monocular visual loss associated with atherosclerosis. Amaurosis fugax was estimated to comprise approximately 25% to 30% of the reported incidence of all transient ischemic attacks. Even using an apparently liberal criterion for atheromatous lesions amenable to carotid surgery (stenosis, with at least 25% reduction of the lumen), the authors state that only 3 of 100,000 cases per year of amaurosis fugax are suitable for carotid surgery. This was the basis for their assertion that surgical treatment of carotid atherosclerotic disease was of limited importance when considered as a preventative measure against stroke for the population at large. It is difficult to surmise how this finding would relate to other populations that might have more prevalent or more severe atherosclerotic disease.

Surgery is also not currently indicated for nonstenotic, ulcerated carotid lesions. Caplan and Pessin are convincing in their assertion that ulcers and plaque hemorrhages have been overemphasized as frequent causes of stroke in patients without severe stenosis.[12] That is not to say that ulcers cannot be embologenic—indeed some studies have reported a higher incidence of stroke in this situation.[13, 14] The presence of ulcers in the carotid artery is highly correlated with stenosis and other risk factors for stroke including hypertension and hypercholesterolemia. Therefore, the extent to which ulcers alone modify the risk for stroke or monocular visual loss has not been determined. In light of this uncertainty, patients should not undergo surgery routinely because of the presence, or suspected presence, of a carotid ulcer.

Two reports emphasized the more benign clinical course of younger patients with transient monocular visual loss as compared to older patients. Tippin et al. reviewed the experience at the University of Iowa in which the majority of the patients with transient monocular blindness experienced headache or orbital pain, suggesting an association with migraine.[15] This retrospective study assessed (only) 51% of the original patients and demonstrated that no patient had suffered a stroke. The longest duration of visual loss was less than 15 minutes for 45 of 72 patients. This finding is an important reminder that the duration of visual loss is not a reliable criterion for distinguishing patients who have significant atherosclerotic disease from those with a benign form of transient visual loss. The benign nature of transient monocular blindness in teenagers was also the subject of a report in a non-ophthalmologic journal.[16] The conclusion of this report is not novel but provides a useful message to physicians who less frequently care for patients with this condition.

A report from Norway on amaurosis fugax echoed the conclusions of many other reports regarding the association of significant carotid artery disease in older patients with this symptom.[17] The authors concluded that patients under 50 years of age generally have a non-atherosclerotic form of disease—"patient's age was the most important factor in predicting the presence of carotid occlusive disease." The report contained two unusual cases. In one, transient monocular blindness was thought to be related to ophthalmic artery stenosis—an association that has been only rarely documented. The other case was associated with occlusion of the brachiocephalic artery, and the patient experienced transient visual loss mainly while using her right arm: a steal syndrome.

One of the most disappointing studies that I reviewed for this chapter proposes a far-reaching hypothesis: that a distinction exists between lesions of the carotid artery that produce amaurosis fugax as opposed to cerebral transient ischemic attacks.[18] The authors suggested that showers of small emboli that enter the retinal circulation cause amaurosis fugax. The study was most seriously flawed in that a meaningful statistical analysis was not applied to the data. For instance, it would have been useful to include the interobserver variability in the diagnosis of atrophy on computed tomography (CT) scans. This is especially important because their conclusions were based on apparent changes in the occurrence of atrophy in small numbers of patients. This points out the need to provide a more comprehensive statistical analysis of results. It would have been useful to examine other factors such as hypertension, raised hematocrit level, cardiac arrhythmias, size of infarcts, something the authors suggested would be useful for future studies to address. I do not accept their conclusions based on the presented material.

As reviewed in the last volume of *Current Neuro-Ophthalmology*,[2] most patients with significant carotid atherosclerotic disease succumb to myocardial infarction within 5 years. This is one of the important considerations when carotid endarterectomy is being considered—this local approach does nothing to reduce the most likely cause of morbidity and mortality. Some current opinions about carotid endarterectomy were presented by a Subcommittee of the American Academy of Neurology.[19] Although it has always been considered prudent to reduce risk factors associated with the increased risk of heart disease in these patients, only recently has there been good evidence that lowering serum cholesterol levels in patients who have already experienced a heart attack reduces the risk for subsequent heart attacks.[20] Hence, modifying this particular risk factor, as well as controlling systemic hypertension,[21, 22] are well-founded strategies to recommend to older patients who experience transient monocular blindness. Furthermore, in a review of the pathogenesis and therapy for atherosclerosis, Yatsu and Fisher recommended a two-pronged approach designed to alter lipoprotein metabolism and avert platelet adhesion and coagulation.[23] A review of the potential benefit of fish oil in reducing atherogenesis was also presented.

Three new studies focused on another important risk factor for stroke: atrial fibrillation.[24–28] At issue was whether therapy, either anticoagulation or aspirin, reduced the risk for stroke in patients with atrial fibrillation (it had been recognized for some time that atrial fibrillation is a very significant risk factor for stroke, especially in older patients). All three studies demonstrated a significantly reduced rate of stroke in the warfarin-treated patients. The most stringent target range for low-dose warfarin therapy in these trials was 1.2 to 1.5 times the control value, and the beneficial effect was accomplished without a significant difference in complications from bleeding between the groups.[27] It remains to be determined whether low-dose warfarin and aspirin are equivalent in reducing the risk of stroke, or how the specifics of the cardiac status (e.g., lone atrial fibrillation vs. that associated with cardiopulmonary disease or hypertension) might modify the risk of stroke or approach to treatment.

Antiphospholipid Antibodies

Antiphosopholipid antibodies are a heterogeneous family of antibodies directed against phospholipids that include the lupus anticoagulant and antibodies to cardiolipin. These antibodies are more commonly discovered in women, in persons under 50 years of age who have experienced stroke or cerebral transient ischemic attack, in persons with a false-positive result in the rapid plasma reagin (RPR) test, a history of thrombotic events, a history of fetal loss, thrombocytopenia, or splinter hemorrhage under the nail beds, and those with a prolonged partial thromboplastin time in the absence of heparin therapy.[29–33] The presence of these antibodies should be suspected in patients with unexplained cerebral infarction, especially multiple small cortical infarcts, and in patients with atypical migraine-like headaches. The mechanism by which these antibodies cause neurologic disease, if indeed they do, has not been determined. The relationship between the presence of these antibodies and progressive optic atrophy seems tenuous in one case report.[34]

Neurologic syndromes most frequently linked to the presence of antiphospholipid antibodies are thrombotic in nature, and include transient ischemic attacks, cerebral infarction, and acute ischemic encephalopathy.[29–33] Cardiogenic brain embolism and migrainous phenomena have also been reported.[30, 33, 35] Reported visual complications include amaurosis fugax, retinal arterial or venous occlusion, and transient diplopia[30, 32, 33] (these are summarized in table form by Kleiner et al.[36]) and occipital ischemia.[30] A single case of recurrent acute ischemic optic neuropathy occurring over a 6-year period was reported by Briley et al., but the lack of clinical detail regarding what would be a highly unusual manifestation of ischemic optic neuropathy weakens this report.[33]

The etiologic role of this family of antibodies in neurologic dysfunction has been controversial. Evidence for and against the role of antiphospholipid antibodies as a cause of ischemic brain disease was discussed by Levine and Welch in a review article.[29] The preponderance of evidence within the past 2 years supports the notion that the coagulant-enhancing properties of these antibodies leads to an increased risk of neurovascular disease, especially among patients under 50 years of age. A recent prospective study of 104 patients demonstrated that anticardiolipin antibodies were significantly more common in a group of patients suffering brain ischemia than in a group with non-ischemic neurologic disorders.[37]

There is no consensus regarding therapy for patients who test positive for these antibodies. Some recommended treatments, including immunosuppression and anticoagulation, have a high risk for serious complication.[31, 33, 36] Strokes have occurred despite treatment with aspirin, or a combination of warfarin and dipyridamole. Digre et al. speculated that treatment with antiplatelet medications or anticoagulants, or both, reduced the frequency of amaurosis fugax.[32]

Other Vascular Diseases

Protein S deficiency was thought to be the cause of central retinal artery occlusion in a single case report.[38] The first documented case of retinal vaso-occlusive disease secondary to procainamide-induced lupus was reported—the role that antiphospholipid antibodies may have played was briefly discussed.[39] There was also a single report of a branch vein occlusion secondary to localized periphlebitis associated with sarcoidosis.[40]

Severe, long-standing carotid occlusive disease may cause retinal arteriovenous communications—this is the first report of such an association.[41] These communications developed proximal to regions of poor retinal perfusion. All three patients had obvious features of ocular ischemia.

A clinicopathologic report of bilateral visual loss in a patient with chronic renal failure proved to be the result of retinal oxalosis.[42] The formation of oxalate crystals in this patient, likely enhanced by the intake of ascorbic acid, hemodialysis, pyroxidine deficiency and increased bowel absorption following resection, resulted in occlusion of retinal blood vessels. Diagnosis of oxalosis depends on examination of the fundus and urine since measurement of serum levels is difficult. A list of additional causes of crystalline retinopathies was provided.

RETINAL DEGENERATION

Two forms of retinopathy associated with neurologic disease have been recently described. Coppeto and Lessell reported a familial syndrome of dystonia, blepharospasm, and pigmentary retinopathy.[43] Their cases were distinctive in that there was prominent extrapyramidal dysfunction and pigmentary change in the retina despite relatively preserved intellect. One patient was deaf, and both patients exhibited signs of pyramidal and cerebellar dysfunction and high-arched palates.

This article included a useful list of neurodegenerative diseases associated with pigmentary retinopathy, to which might be added Lytico-Bodig disease (amyotrophic lateral sclerosis-Parkinsonism-dementia complex of Guam).[44]

Hamilton et al. reported electroretinographic (ERG) evidence of selective involvement of cones in patients with autosomal dominant cerebellar ataxia,[45] which contrasts with some earlier studies in which degeneration of both rods and cones was reported. It is possible that a longer follow-up would have revealed evidence of rod pathology, but interestingly, only one of their four patients showed evidence of progression. They observed supernormal rod b wave amplitudes in two patients; this is not unique to this disease but is a curious finding that lacks explanation (some researchers believe that this ERG pattern might relate to subnormal cyclic guanosine monophosphate levels in photoreceptors). Ultimately, genotypic analysis will more conclusively establish subcategories of hereditary diseases of this type.[46]

Pathologic examination of twins with dominantly inherited olivopontocerebellar atrophy and retinal degeneration showed widespread degeneration of the photoreceptors (cones and rods) that appeared to begin within the central retina.[47] These two cases showed clinical and pathological (i.e., electron microscopic) similarities to the neuronal ceroid lipofuscinoses.

Lambert et al. published a very useful follow-up study of 75 patients with Leber's congenital amaurosis.[48] Forty percent of the diagnoses were revised after the cases were reviewed. The most common revised diagnoses included: congenital stationary night blindness, Joubert's syndrome (an autosomal recessive disorder associated with hypoplasia of the cerebellar vermis), retinitis pigmentosa, achromatopsia, infantile Refsum's disease, Zellweger's syndrome, and Senior's syndrome (retinopathy associated with nephrophthisis). The authors stressed the following points to reduce the likelihood of misdiagnosis: (1) children with known systemic disorders should not be classified as having Leber's congenital amaurosis; (2) children with evidence of developmental delay greater than would be expected for a visually impaired child should undergo laboratory tests to exclude Refsum's disease, Zellwegger's syndrome, and neuronal ceroid lipofuscinosis, and also receive a CT scan of the brain; and (3) the diagnosis of Leber's congenital amaurosis should be made with caution in children with moderately preserved visual acuity. In essence, the diagnosis of Leber's congenital amaurosis should be one of exclusion.

It is worth noting that only 6% of their patients had bone spicule pigmentation of the retina and that these patients were mentally retarded, suggesting that this combination of findings may represent a distinct subgroup. The remainder of the patients with true Leber's congenital amaurosis had normal appearing fundi, except for four who had macular colobomas. The authors suggested that these patients might also represent another subgroup.

The clinical features of ten patients from Honduras with Leber's congenital amaurosis were reported by a group from the Hospital for Sick Childen in Toronto.[49] The variable funduscopic appearance was emphasized, even in patients from the same family. Normal-appearing, pink optic nerves were observed more frequently than optic disk pallor. For the first time, a bull's eye maculopathy was recognized in a patient with Leber's congenital amaurosis.

Degenerative retinopathies usually affect both rods and cones. Three articles described syndromes in which the abnormalities appeared to be more specific. An autosomal dominant condition presented in five members of a family with a preferential involvement of the short-wavelength sensitive cones, producing a tritan-like color defect.[50] The authors stated that this condition could be distinguished from congenital tritanopia partly because there was a mild reduction in visual acuity, yet acuity was 20/20 or better in three of the four patients in whom it was measured. Pigmentary change in the macula was noted in four patients; one had a normal fundus. The normal-appearing optic nerves separated this disorder from autosomal dominant optic atrophy, although the photograph of the optic nerves of patient IV-6 could easily be interpreted as showing optic atrophy (and possibly even increased cupping O.S., which is a recognized feature of autosomal dominant optic atrophy).

Enhanced sensitivity of the short (S) wavelength sensitive cones was described in eight patients who had night blindness, maculopathy (often cystoid), and a characteristic ERG.[51] The ERG showed nearly identical scotopic and photopic responses, and the photopic responses appeared supernormal, among other things. Similar ERG findings observed in earlier reports were thought to represent signals arising from rods (a recent example of which was published by Fishman[52]), but the study by Marmor included a spectral sensitivity analysis that showed an absence of measurable rhodopsin and a spectral analysis of the large photopic ERG responses that were determined to match the spectral properties of the S (blue) cones. A second publication described similar or identical findings in two other patients.[53]

The enhanced S cone syndrome appears to develop in patients with an extremely insensitive rod system, the mechanism of which is not clear. Patients with the enhanced S cone syndrome can be distinguished from patients with congenital stationary night blindness because the former group has pigmentary degeneration in the macular region or cystoid maculopathy, and patients with congenital stationary night blindness show a scotopic ERG with a small or absent b wave, and a cone ERG that is only mildly abnormal.

A tapetal-like sheen appearance of the retina is a distinctive finding that can be associated with a number of disorders that limit vision, a concise review of which was published by Noble.[54] Retinal sheen was also recognized in one family in association with abnormalities of the retinal pigment epithelium of the posterior pole.[55]

A retinal sheen was observed in patients who had progressive cone dystrophy with an unusual X-linked pattern of inheritance.[56] The prolonged latency of visual-evoked potential (VEP) tests in some patients was thought to be evidence that the retinal ganglion cells had degenerated, possibly as a result of a transsynaptic process. While I agree that retinal ganglion cell degeneration can occur together with degeneration of the outer retina,[57] I would hesitate to conclude that the prolonged VEP latencies were necessarily the result of retinal ganglion cell involvement—a selective loss of photoreceptors alone might be sufficient to prolong the neural signal passing into the inner retina. Indeed, the loss of central acuity in patients with retinitis pigmentosa reported by Madreperia may be at least partially the result of concomitant ganglion cell degeneration and not solely related to the loss of central cones, as suggested by the authors.[58]

Retinochoroidal degeneration was reported in association with the infantile form of malignant osteopetrosis.[59] Because of this association, which had been previously reported, it is prudent to obtain an ERG to more accurately assess visual potential prior to performing surgical decompression of the optic foramen. A curious, newly described entity of retinochoroidal degeneration and progressive iris necrosis was reported in a 34-year-old man.[60] This syndrome is a local disease, associated with severe eye pain, in which pathologic examination of the eyes revealed an occlusive vasculopathy. It could not be determined whether the occlusions were primary or secondary phenomena.

A normal fundus (and normal fluorescein angiography of the macula) is not incompatible with the presence of a macular dystrophy and a significant loss of central acuity.[61] Three patients were reported in whom the focal ERG, which reflects the function of cones within the macula, was the only abnormality. The authors cautioned that this disorder could have been misdiagnosed as retrobulbar optic neuritis or amblyopia. A case of unilateral hemianopia that respected the vertical meridian was reported in a patient with sector retinitis pigmentosa.[62]

CANCER-ASSOCIATED RETINOPATHY

The pathologic basis for paraneoplastic involvement of the retina is still unknown. One case report included immunohistochemical staining of a monkey retina with the patient's serum as well as results of a passive immune transfer experiment.[63] In the former, the serum stained all of the cellular layers of the retina, the retinal pigment epithelium, large choroidal blood vessels, and occasional nuclei in the choroid. In the latter, transfer of the patient's serum to a guinea pig resulted in optic nerve demyelination. Plasmaphoresis reduced the antibody titers to retina and optic nerve, but the patient's vision did not improve.

These findings are interesting but do not answer the fundamental question: what caused the loss of vision? To be convincing, a clinico-pathologic study should cogently demonstrate a correlation between a pathologic process and a loss of function consistent with the pathologic process. It is difficult to reconcile, for instance, staining of all of the cells along the foveal outflow pathway and retention of 20/50 acuity. The lack of electrophysiologic recordings further frustrates attempts to understand the basis for visual loss, especially since the transfer experiment demonstrated demyelination. Interestingly, Bogen et al. reported a case of paraneoplastic optic neuritis and encephalomyelitis,[64] a syndrome that could have resulted from an antibody to ganglion cells similar to that described above.

I would certainly agree with the proposed autoimmune basis for the syndrome. Additional studies of the type reported by Thirkill et al.,[63] using basic science techniques in this unusual disease, will be necessary to understand this syndrome more conclusively. The report of Jacobson et al. provided additional evidence that this disorder is autoimmune.[65] They, like some others, reported an improvement in vision following immunosuppressive therapy with corticosteroids. They suggested that the triad of photosensitivity, ring scotomas (albeit the visual fields of patient no. 1 had much more prominent depression of the fields than scotoma formation), and attenuated retinal arterioles was suggestive of this paraneoplastic disorder, although, as they pointed out, none of these features is specific to this disorder.

A different form of paraneoplastic phenomenon was reported in two patients in whom bilateral diffuse uveal melanocytic proliferation developed.[66] The authors suggested that congenital melanocytosis of the uveal tract might exhibit limited growth and melanin production in response to certain hormone-producing visceral carcinomas (e.g., those of reproductive organs in women, and those of the retroperitoneum and lungs in men). The characteristic funduscopic appearance antedated signs and symptoms of the carcinomas by 3 and 12 months, emphasizing the value of early diagnosis. This condition may be accompanied by severe visual loss, the reason for which is not immediately apparent.

Two patients with metastasis to the retina were reported.[67] This rare occurrence, compared to the relatively common metastasis to the choroid, was the result of an oat-cell carcinoma of the lung in one case and breast carcinoma in the other. When the metastatic tumor is solitary, as occurred in one patient, the early findings may be difficult to distinguish from a retinal infarct—this has also been my experience. Seeding of the vitreous body may give the mistaken impression that the process is inflammatory.

OTHER RETINOPATHIES

Big Blind Spot Syndrome

Fletcher et al. reported a new syndrome of enlargement of the blind spot in the absence of optic disk edema secondary to a focal peripapillary retinopathy.[68] Of the seven cases reported, four were associated with positive visual phenomena in the region of the scotoma, and all exhibited absolute scotomas with steep margins and geographic features that centered on the blind spot. Multifocal electroretinography, a novel technique for which specific methods have not yet been published, showed abnormalities interpreted as demonstrating focal retinal dysfunction. Central acuity and color vision were not affected by the process; two patients had a mild afferent pupillary defect. Follow-up examinations performed on five of the patients showed resolution of the field defects. Interestingly, two of the patients had experienced prior episodes of blind spot enlargement that resolved.

One year later, two others patients were reported who had blind spot enlargement with features similar to those described by Fletcher, as well as funduscopic findings in the acute phase that were characteristic of the multiple evanescent white dot syndrome (MEWDS).[69] This latter syndrome, described in 1984, can be recognized by the characteristic small, white spots deep to the retina and related fluorescein angiographic findings. The authors convincingly described the similarities between these disorders. For instance, swelling of the optic nerve head, enlargement of the blind spot, and ERG abnormalities had been previously reported in some patients with MEWDS. It may be that for some patients the evanescent funduscopic abnormalities vanish prior to the evaluation that leads to the diagnosis of the big blind spot syndrome. The association of optic neuropathy in MEWDS was later stressed by Dodwell et al. in a series of five patients who were initially misdiagnosed as having optic neuritis, retrobulbar neuritis, and optic nerve edema and vitreitis.[70]

MEWDS has also occurred together with the acute macular neuroretinopathy syndrome.[71] This latter condition presents as an acute change in vision, sometimes progressive, with dense parafoveal scotomas and characteristic dark lesions visible on funduscopy that correspond to the location of the field defect(s).[72]

The etiology of these three syndromes is not known, but a virus has been suspected because of the occurrence in some patients of an antecedent viral illness and evidence of immune disturbance. Women are more often affected than men.

Leukemia

A prospective evaluation of ophthalmologic manifestations of leukemia was performed in 117 patients on the one hand, and 120 patients on the other hand: representing an egregious example of double-reporting.[73, 74] Amalgamating the reports, the salient conclusions were as follows: thrombocytopenia was the most important hematologic factor associated with intraretinal hemorrhage, hematocrit level was related to the likelihood of formation of white-centered hemorrhages, hematologic parameters were generally not associated with cotton-wool spots, children were less likely than adults to have retinopathy, and retinopathy was more common in patients with myeloid (as opposed to lymphoid) leukemia.

An autopsy study of 135 eyes in patients with leukemia revealed involvement in 31% of them, with the choroid being the most commonly affected site.[75] Using the agonal hematologic profile for analysis, the authors reported a lack of correlation between intraretinal hemorrhage and thrombocytopenia. They did not find a difference in the frequency of ocular involvement between acute and chronic forms of leukemia. Most of the patients with leukemic infiltrates of the central nervous system also had infiltration of the optic nerve. Although most cases of optic nerve involvement were seen in patients who had acute leukemia, Currie et al. stressed that optic neuropathy may occur in patients with chronic lymphocytic leukemia.[76]

Vascular Malformations of the Retina

Hemangioma-like masses of the retina resembling those seen in von Hippel-Lindau disease were observed in five patients.[77] The older age of onset, absence of radiologic evidence of systemic tumors, and absence of retinal or systemic abnormalities in family members were features that contrasted these patients from those with the hereditary retinal-neurologic syndrome of von Hippel-Lindau. The lesions reported in this nonfamilial entity were large, associated with exudate, and located in the posterior pole in three patients. There was evidence that the lesions were acquired and, in one case, that the lesion enlarged during the period of observation. Vision was variably affected as a consequence of leakage from the vascular mass.

Twenty patients with hereditary hemorrhagic telangiectasia (Rendu-Osler-Weber disease) were examined. Two of them had retinal vascular malformations, and seven had conjunctival telangiectasia. The conjunctival lesions can result in bloody tears.[78]

Other Disorders

The neuro-ophthalmologic manifestations of Lyme disease were reviewed by Lesser et al.,[79] and their cases included one patient who presented with funduscopic findings of neuroretinitis (i.e., blurred optic disks and exudate in the maculae). This article provided a useful review of the value of various laboratory tests in the diagnosis of this sometimes elusive disease. Neuroretinitis was also reported in an adolescent with mumps, a coincidence which in the future may be recognized more commonly since the incidence of mumps has substantially increased in recent years.[80]

Two patients were reported who presented with chronic intraocular inflammatory disease of unknown origin, manifested initially by bilateral optic disk swelling and retinal vasculitis. Years later they developed funduscopic findings that were characteristic of birdshot retinochoroidopathy.[81] These cases were remarkable in that the funduscopic features of birdshot retinochoroidopathy generally occur together with the onset of visual symptoms. The presence of the HLA-A29 antigen can be helpful in establishing the diagnosis in those cases of chronic posterior uveitis of unknown cause.

A case of acute retinal necrosis (ARN) syndrome was heralded by a presumed focal infection of the retina that resulted in a peculiar arcuate band of retinitis that conformed to the course of the parafoveal nerve fiber bundle.[82] Papillitis was also present. Two weeks later, the patient developed retinoscopic features of the ARN syndrome, including confluent retinal whitening and retinal vasculitis.

RETINAL CHANGES ASSOCIATED WITH OPTIC NERVE PITS

Serous retinal detachment is a well-recognized finding in association with optic nerve pits. Lincoff et al. used magnified stereoscopic fundus photographs and recognized that schisis-like separation of the inner layers of the retina was present in the maculas of 12 of 14 patients with optic nerve pits.[83] The authors suspected that the separation of the outer retina (i.e., serous detachment) was secondary to the formation of a schisis cavity and that macular holes would also develop after the intraretinal fluid had been present for some time: 14 of the 15 eyes that they examined developed macular holes. Anatomic disruption largely confined to the inner retina would explain why therapy directed at reattaching the presumed detached retina might appear to be unsuccessful in some cases. It is interesting to note, as the authors did, that an absolute scotoma was not present—scotomas are absolute in cases of peripheral retinal schisis because of the discontinuity that develops between the inner and outer layers of the retina. However, in the macula, a separation in the inner retina may not necessarily disrupt the anatomic connection between inner and outer retina because the nerve fiber layer of Henle allows the retina to stretch vertically without actually splitting.

The findings of the Lincoff study are persuasive—the authors were probably able to recognize the schisis cavity because of their attention to detail and their careful methods. Interestingly, Sobol et al. did not describe a schisis cavity in any of the 15 eyes studied as part of a retrospective review of visual function in patients with serous retinal detachment of the macula in association with a pit of the optic nerve.[84] They stated that visual loss occurred within 6 months of the serous detachment, and that improvement in vision thereafter was very unusual. Accordingly, the authors recommended early treatment to surgically eliminate the detachment. Obviously, the discrepancy between the observations of Lincoff and others (is the primary retinal process one of schisis formation) must be reconciled before the need for therapy and options can be better defined.

TOXICITY

Synthetic retinoids, now in wide use for acne vulgaris, may cause a reduction in amplitude of the a wave of the ERG. A prospective, pilot study included 12 patients who were given retinoids for dermatologic conditions: 7 patients were available for assessment before and 3 months after treatment was begun.[85] Although not explicitly stated, I surmise that no patient reported a change in vision. Vision was not detailed other than with electrophysiologic and dark adaptation testing. The authors suggested that patients receiving retinoids who report a change in night or color vision be evaluated for possible photoreceptor dysfunction.

There was an interesting case report of acute quinine toxicity from London.[86] The patient exhibited total blindness after she awoke and retinal edema was evident over both posterior poles. The visual fields became normal and central acuity improved to 20/60 bilaterally over the ensuing 2 months. Despite these encouraging features, she developed optic nerve pallor, attenuated retinal arteries, and ERG amplitudes that were lower than those recorded within 24 hours of the overdose—the paradox of quinine. Therapeutic considerations were briefly discussed; basically there is no evidence that any form of therapy improves visual outcome. The authors put forth a hypothesis that quinine blocks cholinergic transmission within the inner plexiform layer of the retina, a supposition based largely, or almost exclusively, on the known curare-like effects of quinine and the known localization of cholinergic cells and synapses within the inner retina rather than from any specific features of their case. As the authors discussed, the abnormal electro-oculogram was evidence that the outer retina must have also been involved.

Niacin is known to cause a reversible cystoid maculopathy (Gass, 1973). This maculopathy occurs as a result of high daily doses, usually taken as therapy for hypercholesterolemia. Millay et al. described 4 patients who experienced visual symptoms associated with niacin therapy; cystoid maculopathy without leakage on fluorescein angiography was recognized in three of the patients.[87] Patients reported foggy/blurred vision, and spokes or radiations around lights. Examination of 15 visually asymptomatic patients receiving high-dose niacin revealed no abnormalities, prompting the authors to suggest that only visually symptomatic patients need eye examinations. The authors stated that only 0.67% of patients receiving high doses of niacin will develop maculopathy; the justification for this figure is not given, other than to remark that only 2 cases of definite cystoid maculopathy were observed in the 300 patients treated at their institution. It is not stated whether all 300 patients underwent eye examinations, or what proportion received fluorescein angiography, etc. Fortunately, visual symptoms apparently develop quickly after starting on a high dose of niacin and appear to be reversible.

REFERENCES

1. Curcio C, Sloan KR, Packer O, et al: Distribution of cones in human and monkey retina: Individual variability and radial asymmetry. *Science* 1987; 236:579–582.

2. Rizzo J: The retina, in Lessell S, Van Dalen JTW (eds): *Current Neuro-Ophthalmology,* vol 2. Chicago, Year Book Medical Publishers, 1990, pp 223–238.

3. Mikelberg FS, Drane SM, Schulzer M, et al: The normal human optic nerve. Axon count and axon diameter distribution. *Ophthalmology* 1989; 96:1325–1328.

4. Jonas JB, Müller-Bergh JA, et al: Histomorphometry of the human optic nerve. *Invest Ophthalmol Vis Sci* 1990; 31:736–744.

5. Repka MX, Quigley HA: The effect of age on normal human optic nerve fiber number and diameter. *Ophthalmology* 1989; 96:26–32.

6. Balazi AG, Rootman J, Drance SM, et al: The effect of age on the nerve fiber population of the human optic nerve. *Am J Ophthalmol* 1984; 97:760–766.

7. Kuritzky S: Nitroglycerin to treat acute loss of vision. *N Engl J Med* 1990; 323:1428.

8. Miller Fisher C: Transient monocular blindness versus amaurosis fugax. *Neurology* 1989; 39:1622–1624.

9. The Amaurosis Fugax Study Group: Current management of amaurosis fugax. *Stroke* 1990; 21:201–298.

10. Bernstein EF, Browse NL: The CHAT classification of stroke. *Ann Surg* 1989; 209:242–248.

11. Anderson CU, Marquardsen J, Mikkelsen B, et al: Amaurosis fugax in a Danish community: A prospective study. *Stroke* 1988; 19:196–199.

12. Caplan LR, Pessin MS: Symptomatic carotid artery disease and carotid endarterectomy. *Ann Rev Med* 1988; 39:273–299.

13. Moore WS, Boren C, Malone J, et al: Natural history of nonstenotic asymptomatic ulcerative lesions of the carotid artery. *Arch Surg* 1978; 113:1352–1359.

14. Dixon S, Pais O, Raviola C, et al: Natural history of nonstenotic, asymptomatic ulcerative lesions of the carotid artery. *Arch Surg* 1982; 117:1493–1498.

15. Tippin J, Corbett JJ, Kerber RE, et al: Amaurosis fugax and ocular infarction in adolescents and young adults. *Ann Neurol* 1989; 26:69–77.

16. Appleton R, Farrell K, et al: Amaurosis fugax in teenagers. A migraine variant. *Am J Dis Child* 1988; 142:331–333.

17. Aasen J, Kerty E, Russell D, et al: Amaurosis fugax: Clinical, Doppler, and angiographic findings. *Acta Neurol Scand* 1988; 77:450–455.

18. Grigg MJ, Papadakis K, Nicolaides AN, et al: The significance of cerebral infarction and atrophy in patients with amaurosis fugax and transient ischemic attacks in relation to internal carotid artery stenosis: A preliminary report. *J Vasc Surg* 1988; 7:215–222.

19. Report of the American Academy of Neurology, Therapeutics and Technology Assessment Subcommittee: Interim assessment: Carotid endarterectomy. *Neurology* 1990; 40:682–683.

20. Rossouw JE, Lewis B, et al.: The value of lowering cholesterol after myocardial infarction. *N Engl J Med* 1990; 323:1112–1119.

21. Hypertension Detection and Follow-up Program Cooperative Group: Five year findings of the hypertensive detection and follow-up program. III. Reduction in stroke incidence among persons with high blood pressure. *JAMA* 1982; 247:663–683.

22. Whelton PK: Declining mortality from hypertension and stroke. *South Med J* 1982; 75:33–38.

23. Yatsu FM, Fisher M: Atherosclerosis: Current concepts on pathogenesis and interventional therapies. *Ann Neurol* 1989; 26:3–12.

24. Petersen P, Boysen G, Godtfredsen J, et al: Placebo controlled, randomized trial of warfarin and aspirin for prevention of thromboembolic complications in chronic atrial fibrillation: The Copenhagen AFASAK study. *Lancet* 1989; 1:175–179.

25. Petersen P, Boysen G: Prevention of stroke in atrial fibrillation. *N Engl J Med* 1990; 323:482.

26. Stroke Prevention in Atrial Fibrillation Study Group Investigators: Preliminary report of the stroke prevention in atrial fibrillation study. *N Engl J Med* 1990; 322:863–868.

27. The Boston Area Anticoagulation Trial for Atrial Fibrillation Investigators: The effect of low-dose warfarin on the risk of stroke in patients with non-rheumatic atrial fibrillation. *N Engl J Med* 1990; 323:1505–1511.

28. Chesebro JH, Fuster V, Halperin JL: Atrial fibrillation—risk marker for stroke. *N Engl J Med* 1990; 323:1556–1558.

29. Levine SR, Welch KMA: Antiphospholipid antibodies. *Ann Neurol* 1989; 26:386–389.

30. Levine SR, Deegan MJ, et al: Cerebrovascular and neurological disease associated with antiphospholipid antibodies: 48 cases. *Neurology* 1990; 40:1181–1189.

31. Brey RL, Hart RG, et al: Antiphospholipid antibodies and cerebral ischemia in young people. *Neurology* 1990; 40:1190–1196.

32. Digre KB, Durcan FJ, Branch DW, et al: Amaurosis fugax associated with antiphospholipid antibodies. *Ann Neurol* 1989; 25:228–232.

33. Briley DP, Coull BM, Goodnight SH: Neurological disease associated with antiphospholipid antibodies. *Ann Neurol* 1989; 25:221–227.

34. Gerber SL, Cantor LB: Progressive optic atrophy and the primary antiphospholipid antibody syndrome. *Am J Ophthalmol* 1990; 110:443–444.

35. Young SM, Fisher M, et al: Cardiogenic brain embolism and lupus anticoagulant. *Ann Neurol* 1989; 26:390–392.

36. Kleiner RC, Najarian LV, Schatten S, et al: Vaso-occlusive retinopathy associated with anti-phospholipid antibodies (lupus anticoagulant retinopathy). *Ophthalmology* 1989; 96:896–904.

37. Kushner MJ: Prospective study of anticardiolipin antibodies in stroke. *Stroke* 1990; 21:295–298.

38. Golub BM, Sibony PA, et al: Protein S deficiency associated with central retinal artery occlusion. *Arch Ophthalmol* 1990; 108:918.

39. Nichols CJ, Mieler WF: Severe retinal vaso-occlusive disease secondary to procainamide-induced lupus. *Ophthalmology* 1989; 96:1535–1540.

40. Kimmel AS, McCarthy MJ, et al: Branch retinal vein occlusion in sarcoidosis. *Am J Ophthalmol* 1989; 107:561–562.

41. Bolling JP, Buettner H: Acquired retinal arteriovenous communications in occlusive disease of the carotid artery. *Ophthalmology* 1990; 97:1148–1152.

42. Wells CG, Johnson RJ, Qingli L, et al: Retinal oxalosis. A clinicopathologic report. *Arch Ophthalmol* 1989; 107:1638–1643.

43. Coppeto J, Lessell S: A familial syndrome of dystonia, blepharospasm, and pigmentary retinopathy. *Neurology* 1990; 40:1359–1363.

44. Cox TA, McDarby JV, Lavine L, et al: A retinopathy on Guam with high prevalence in Lytico-Bodig. *Ophthalmology* 1989; 96:1731–1735.

45. Hamilton SR, Chatrian GE, Mills RP, et al: Cone dysfunction in a subgroup of patients with autosomal dominant cerebellar ataxia. *Arch Ophthalmol* 1990; 108:551–556.

46. Rosenberg RN: Autosomal dominant cerebellar phenotypes: The genotype will settle the issue. *Neurology* 1990; 40:1329–1331.

47. Traboulsi EI, Maumenee IH, Green WR, et al: Olivopontocerebellar atrophy with retinal degeneration. A clinical and ocular histopathologic study. *Arch Ophthalmol* 1988; 106:801–806.

48. Lambert SR, Kriss A, Taylor D, et al: Follow-up and diagnostic reappraisal of 75 patients with Leber's congenital amaurosis. *Am J Ophthalmol* 1989; 107:624–631.

49. Smith D, Oestreicher J, Musarella MA: Clinical spectrum of Leber's congenital amaurosis in the second to fourth decades of life. *Ophthalmology* 1990; 97:1156–1161.

50. Bresnick GH, Smith VC, Pokorny J: Autosomal dominantly inherited macular dystrophy with preferential short-wavelength sensitive cone involvement. *Am J Ophthalmol* 1989; 108:265–276.

51. Marmor MF, Jacobson SG, Foerster MH, et al: Diagnostic clinical findings of a new syndrome with night blindness, maculopathy, and enhanced S cone sensitivity. *Am J Ophthalmol* 1990; 110:124–134.

52. Fishman GA, Peachey NS: Rod-cone dystrophy associated with a rod system electroretinogram obtained under photopic conditions. *Ophthalmology* 1989; 96:913–918.

53. Keunen JEE, Van Meel GJ, Van Norren D: Rod densitometry in night blindness. A review and two puzzling cases. *Doc Ophthalmol* 1988; 68:375–387.

54. Noble KG, Margolis S, Carr RE: The golden tapetal sheen reflex in retinal disease. *Am J Ophthalmol* 1989; 107:211–217.

55. Noble KG, Sherman J: Central pigmentary sheen dystrophy. *Am J Ophthalmol* 1989; 108:255–259.

56. Jacobson DM, Thompson HS, Bartley JA: X-linked progressive cone dystrophy. *Ophthalmology* 1989; 96:885–895.

57. Newman NM, Stevens RA, Heckenlively JR: Nerve fiber layer loss in diseases of the outer retinal layer. *Br J Ophthalmol* 1987; 71:21–26.

58. Madreperia SA, Palmer RW, et al: Visual acuity loss in retinitis pigmentosa. Relationship to visual field loss. *Arch Ophthalmol* 1990; 108:358–361.

59. Ruben JB, Morris RJ, Judisch GF: Chorioretinal degeneration in infantile malignant osteopetrosis. *Am J Ophthalmol* 1990; 110:1–5.

60. Margo CE, Friedman SM, et al: Retinochoroidal degeneration associated with progressive iris necrosis. *Arch Ophthalmol* 1990; 108:989–992.

61. Miyake Y, Ichikawa K, Shiose Y, et al: Hereditary macular dystrophy without visible fundus abnormality. *Am J Ophthalmol* 1989; 108:292–299.

62. Johnson LN, Rabinowitz YS, Hepler RS: Hemianopia respecting the vertical meridian and with foveal sparing from retinal degeneration. *Neurology* 1989; 39:872–873.

63. Thirkill CE, Fitzgerald P, Sergott RC, et al: Cancer-associated retinopathy (CAR syndrome) with antibodies reacting with retinal, optic nerve, and cancer cells. *N Engl J Med* 1989; 321:1589–1594.

64. Bogen D, Sebag M, Michaud J: Paraneoplastic optic neuritis and encephalomyelitis. Report of a case. *Arch Neurol* 1988; 45:353–356.

65. Jacobsen DM, Thirkill CE, Tipping SJ: A clinical triad to diagnose paraneoplastic retinopathy. *Ann Neurol* 1990; 28:162–167.

66. Gass JDM, Gieser RG, Wilkinson CP, et al: Bilateral diffuse uveal melanocytic proliferation in patients with occult carcinoma. *Arch Ophthalmol* 1990; 108:527–533.

67. Leys AM, Van Eyck LM, Nuttin BJ, et al: Metastatic carcinoma to the retina. Clinicopathologic findings in two cases. *Arch Ophthalmol* 1990; 108:1448–1452.

68. Fletcher WA, Imes RK, Goodman D, et al: Acute idiopathic blind spot enlargement. A big blind spot syndrome without disc edema. *Arch Ophthalmol* 1988; 106:44–49.

69. Hamed LM, Glaser JS, et al: Protracted enlargement of the blind spot in multiple evanescent white dot syndrome. *Arch Ophthalmol* 1989; 107:194–198.

70. Dodwell DG, Jampol LM, et al: Optic nerve involvement associated with the multiple evanescent white-dot syndrome. *Ophthalmology* 1990; 97:862–868.

71. Gass JD, Hamed LM: Acute macular neuroretinopathy and multiple evanescent white dot syndrome occurring in the same patients. *Arch Ophthalmol* 1989; 107:189–193.

72. Miller MH, Spalton DJ, et al: Acute macular neuroretinopathy. *Ophthalmology* 1989; 96:265–269.

73. Guyer DR, Schachat AP, Vitale S, et al: Leukemic retinopathy. Relationship between fundus lesions and hematologic parametetrs at diagnosis. *Ophthalmology* 1989; 96:860–864.

74. Schachat AP, Markowitz JA, Guyer DR, et al: Ophthalmologic manifestations of leukemia. *Arch Ophthalmol* 1989; 107:697–700.

75. Leonardy NJ, Rupani M, et al: Analysis of 135 autopsy eyes for ocular involvement in leukemia. *Am J Ophthalmol* 1990; 109:436–444.

76. Currie JH, Lessell S, Lessell I, et al: Optic neuropathy in chronic lymphocytic leukemia. *Arch Ophthalmol* 1988; 106:654–660.

77. Campochiaro PA, Conway BP: Hemangiomalike masses of the retina. *Arch Ophthalmol* 1988; 106:1409–1413.

78. Brant AM, Schachat AP, White RI: Ocular manifestations in hereditary hemorrhagic telangiectasia (Rendu-Osler-Weber disease). *Am J Ophthalmol* 1989; 107:642–646.

79. Lesser RL, Kornmehl EW, Pachner AR, et al: Neuro-ophthalmologic manifestations of Lyme disease. *Ophthalmology* 1990; 97:699–706.

80. Foster RE, Lowder CY, Meisler DM, et al: Mumps neuroretinitis in an adolescent. *Am J Ophthalmol* 1990; 110:91–93.

81. Soubrane G, Bokobza R, Coscas G: Late developing lesions in birdshot retinochoroidopathy. *Am J Ophthalmol* 1990; 109:204–210.

82. Margolis T, Irvine AR, et al: Acute retinal necrosis syndrome presenting with papillitis arcuate neuroretinitis. *Ophthalmology* 1988; 95:937–940.

83. Lincoff H, Lopez R, Kreissig I, et al: Retinoschisis associated with optic nerve pits. *Arch Ophthalmol* 1988; 106:61–67.

84. Sobol WM, Blodi CF, et al: Long-term visual outcome in patients with optic nerve pit and serous retinal detachment of the macula. *Ophthalmology* 1990; 97:1539–1542.

85. Brown RD, Grattan CEH: Visual toxicity of synthetic retinoids. *Br J Ophthalmol* 1989; 73:286–288.

86. Canning CR, Hague S: Ocular quinine toxicity. *Br J Ophthalmol* 1988; 72:23–26.

87. Millay RH, Klein ML, Illingworth DR: Niacin maculopathy. *Ophthalmology* 1988; 95:930–936.

PART FIVE

THE ORBIT

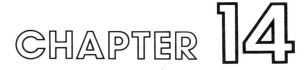

CHAPTER 14

The Orbit

Peter J. Savino, M.D.

Director, Neuro-Ophthalmology Service, Wills Eye Hospital, Philadelphia, Pennsylvania

In this edition of *Current Neuro-ophthalmology*, I plan to review some of the more recent contributions to several orbital processes. As in previous years, I will make no attempt to be all-inclusive but highlight only selected orbital problems.

OPHTHALMOPATHY OF GRAVES' DISEASE

The ophthalmopathy of Graves' disease is the most frequent orbital process that will be encountered by the ophthalmologist. It seems that the harder one looks for signs of ophthalmopathy in the patient with Graves' disease, the more likely these signs will be found. It has been estimated that clinically obvious ophthalmopathy from Graves' disease may be seen in 40% of patients with Graves' disease.[1]

Natural History of the Ophthalmopathy

Several studies have demonstrated the temporal relationship between the thyroid gland abnormality and the ophthalmopathy from Graves' disease. Wiersinga et al.[2] reviewed 125 consecutive patients with ophthalmopathy from Graves' disease and found that 99 (79%) had thyroid gland dysfunction: only 3 had hypothyroidism, the remainder had hyperthyroidism. In these patients, the thyroid gland disease preceded the eye signs in 37 patients, appeared simultaneously with the eye disease in 39 patients, and was detected only after the eye disease appeared in 23 patients. While the eye signs occurred with the same frequency before or after thyroid gland dysfunction was detected, ophthalmopathy from Graves' disease was closely related temporally to thyroid gland dysfunction appearing during the year before or after the appearance of hyperthyroidism in 75% of patients.

It has often been speculated, without statistical proof, that certain types of treatment for the underlying thyroid gland dysfunction might predispose to the development of ophthalmopathy more than other treatments. Siridama et al.[1] prospectively examined 426 patients with Graves' disease treated with either ^{131}I, surgery, or drugs. They found that patients free of ophthalmopathy at the time of thyroid treatment developed ophthalmopathy in approximately the same ratio independent of the type of primary treatment used (4.9% to 7.1%). In addition, those who already had ophthalmopathy had equal progression of eye signs, independent of the type of primary treatment used (19.2% to 22.7%). Likewise, there was an equal degree of improvement of the ophthalmopathy with all treatment modalities (12.3% to 14.1%). It therefore appears that the development, worsening, or improvement of ophthalmopathy is independent of the type of treatment directed at the underlying thyroid gland disease. This article points out, and it is further substantiated by the report of Prummel et al.,[3] that returning patients to the euthyroid state may in fact improve some signs of ophthalmopathy due to Graves' disease.

These studies emphasize that the natural history of Graves' ophthalmopathy is variable. They should caution readers and investigators to consider treatment of ophthalmopathy due to Graves' disease with manipulation of the underlying thyroid states when considering the efficacy of specific regimens for treatment of the ophthalmopathy itself.

Immunology

It is commonly accepted that ophthalmopathy from Graves' disease is an immunologic disorder. The exact mechanism by which the host becomes immunized and the precise antigenic tissue(s) involved remain the subject of intensive investigation. Since this terrain is still uncertain and ever-changing, specifics of immunologic debates will not be considered here.

For the reader interested in a detailed state-of-the-science review of current immunologic research in Graves' disease, a symposium entitled, Advances in Endocrine Ophthalmopathy of Graves' Disease—Immunology and Treatment[4] is recommended.

Another excellent review of the autoimmunity in Graves' disease is provided by Weetman.[5] What is known now about the immunohistopathologic state of Graves' disease is that a stimulus causes lymphocytic infiltration of the retrobulbar tissue (extraocular muscle). Fibroblasts enlarge and proliferate and produce glycosaminoglycans (GAG), which are hydrophilic. Finally, the enlarged muscle becomes fibrosed and then atrophies. It seems that the major damage to the extraocular muscle is produced by the mucopolysaccharide production and not by the direct effect of the lymphocyte.

Weetman[5] also posed the pertinent questions that still remain unanswered in the immunology of ophthalmopathy due to Graves' disease: 1) are there shared antigenic determinates between thyroid and eye; if so, what are they? 2) is any retroocular/bulbar tissue antigenically unique so that localization of disease can be explained? Until these two questions are answered, the underlying process resulting in ophthalmopathy due to Graves' disease must remain speculative.

Treatment

The appearance of ophthalmopathy due to Graves' disease in the First Lady of the United States caused this disorder to obtain wide coverage in the lay press. The underlying dilemmas in the treatment of ophthalmopathy from Graves' disease were exposed, and it became obvious that a consensus on this subject does not exist in the American medical community. Recent information regarding treatment modalities in ophthalmopathy from Graves' disease include immunosuppressive therapy, radiation therapy, and orbital surgery.

Immunosuppression Therapy

Prednisone is the mainstay of immunosuppression therapy in ophthalmopathy due to Graves' disease. Prummel et al.[6] divided patients with ophthalmopathy from Graves' disease into two groups, each containing 18 patients. In group I, the patients were treated with prednisone, 60 mg a day tapered to 20 mg daily. In group II, cyclosporin, 7.5 mg/kg/day was used. The patients were treated for 12 weeks, and in group I, 11 (61%) patients improved, while in group II, only 4 (22%) improved. The nonresponders in each group were then treated with a combination of both drugs for another 12 weeks. Of the original 9 nonresponders in group I, 5 (56%) improved, while 8 (62%) of the 13 nonresponders in group II improved. It appears therefore if one immunosuppressive drug is to be used, it should be prednisone. For those who do not respond, a combination of prednisone and cyclosporin deserves consideration.

The routine use of systemic prednisone treatment at the time of treatment of the primary thyroid gland dysfunction to prevent ophthalmopathy remains controversial. Bartalena et al.[7] randomized 52 patients into two groups. In group I, 26 patients were treated with ^{131}I, while in group II, another 26 patients were treated with ^{131}I and concomitant prednisone therapy for 4 months. In group I, 10 patients who did not have ophthalmopathy at the time of treatment did not develop eye signs following treatment. Sixteen patients in whom the eye signs were present either did not experience any eye change (44%) or worsened (56%). In group II, the 5 patients with no ophthalmopathy did not develop eye signs, while of the 21 patients with ophthalmopathy from Graves' disease at the time of initial treatment, 52% improved and 48% did not experience any change. No patient treated with the concomitant ^{131}I, prednisone regimen showed worsening of ophthalmopathy from Graves' disease. This is an extremely small study, and further data are required before subjecting all patients treated for thyroid dysfunction to 4 months of systemic prednisone.

Other immunosuppressive or immunomodulating agents have been investigated in the treatment of ophthalmopathy due to Graves' disease. Ciamexone was administered to patients with ophthalmopathy from Graves disease.[8] Two groups were formed, one treated with placebo, the other with ciamexone. The subjective and objective clinical findings, ultrasonographic data, and computed tomography (CT) scan differences between the groups were compared. There was no difference between the placebo group and the group treated with ciamexone. It should be noted that all patients in this study were treated with corticosteroids for 4 weeks. It does appear, however, that ciamexone has no role in the treatment of thyroid gland ophthalmology.

Azathioprine was also investigated in the treatment of ophthalmopathy due to Graves' disease.[9] Ten patients were treated with azathioprine while ten patients were control subjects. There was no apparent difference in the grading of the ophthalmopathy from Graves' disease between the two groups, and the authors state that azathioprine is not useful in the treatment of moderately severe thyroid ophthalmopathy.

Manipulation of the immune system by plasma exchange has also been recommended for the treatment of ophthalmopathy due to Graves' disease. Glinder et al.[10] treated 15 patients with a combination of plasma exchange and immunosuppression. All patients in the study received prednisone, 40 mg a day and azathioprine, 100 mg a day after plasmapheresis. While the authors note clinical improvement in almost all patients and improvement of transverse muscle thickness and density on CT scan, recurrence of ophthalmopathy occurred in one third of their patients when immunosuppression was discontinued. It appears that plasma exchange can be useful in the treatment of resistant ophthalmopathy, but it should not be used as a first-line treatment in this disorder.

Radiation Therapy

The role of radiation therapy was championed again by Kriss et al.,[11] who presented their institution's 20-year experience in the treatment of 311 patients, 275 of whom had been followed up for at least a year, or until eye surgery was performed. These authors concluded that radiation therapy was effective; the ophthalmopathy due to Graves' disease was worse in only 29 of 1,025 observations collected. Thirty percent of their patients did require eye muscle surgery after radiation therapy. These authors state that radiation therapy was less effective in men, patients over 60 years of age, or in patients who were never thyrotoxic or were being treated concomitantly for hyperthyroidism.

While Sandler et al.[12] agreed that radiation therapy was indeed effective in the treatment of ophthalmopathy due to Graves' disease, they disagreed with Kriss et al.[11] in that they found the treatment response was not influenced by age, sex, or the hyperthyroid or euthyroid state of the patient.

Radiation therapy for acute ophthalmopathy due to Graves' disease is very viable and may be used as primary treatment. Complications of radiation therapy are rarely reported and can almost always be traced to errors in technique, which may be avoided if performed at institutions familiar with this specific type of therapy.

Surgery

Orbital surgery for the treatment of ophthalmopathy due to Graves' disease continues to occupy a significant portion of the ophthalmic literature. Within the past 2 years, several modifications of orbital decompressive surgery have been proposed.

Ronecevic and Jackson[13] recommend a surgical approach to the patient with exophthalmos that includes three skin incisions and the removal of orbital fat. The first incision is performed in the upper lid and is designed to remove fat and to split the levator aponeurosis. They also advise to remove as much fat as possible. An incision is then made medially, and the medial wall (ethmoidal section) is removed as well as more fat. A third incision is made inferiorly through which the posterior portion of the orbital floor and the zygomatic portion of the lateral wall are removed along with more orbital fat. This technique purportedly provides a more symmetric decompression and one that is adequate, although the millimeters of average decompression obtained is not recorded. It is speculated that the superior incision relieves lid retraction by both the division of the levator aponeurosis and the superior removal of fat.

Leone et al.[14] recommended an orbital decompressive procedure using a lateral skin incision and a medial skin incision. In the eight patients they describe, a range of 4 to 7 mm of decompression was obtained. However, two skin incisions are required.

Mourits et al.[15] describe their experience in 60 consecutive patients who underwent orbital decompression with inferomedial, inferomedial plus lateral, and a coronal approach. They found that all three approaches resulted in improvement of visual function, there was no net change in the amount of diplopia with any procedure, and the complication rate was the same (approximately 10%) with each procedure. The conclusion is that decompression is safe and effective, independent of the surgical approach used.

In addition to decompressing the orbit, some authors have added another wrinkle, that of advancement of the lateral wall.[16] These authors describe the three-wall decompression (lateral, medial, floor) combined with an anterior 4-mm and an outward 2-mm displacement of the lateral wall. They describe nine patients and believe that lateral wall advancement is beneficial because it expands the size of the orbit and provides better postoperative upper and lower lid position.

Despite this series of articles, I still maintain my bias, which is:

1. For ophthalmopathy due to Graves' disease without an optic neuropathy, an anterior decompression is adequate.
2. For optic neuropathy, posterior decompression, especially on the medial wall, is essential.
3. From a cosmetic standpoint, an admirable goal is to avoid or reduce the number of skin incisions.

My method of treating patients with optic neuropathy from Graves' disease remains surgical. I believe that orbital decompressive surgery is, in competent hands, the quickest, surest, and safest way to attack the optic neuropathy due to Graves' disease.

ORBITAL INFLAMMATORY DISEASE

Idiopathic

The terms idiopathic orbital inflammatory disease and orbital pseudotumor are used synonymously.

The diagnosis of orbital inflammatory disease remains largely a clinical one. When the extraocular muscles are enlarged on images, the distinction between myositis and ophthalmopathy due to Graves' disease is said to be a clear one. However, Patrinely et al.[17] have shown that orbital pseudotumor may mimic Graves' disease more than previously appreciated. The signs of myositis were often bilateral (40%), and the myositic muscle may have less tendinous involvement than previously described (47%). Since these signs, i.e., bilaterality and sparing of the tendon, are thought to be typical of thyroid ophthalmopathy, it appears now that they, although present in ophthalmopathy due to Graves' disease, are signs that are less than pathognomonic.

While many instances of orbital pseudotumor are idiopathic, underlying disease may be found. Two articles described an association between optic neuropathy and inflammatory orbital and sinus disease in patients who chronically used intranasal cocaine.[18, 19] They pointed out that the typical findings of long-standing cocaine abuse, chronic osteolytic sinusitis, and optic neuropathies are due to a contiguous orbital inflammation from the primary sinus disease due to intranasal cocaine abuse.

A patient is described who was said to have orbital myositis as a result of giant cell arteritis.[20] However, in this paper the CT scan was said to show normal extraocular muscles and paranasal sinuses. The patient had proptosis and decreased motility, which improved with 80 mg of prednisone in 24 hours. However, with normal neuro-imaging (not shown in the article), other causes of the clinical signs should be considered, particularly ischemia of the extraocular muscles as described by Barricks et al.[21]

Corticosteroid or radiation therapy is the customary treatment for orbital inflammatory disease. An unusual case required emergency surgery when the idiopathic inflammatory orbital disease was associated with a spontaneous orbital hemorrhage.[22]

Noble et al.[23] describe a patient who refused a second course of oral corticosteroids for orbital myositis. This patient was given indomethacin, 75 mg twice a day, and the orbital inflammation resolved in 3 weeks. The patient, however, was also receiving topical steroids. If this isolated case report proves to be reproducible in other patients with orbital pseudotumor, indomethacin would be a welcome addition and substitution for systemic steroid therapy.

Lymphoid Inflammation/Lymphoma

The debate regarding the use of immunohistologic techniques to distinguish between inflammatory lymphoid pseudotumors, reactive hyperplasia, and lymphomas continues. Medeiros et al.[24] reviewed 61 patients with orbital and conjunctival lymphoid infiltrates and determined the prognostic significance of monotypic immunoglobulin expression. They divided their patients into three groups histologically: group I, malignant in 20 patients; group II, benign in 14 patients, including both inflammatory pseudotumor and reactive follicular hyperplasia; and group III, indeterminate in 27 patients. They then, on the basis of immunologic testing, reclassified all the lesions that expressed monotypic immunoglobulins as malignant lymphomas and those that expressed polytypic immunoglobulins as benign. The group with malignant lesions comprised 40 patients, 20 of whom were previously classified as having malignant lesions histologically. This represented all of those classified histologically as malignant. Twenty of the 27 patients with lesions that were histologically indeterminate were reclassified as malignant on the basis of immunologic testing. The second large group, classified as benign, included all 14 patients with lesions that were histologically classified as benign as well as 7 patients from the indeterminate group. Patients with cytologically atypical (malignant) lesions had an 80% risk of dissemination in 5 years compared with 45% in the indeterminate group. No patient with a histologically benign lesion had dissemination. Patients with localized monotypic infiltrates had a 50% risk of dissemination compared with no patient with polytypic lesions showing dissemination. For the patients with histologically indeterminate lesions, there was a 62% probability of dissemination within 5 years if the immunologic testing showed a monotypic response. No dissemination was found with a polytypic infiltrate. For all patients, monotypic immunoglobulin expression correlated with reduced survival. However, the survival was good, indicating that these monotypic small infiltrates behaved like other low-grade B-cell lymphomas showing a relatively indolent clinical course.

The authors then addressed why their findings differed from those of Jakobiec et al.[25] They speculate it was due to the different methods used in the two studies.

This article shows that we should continue performing immunologic testing on patients with orbital inflammatory disease, but it again demonstrates that histologic evaluation of the lesion remains crucial.

ORBITAL MASS LESIONS

Orbital Tumors

A large series of one institution's experience with orbital mass lesions appeared. One was a review article of metastatic tumors to the orbit, which included a review of a personal series and the literature.[26] These authors found that metastatic lesions represented 1.5% to 3.3% of all orbital disease, but about 10% of all orbital tumors. The locations of the primary lesions were breast, lung, prostate gland, and skin. The localization for metastatic disease was most frequent in the lateral orbit (39%), followed by the superior orbit (32%), medial orbit (20%), and finally the inferior orbit (12%). A striking figure is that in 42% of the combined cases reviewed, the orbital presentation heralded the declaration of the presence of a primary malignancy. Survival in this group averaged 9.3 months for all cases. In a second report, these authors remind us that enophthalmos is frequently encountered with orbital metastasis (25% of their 38 patients).[27]

A particularly insidious type of orbital tumor that is frequently difficult to diagnose presents with ophthalmoplegia and orbital pain. This syndrome, as described in the five patients of Clouston et al.,[28] represents perineural infiltration from cutaneous squamous cell carcinoma and may occur years after excision of these skin cancers. These tumors spread along the branches of cranial nerves V and VII and even superb orbital imaging may be normal until the tumor forms a mass lesion that becomes obvious. While squamous cell carcinoma is the most frequent cause of this syndrome, other cutaneous cancers, e.g. melanoma, may also be responsible.[29] This is an important syndrome, not because it is frequent, but because it will often occur years after the primary skin tumor is apparently "successfully" removed. The patient may completely forget the relatively insignificant removal of this tumor and the diagnosis may be delayed. The treatment of these patients is a problem, and I agree that radiation therapy and chemotherapy have little role. Clouston et al.[28] recommend extensive surgery to remove the tumor, but usually by the time the diagnosis is made, this type of radical surgery is not feasible.

Orbital tumors, and particularly metastatic disease, may not present as an isolated mass in the orbit. While the so-called "fat muscle" seen on a CT scan is most often a sign of idiopathic inflammatory disease or Graves' disease, it may be a sign of tumor. In one series of 60 patients with non-thyroid enlargement of extraocular muscles,[17] the most frequent cause was a tumor. While this series is almost assuredly biased toward unusual causes of fat muscles, it does make the point that tumors should be considered when this imaging picture is encountered.

Capone and Slamovits[30] describe the specific CT characteristics of metastatic solid tumors to the extraocular muscles. In their five patients, one muscle was involved in two patients and bilateral multiple muscles were involved in three. In two of the five patients, this orbital metastasis was the first sign of a systemic cancer with breast cancer being the most frequent primary site. The authors also provide a useful table of other causes of extraocular muscle enlargement found on imaging.

Hematic Cysts

The advent of magnetic resonance imaging (MRI) and its application to the orbit has made the diagnosis of blood within the orbital contents relatively straightforward. As described in a photo essay in the *Archives of Ophthalmology,* the MRI signal for hematic cyst is typically high on both T1- and T2-weighted images.[31] In the neuroradiologic literature, it has been shown that even with chronic hematic cysts of up to 10 years duration, the MRI signal remains high on both T1- and T2-weighted images.[32]

An interesting article appeared that described eight patients with hematic cysts, but only two of these patients underwent MRI.[33] The MRI images were fascinating in that the signal on T1-weighted images was low and not high as expected. The cysts were both in young people, were intraconal, and nontraumatic. In the first case, no time was given from the onset of the symptoms to MRI, but in the second patient, the time was 3 weeks. The authors state that they have seen a low T1 signal and a high T2 signal in other patients with hematic cysts. This finding is remarkably unlike previous experience with the detection of blood in the orbit or intracranially. The authors do not speculate as to why blood should have a low signal on a T1-weighted image. This finding was so unexpected that I reviewed this paper with one of the authors (RAZ) of the seminal paper regarding MRI findings of blood.[34] He speculates that this low signal may be caused by a major concentration of a proteinacious fluid in the so-called hematic cyst. This could occur with cysts of long duration, or with acute cyst whose major component is not blood. In the first patient, the interval from the symptoms to MRI seems too short to explain signs of chronicity. In the second patient, there was a 6-year history of orbital disease, so that chronicity might be invoked as the explanation.

SINUS DISEASE

Orbital Complications of Sinus Disease

Since the orbit is surrounded on several sides by the paranasal sinuses, sinus diseases or surgical correction of these diseases can produce orbital syndromes.

It is well known that infectious sinusitis may cause a variety of orbital signs and symptoms. One patient with ethmoid sinusitis developed a subperiosteal orbital hematoma.[35] The authors speculate that this unusual finding may be a stage preceding the development of a subperiosteal abscess. Two children were described with ethmoid sinusitis and the onset of acute diplopia and the pattern of acute Brown's syndrome.[36] The Brown's syndrome resolved with antibiotics alone in one child, and partially resolved in the other.

Sphenoid sinusitis, which is less frequent, was reviewed by Kibblewhite et al.[37] Fourteen patients with sphenoid sinusitis were described, and five patients had ophthalmic signs including chemosis, proptosis, diplopia, ophthalmoplegia, and decreased vision. The authors stress that imaging is the best way to detect this abnormality. In this day and age, most clinicians have a relatively low threshold for imaging in patients with orbital signs, yet a report appeared which described a patient with sphenoid sinusitis and orbital cellulitis with negative plain x-rays as interpreted by an experienced radiologist. The correct diagnosis was made when CT was performed.[38] This again stresses the fact, I believe, that plain skull x-rays have no role in the investigation of patients with visual or orbital disease. CT and/or MRI should be the only procedures performed.

Complications of Sinus Surgery

Intranasal surgery, particularly rhinoplasty, has been associated with intraorbital complications. Four patients presented with visual loss following apparently uncomplicated nasal surgery. These patients had ischemic optic neuropathy, branch retinal artery occlusion, central retinal artery occlusion, and one was said to have a retrobulbar ischemic optic neuropathy.[39] Three different surgical procedures were performed on the four patients, but the one thing that all the surgeries had in common was a submucosal injection of local anesthetic with a vasoconstrictive agent. Since no particulate matter, e.g. corticosteroid suspension, was injected, the proposed mechanism of the visual loss is intraorbital vasospasm.

Dental surgery may also cause orbital problems[40] as described in a patient with extraction of a mandibular molar with a high-speed, air-driven drill. During the surgery, she developed lid edema and later subcutaneous emphysema. The emphysema involved the orbit and resulted in an optic neuropathy (disk pallor, visual field loss, and relative afferent pupillary defect). The suspected cause was the high-speed, air-driven drill.

Orbital hemorrhage may occur with a variety of surgical procedures and represents an opthalmic emergency. Sacks et al.[41] described four patients who had orbital hemorrhage following dacryocystorhinostomy, external frontal ethmoidectomy, trauma with a blowout fracture, and after anterior ethmoid artery ligation for epistaxis. All of these patients were treated with orbital decompression via a transantral external ethmoidectomy approach. Interestingly, two of four patients had anterior chamber paracentesis despite the orbits being described as tight and with intraocular pressures only in the 40s. Two other instances of orbital hemorrhage are described,[42] one during a medial maxillectomy and one during a transethmoid sphenoidectomy.[42]

Buus et al.[43] described seven patients who had complications of sinus surgery. Three had intraorbital hemorrhages, one resulted in permanent blindness following ethmoidectomy. Two patients had diplopia, one attributed to superior oblique injury during a transantral ethmoidectomy, and one to a medial rectus injury during an intranasal ethmoidectomy. One unfortunate patient had bilateral optic nerve transection during intranasal endoscopic ethmoidectomies. In this patient, the pathologic specimen clearly shows the optic nerves! In a discussion of this paper, Shore[44] adds his experience with similar complications and includes brain biopsy, bilateral superior oblique paralyses, orbital hemorrhage, incarceration of tissue medially with both abduction and adduction deficits, and dacryostenosis presumably occurring during maxillary ostium enlargement.

Of importance in this article is the recommendation for the treatment of orbital hemorrhage. The authors state that treatment should be initiated without delay and recommend the following:

1. Remove any sinus packing.
2. Normalize systemic blood pressure.
3. Identify bleeding source and control it intraoperatively.
4. Open the periorbita medially for decompression and drainage into the sinus.
5. Add a topical β blocker, intravenous acetazolamide, and mannitol if the intraocular pressure is elevated. If this does not resolve the situation, perform a lateral canthotomy and inferior cantholysis.
6. As a last resort, perform orbital decompression.

Shore[44] agrees with these recommendations but also adds intravenous steroids.

I also agree with these recommendations and do not believe paracentesis of the anterior chamber plays any role in the face of increased orbital pressure.

REFERENCES

1. Sridama V, De Groot LJ: Treatment of Graves' disease and the course of ophthalmopathy. *Am J Med* 1989; 87:70–73.
2. Wiersinga WM, Smit T, van der Gaag R, et al: Temporal relationship between onset of Graves' ophthalmopathy and onset of thyroidal Graves' disease. *J Endocrinol Invest* 1988; 11:615–619.
3. Prummel MF, Wiersinga WM, Mourits MP, et al: Amelioration of eye changes of Graves' ophthalmopathy by achieving euthyroidism. *Acta Endocrinol (Copenh)* 1989; 121:185–189.

4. Lamberg B-A, Välimäki M: Advances in endocrine ophthalmopathy of Graves' disease—Immunology and treatment. *Acta Endocrinol (Copenh)* 1989; 121:1–131.

5. Weetman AP: Autoimmunity in Graves' ophthalmopathy: A review. *J R Soc Med* 1989; 82:153–158.

6. Prummel MF, Mourits MP, Berghout A, et al: Prednisone and cyclosporin in the treatment of severe Graves' ophthalmopathy. *N Engl J Med* 1989; 321:1353–1359.

7. Bartalena L, Marcocci C, Bogazzi F, et al: Use of corticosteroids to prevent progression of Graves' ophthalmopathy after radioiodine therapy for hyperthyroidism. *N Engl J Med* 1989; 321:1349–1352.

8. Kahaly G, Lieb W, Müller-Forell W, et al: Ciamexone in endocrine orbitopathy. *Acta Endocrinol (Copenh)* 1990; 122:13–21.

9. Perros P, Weightman DR, Crombie AL, et al: Azathioprine in the treatment of thyroid-associated ophthalmopathy. *Acta Endocrinol (Copenh)* 1990; 122:8–12.

10. Glinder D, Schrooyen M: The treatment of severe Graves' ophthalmopathy with plasma exchange and immunosuppression. *Acta Endocrinol (Copenh)* 1989; 121:149–153.

11. Kriss JP, Petersen IA, Donaldson SS, et al: Supervoltage orbital radiotherapy for progressive Graves' ophthalmopathy: Results of a twenty-year experience. *Acta Endocrinol (Copenh)* 1989; 121:154–159.

12. Sandler HM, Rubenstein JH, Fowble BL, et al: Results of radiotherapy for thyroid ophthalmopathy. *Int J Radiat Oncol Biol Phys* 1989; 17:823–827.

13. Ronecevic R, Jackson IT: Surgical treatment of thyrotoxic exophthalmos. *Plast Reconstr Surg* 1989; 84:754–760.

14. Leone CR Jr, Piest KL, Newman RJ: Medial and lateral wall decompression for thyroid ophthalmopathy. *Am J Ophthalmol* 1989; 108:160–166.

15. Mourits MP, Koornneerf L, Wiersinga WM, et al: Orbital decompression for Graves' ophthalmopathy by inferomedial, by inferomedial plus lateral, and by coronal approach. *Ophthalmology* 1990; 97:636–641.

16. Wulc AE, Popp JC, Bartlett SP: Lateral wall advancement in orbital decompression. *Ophthalmology* 1990; 97:1358–1369.

17. Patrinely JR, Osborn AG, Anderson RL, et al: Computed tomographic features of nonthyroid extraocular muscle enlargement. *Ophthalmology* 1989; 96:1038–1047.

18. Goldberg RA, Weisman JS, McFarland JE, et al: Orbital inflammation and optic neuropathies associated with chronic sinusitis of intranasal cocaine abuse. *Arch Ophthalmol* 1989; 107:831–835.

19. Newman NM, DiLoretto DA, Ho JT, et al: Bilateral optic neuropathy and osteolytic stinusitis: Complications of cocaine abuse. *JAMA* 1988; 259:72–74.

20. Laidlaw DAH, Smith PEM, Hudgson P: Orbital pseudotumor secondary to giant cell arteritis: An unreported condition. *Br Med J* 1990; 300:784.

21. Barricks ME, Traviesa DB, Glaser JS, et al: Ophthalmoplegia in cranial arteritis. *Brain* 1977; 100:209–221.

22. Linberg JV, Mayle M: Spontaneous orbital hemorrhage associated with idiopathic inflammatory pseudotumor. *Am J Ophthalmol* 1990; 109:103–104.

23. Noble AG, Tripathi RC, Levine RA: Indomethacin for the treatment of idiopathic orbital myositis. *Am J Ophthalmol* 1989; 108:336–338.

24. Medeiros LJ, Harmon DC, Linggood RM, et al: Immunohistologic features predict clinical behavior of orbital and conjunctival lymphoid infiltrates. *Blood* 1989; 74:2121–2129.

25. Jakobiec FA, Neri A, Knowles DM II: Genotypic monoclonality in immunophenotypically polyclonal orbital lymphoid tumors. *Ophthalmology* 1987; 94:980–994.

26. Goldberg RA, Rootman J, Cline RA: Tumors metastatic to the orbit: A changing picture. *Surv Ophthalmol* 1990; 35:1–24.

27. Goldberg RA, Rootman J: Clinical characteristics of metastatic orbital tumors. *Ophthalmology* 1990; 97:620–624.

28. Clouston PD, Sharpe DM, Corbett AJ, et al: Perineural spread of cutaneous head and neck cancer. Its orbital and neurologic complications. *Arch Neurol* 1990; 47:73–77.

29. Hufnagel TJ, Savino PJ, Zimmerman RA, et al: Painful ophthalmoplegia caused by neurotropic malignant melanoma. *Can J Ophthalmol* 1990; 25:38–41.

30. Capone A Jr, Slamovits TL: Discrete metastasis of solid tumors to extraocular muscles. *Arch Ophthalmol* 1990; 108:237–243.

31. Loeffler M, Hornblass A: Hematic cyst of the orbit. *Arch Ophthamol* 1990; 108:886–887.

32. Wiot JG, Pleatman C: Chronic hematic cysts of the orbit. *Am J Neuroradiol* 1989; 10:537–539.

33. Travis RC, Murray PI, Moseley IF, et al: Orbital intraconal haematic cysts in young people: Computed tomography and magnetic resonance imaging. *Br J Radiol* 1989; 62:521–525.

34. Gomori JM, Grossman RI, Goldberg HI, et al: Intracranial hematomas: Imaging by high-field MR. *Radiology* 1985; 157:87–93.

35. Choi S, Lawson W, Urken ML: Subperiosteal orbital hematoma. An unusual complication of sinusitis. *Arch Otolaryngol Head Neck Surg* 1988; 114:1464–1466.

36. Saunders RA, Stratas BA, Gordon RA, et al: Acute onset Brown's syndrome associated with pansinusitis. *Arch Ophthalmol* 1990; 108:58–60.

37. Kibblewhite DJ, Cleland J, Mintz DR: Acute sphenoid sinusitis: Management strategies. *J Otolaryngol* 1988; 17:159–163.

38. Roberts C, Nylander AE, Jayaramachandran S: Orbital cellulitis complicating isolated sphenoid sinusitis: Importance of the CT scan. *Br J Ophthalmol* 1989; 73:769–770.

39. Savino PJ, Burde RM, Mills RP: Visual loss following intranasal anesthetic injection. *J Clin Neuro-ophthalmol* 1990; 10:140–144.

40. Buckley MJ, Turvey TA, Schumann SP, et al: Orbital emphysema causing vision loss after dental extraction. *J Am Dent Assoc* 1990; 120:421–424.

41. Sacks SH, Lawson W, Edelstein D, et al: Surgical treatment of blindness secondary to intraorbital hemorrhage. *Arch Otolaryngol Head Neck Surg* 1988; 114:801–803.

42. Thompson RF, Gluckman JL, Kulwin D, et al: Orbital hemorrhage during ethmoid sinus surgery. *Otolaryngol Head Neck Surg* 1990; 102:45–50.

43. Buus DR, Tse DT, Farris BK: Ophthalmic complications of sinus surgery. *Ophthalmology* 1990; 97:612–619.

44. Shore JW: Discussion. *Ophthalmology* 1990; 97:619.

PART SIX

OCULAR MANIFESTATIONS OF NEUROLOGIC DISEASE

CHAPTER 15

Myasthenia Gravis

Dieter Schmidt, M.D.

Professor, Universitäts-Augenklinik Freiburg, Germany

Myasthenia gravis (MG) is one of the best models of autoimmune disease in human neurology. With accurate diagnosis and selective use of current therapies, the vast majority of cases of MG can be stabilized or improved.[1] New clinical and immunologic observations on this puzzling disorder are continually being reported. To gain an overview of the essential problems of MG, papers by Pachner,[2] Newsom-Davis,[3] Eymard,[4] Breucking,[5] Gajdos,[6] and Christadoss[7] are recommended for additional information.

OCULAR MYASTHENIA

The diagnosis of ocular myasthenia depends mainly on clinical data: ptosis, external ophthalmoplegia, and/or weakness of the orbicularis oculi muscle, with spontaneous fluctuations, remissions, and relapses—even after a delay of years.

Ultrastructural Eye and Eyelid Muscles and Eye Motility Disorders

The extraocular muscles are quite different from the true skeletal muscles. Six distinct fiber types with the most important differences between fast-twitch and slow-tonic fiber types were found.[8, 9] The variability of saccadic eye movements

273

reflects the many factors that contribute to the pulse transmission at the neuromuscular junction. Changes in the paretic myasthenic eye muscle are due to a varying involvement of the fast-twitch and slow-tonic fibers as well as to the central adaptation of an existing peripheral deficit (paresis). The multiple innervation of the muscle fiber types seems to be characteristic of the rectus and oblique extraocular muscles, in contrast to the levator palpebrae superioris, which is considered to contain only singly innervated muscle fibers. Muscles with a predominantly tonic innervation (like the levator palpebrae muscle) fatigue more readily during the day than the extraocular muscles. Iwasaki and Kinoshita[10] encountered bilateral blepharoptosis due to myasthenia without ophthalmoplegia in a 62-year-old woman. Evoli et al.[11] investigated 48 patients with ocular myasthenia. In 5 patients (10%), ptosis was the only clinical sign; in 43 patients (90%), ptosis and diplopia occurred; and in 12 patients (25%), weakness of the orbicularis oculi muscle was diagnosed. The investigation of the morphology of the levator palpebrae superioris muscle (Porter et al.[12]) revealed three types of singly innervated muscle fibers, found in the global layer of other extraocular muscles, and an additional, unique slow-twitch fiber type. By contrast, the orbicularis muscle exhibited three distinct fiber types: one slow-twitch and two fast-twitch fiber types. On the basis of oxidative enzyme profiles and mitochondrial content, the majority of the orbicularis oculi fibers would be fatigue-prone. This morphologic finding explains the clinical observation of facial weakness due to myasthenic fatigue (like the afternoon ectropion, Walsh and Hoyt[13]). The occurrence of unilateral and isolated weakness of the orbicularis oculi muscle with sparing of the ipsilateral facial muscles in 2 patients, a 39-year-old woman and a 25-year-old man, was described by Gangadhar et al.[14] The woman also showed periodic lid retraction, Cogan's lid twitch sign, and quiver eye movements. Chia[15] saw a 20-year-old woman with facial weakness due to MG, without paresis of the extraocular muscles. This finding is very unusual.

Porter et al.[9] investigated the denervation of extraocular muscles in the monkey. Histopathologic changes were most apparent in the orbital singly innervated fiber type and its global layer counterpart. The essential findings indicated that the extraocular muscles exhibited a "resilience" to denervation, and the total number of fibers was not significantly changed. The extensive myofilament loss that usually follows skeletal muscle denervation did not occur in the extraocular muscles. Singly innervated fibers with the highest mitochondrial content exhibited the most severe changes. These ultrastructural findings corroborate the clinical observation in myasthenic pareses that ocular motility disturbances are quite different from those of true skeletal muscles.

In patients with MG, a faster than normal initial segment of a saccade, which cannot be sustained, often occurs. This means that the fast-twitch fibers of the muscles are intact, although the tonic fibers that are responsible for holding the eye in a sideward position are weak. The central gain of a saccade is increased in response to the paretic extraocular muscle. The supernormal saccadic velocities, especially of the small saccades, despite the muscle paresis, support the conclusion that phasic muscle fibers are relatively spared in myasthenia. The central gain increase is manifest when the muscle defect is transiently alleviated by edrophonium. Hypermetria and increased saccadic gain result after the injection of the pharmacologic agent or after maintained gaze to one side. The high-gain instability of the saccadic system in a 52-year-old man, who had a long-standing, myasthenic incomplete ophthalmoplegia of both eyes, was apparent immediately after the administration of edrophonium chloride: both eyes showed macro-saccadic oscillations for several minutes, as a sign of unmasking the increased central gain. Even in the primary position, gaze-holding on the target was completely impossible.[16]

Ocular myasthenia might be considered to be a separate type of myasthenia gravis because of the highly restricted symptoms, predominance of affected men, good response to steroids, and relatively poor response to anticholinesterase drugs. Two forms of ocular myasthenia have been postulated: an acetylcholine receptor (AChR) antibody (ab)-positive form associated with women, thymus hyperplasia or thymoma, other autoantibodies, and positive electromyography (EMG) findings, and an AChR ab-negative form, more often associated with men, a normal thymus, absence of autoantibodies, and negative EMG findings.

The results of an immunologic study on patients with ocular myasthenia[17] showed that the AChR abs were found in only 22 of the 48 patients investigated. (AChR ab—binding and blocking—were assayed with radioimmunoassay with human antigen.) Nine men and 13 women were found in the AChR-ab positive group; in the negative group, there were 19 men and 7 women. Morel et al.[18] found that more than half of the patients with ocular myasthenia had negative or limited values of anti-AChR titers, regardless of age and sex. Patients with ocular myasthenia generally had low titers of anti-AChR abs. The ocular disease occurred almost equally among men and women. Tsujihata et al.[19] investigated 19 patients with ocular myasthenia, all of whom improved after the injection of edrophonium chloride. Circulating anti-AChR abs were absent in 6 of the 16 patients investigated, but the motor end plate fine structure of the postsynaptic region from the biceps brachii muscles was abnormal in all 16 patients. Deposits of the immune complexes IgG, C3, and C9 were detected at the motor endplates of these muscles in 16 of 19 patients. Repetitive nerve stimulation disclosed a decremental response in the orbicularis oculi muscles of 2 of 17 patients. Single-fiber EMG revealed no abnormality in 8 of 13 patients studied.

Different Immunologic Types of MG

Mossman et al.[20] reported a special form of MG without acetylcholine receptor antibodies. In 8 patients with clinical features of a generalized or an ocular MG, no serum antibody against acetylcholine receptor could be detected. Immunoglobulin preparations from the 8 patients were injected intraperitoneally into mice.

Neuromuscular transmission was significantly impaired in comparison with mice receiving control human immunoglobulin. This form of MG is immunologically and physiologically distinct from the AChR ab-positive form. Hayashi et al.[21] studied the binding characteristics of AChR ab in sera of 9 patients with MG. The comparison between the sera of 5 patients with ocular myasthenia and the sera of 4 patients with generalized MG showed that polyclonal or heterogeneous AChR abs occurred in the sera, which did not help to explain the clinical difference between ocular and generalized MG. Evoli et al.[22] studied the clinical and immunologic characteristics of patients with MG who had no detectable anti-AChR abs. Sixty patients with negative anti-AChR abs were compared with 287 patients with positive anti-AChR abs. Significant differences were found with regard to sex incidence, disease severity, and thymic pathology. However, no difference was found in patients with ocular or severe generalized MG as far as both groups of positive and negative antibody titer were concerned.

Diagnostic Tests

Sleep Test

A new diagnostic procedure was recommended by Winterkorn et al.[23] They used the sleep test as a safe alternative to the Tensilon (edrophonium) test for the diagnosis of MG. Sometimes edrophonium is medically undesirable, or the test is difficult to perform or refused by the patient. A temporary remission of ptosis and muscle paresis after a rest of approximately 30 minutes in a quiet, dark room is helpful in diagnosis. Photographs of the palpebral fissures and eye movements are taken before and after sleep for demonstrating the recovery of the eye muscle paresis. Additional prospective investigations should be performed to evaluate this new test as an alternative to other examinations like the Tensilon test.

Morning/Evening Comparison Test

Another simple and also relatively safe test for the diagnosis of myasthenic pareses was suggested and involves measuring the difference in the width of the palpebral fissure between morning and night.[16] The advantage of this test is the observation of fatigue-dependent paresis at night in comparison with the recovery from paresis in the morning, immediately after sleep. Therefore, in this test, the difference of the eye muscle paresis is more pronounced. Photographs of the palpebral fissure and the eye muscle paresis should be obtained at different times during the day. We have used this test for years in several patients who had questionable eye muscle paresis and/or ptosis. This test was always very helpful in diagnosis and was carried out in the ward.

Tensilon Test

A transient improvement of paresis with edrophonium chloride is considered to be a fundamental test in the diagnosis of MG. Since Osserman's introduction of the edrophonium test (1952), it has been regarded as the most reliable diagnostic test for MG. Evoli et al.[11] stated that ptosis responded better than diplopia to the anticholinesterase drug. In 48 patients with purely ocular myasthenia, the edrophonium chloride test was positive in 46 patients (95%). In 15 of 43 patients (35%) who had ptosis and diplopia, only relief of the ptosis occurred. Oh and Cho[24] observed an unequivocal positive edrophonium test, both clinically and electrophysiologically, in a 57-year-old woman with the characteristic features of the Lambert-Eaton syndrome. The authors point out that an unequivocal positive edrophonium test alone is not necessarily pathognomonic for MG. A positive edrophonium test has been also described in botulism, the Guillain-Barré syndrome, amyotrophic lateral sclerosis, lesions of the cavernous sinus, and in congenital myasthenic syndromes. Additionally, patients with neurasthenia may also have a temporary improvement in strength that cannot be fully distinguished by double-blind testing.[25] The diagnosis of MG should be based on the clinical features, edrophonium-responsiveness, and other laboratory findings.

Rodgin[26] mentioned the possibility of giving different amounts of edrophonium chloride at different times. A high dose of edrophonium chloride can be dangerous because of side effects. In such a situation, atropine also should be given as in the neostigmine test. The author reports on the history of a 58-year-old man with diplopic episodes, for one of which he was hospitalized at the age of 25. This was followed by remission. He had had intermittent shortness of breath and/or fatigue since he was 49. In 1984, he presented with fluctuating ptosis. Successive visits over the next 5 years showed varying amounts of ptosis and diplopia. In 1985, a severe bout of meningitis resulted in residual diplopia. The anti-AChR abs were elevated. Two edrophonium chloride tests were performed: the first test showed a negative result, the second test was positive.

Electrophysiologic Methods

Evoli et al.[11] found that 24 of 48 patients (50%) with purely ocular myasthenia showed a decremental response in the EMG from the limb muscles. Gilchrist and Sanders[27] stressed that a U-shaped decremental response to repetitive stimulation of a peripheral nerve, which is characteristic of MG, can also occur as a sign of denervation of motor units in cervical radiculopathy. Negative results of repetitive stimulation in patients with MG during an EMG investigation may also occur, as has been reported by Scoppetta et al.[28]

Single fiber electromyography (SFEMG) is a sensitive method for detecting neuromuscular transmission disorders. The investigation of the extensor digitorum communis muscle with SFEMG in 20 patients with ocular myasthenia revealed 17 patients with elongated jitter. This finding means that, even in ocular myasthenia, there is subclinical generalizition of the disease.[29] (The time between two potentials, the interpotential interval, varies from discharge to discharge. This variability is called the electromyographic jitter.[30]) An increased amount of jitter on SFEMG is a nonspecific measure of neuromusclar dysfunction. Trontelj et al.[31] found with this method that, in patients with MG, the orbicularis oculi muscle was more often abnormal than the frontalis muscle. In a group of 19 healthy volunteers, the normal values of the jitter of the stimulated orbicularis oculi muscle were measured and the upper normal limits determined statistically. In addition, Jabre et al.[32] investigated the jitter and determined normal SFEMG values in the extensor digitorum communis muscle of 8 healthy subjects. In 4 patients with MG who were treated with pyridostigmine, Massey et al.[33] found normal jitter measurements in the frontalis and orbicularis oculi muscles, but the jitter became abnormal 2 to 14 days after the medication was discontinued. It is concluded that cholinesterase inhibitors may mask the electrophysiologic abnormality in myasthenia.

Antibodies to the nicotinic acetylcholine receptor (anti-AChR abs) were detected in 20 of 44 patients (45.5%) with ocular myasthenia[11]; in the presence of positive results, the mean antibody titer was significantly lower (7.8 nM) than that found in patients with generalized MG (47.9nM).[11] Oosterhuis[34] found that antibodies to AChR were present in 34% of cases of ocular MG and in 92% of cases of generalized MG.

Differential Diagnosis

Davis and Lavin[35] described eye muscle paresis in ocular myasthenia mimicking the one-and-a-half syndrome of brain stem disease. A 65-year-old man with a history of hypertension and diabetes mellitus was unable to look to the left and on attempted right gaze he had a slow and incomplete adduction of the left eye. Two edrophonium tests were negative or equivocal, but after 1 week, ptosis was relieved completely and ocular motility was improved by the injection of edrophonium.

Exercise-induced diplopia is characteristic of myasthenia. However, this phenomenon has also been described as diagnostic of a midline cerebral tumor, an astrocytoma, in a 22-year-old man.[36] Diplopia was noticed twice while the patient was playing football and once while undergoing physical training. It lasted between 15 and 90 minutes, and the symptoms subsided 5 minutes after the cessation of exercise.

Experienced clinicians[37] made the diagnosis of ocular myasthenia in these eight patients (Table 1)[37, 38] predominantly on the basis of clinical features, response to anticholinesterase agents, and some additional laboratory tests. All these patients were eventually found to have a parasellar mass. Retrospective review suggests, according to the authors, that four of these patients probably had only an intracra-

TABLE 1.

Ocular Pseudomyasthenia*

Age (yr), Sex	Eye Signs at the First Visit; Tensilon Test	Follow-up	Computed Tomography (CT) and/or Arteriographic Findings	Final Diagnosis
Patient 1: 51, F	Horizontal diplopia due to weakness of elevation, depression, and adduction of the right eye, ptosis (right), orbicularis oculi muscles weak, occasional dilation right pupil, Cogan's lid twitch sign, Tensilon test positve, pyridostigmine: improvement of paresis	1 year later: increasing ptosis, orbicularis oculi weakness more marked on the right side. 2 months later: dilation of the right pupil, complete absence of right medial, superior, inferior rectus function	CT: mass in the region of the right sphenoid ridge	Craniotomy: meningioma of the right sphenoid ridge
Patient 2: 77, F	Sudden onset of double vision, intermittent right ptosis, marked limitation of elevation and adduction of right eye, neostigmine test positive	2 years later: worsening of diplopia. 2 ½ years later: increasing headaches, ptosis, diplopia. Right pupil contracted only minimally to direct light, Tensilon test negative	CT: large mass in right cavernous sinus with encroachment on the superior orbital fissure, no arteriography	No surgery
Patient 3: 16, M	1-month history of diplopia, episodes of variable right ptosis, right temporal headaches. Examination: ptosis (right) after sustained upgaze, decreased abduction of right eye, worse with fatigue, Tensilon test: improvement of variable degree.	Treatment with prednisone: symptoms were thought to be stabilized	3 months later: CT: large calcified mass in the region of the right cavernous sinus.	Surgery: Chondrosarcoma involving the right cavernous sinus
Patient 4: 77, F	Mild ptosis, limitation of adduction (right eye), Tensilon test positive, pyridostigmine: at first some improvement	Effect of pyridostigmine was incomplete	2 months later: CT: right parasellar mass with rim calcification, suggestive of a meningioma; angiogram: meningioma	Surgery was refused

(Continued.)

TABLE 1 (cont.).

Ocular Pseudomyasthenia*

Age (yr), Sex	Eye Signs at the First Visit; Tensilon Test	Follow-up	Computed Tomography (CT) and/or Arteriographic Findings	Final Diagnosis
Patient 5: 70, M	10 and 2 years earlier he had transient diplopia. He had now horizontal and vertical diplopia, left ptosis of 2 years' duration. Edrophonium test equivocal	10 months later: vertical diplopia and variable ptosis, fatigue-dependent, abnormal lid twitch sign on the left, limitation of abduction and adduction of the left eye, more marked on upward gaze. Tensilon test positive, another examination: additional proptosis was noted and a decreased sensation of the territory of the left ophthalmic nerve	CT: left parasellar calcified mass with a thickened tortuous left optic nerve, consistent with meningioma	No surgery
Patient 6: 53, M	Left ptosis, intermittent diplopia, Tensilon test negative	10 months later: left ptosis with questionable lid twitch, deficits of ocular motility on elevation, depression, and adduction of the left eye. Tensilon test positive (on two occasions)	3 years later: CT: left parasellar lesion, consistent with meningioma	No surgery, treatment with radiation
Patient 7: 77, M	Intermittent right ptosis of 6 years' duration; 5 years previously a right sphenoid ridge meningioma was resected; 1 year later, recurrence of the right ptosis and left ptosis, elevation and adduction were impaired, Tensilon test positive, pyridostigmine: good improvement		2 years later: CT showed a mass attached to the right carotid artery: cerebral angiogram: 5 cm tumor blush: recurrent tumor	No further surgery

Patient 8: 65, F	18-month history of right ptosis, fatigue-dependent, 6 months history of transient diplopia on right gaze, examination: right ptosis, Cogan's lid twitch sign, limitation of elevation, adduction, abduction of the right eye. Tensilon test positive, cerebrospinal fluid: 78 mg/dL protein, pyridostigmine: improvement	5 years later: headache, nausea, vomiting, dizziness, lethargy	CT and angiogram: mass in the right cavernous sinus, parasellar and suprasellar region: meningioma	No surgery, radiation therapy
Patient 9: 74, F	6-month history of variable intermittent diplopia; occasional generalized headache; on sustained upgaze or right, a right hypertropia developed; on sustained downgaze or left, a left hypertropia developed. Tensilon test negative; Anti-AChR abs: negative; EMG normal	After CT investigation, the patient was followed up for the next 3 years with no change in hormone or visual status	CT: enhancing sellar-parasellar mass; arteriography: bilateral intracavernous carotid aneurysms, serum prolactin level was elevated	Bilateral intracavernous carotid aneurysms
Patient 10: 65, F	3 years prior: onset of intermittent diplopia; occasional headaches above the left eye; 1½ years prior: intermittent exotropia (right), intermittent ptosis (left). Investigation: bilateral ptosis, horizontal and vertical diplopia, left eye only had lateral movements; Tensilon test positive; Anti-AChR abs: negative; EMG normal	Treatment with pyridostigmine had a good response, but during the next year she required increasing doses of pyridostigmine. Thymectomy: involuted thymus. 6 months later: ptosis (right) increased, visual acuity fell to 20/400 (right), pallor of right disk. Bypass operation.	CT: prominent venous sinuses. 3 years after initial symptoms, CT: bilateral intracavernous carotid aneurysms	Bilateral intracavernous carotid aneurysms

*Information for patients 1 through 8 is adapted from Moorthy G, Behrens MM, Drachman DB, et al: *Neurology* 1989;39:1150–1154; information for patients 8 and 9 is adapted from Mindel JS, Charney IZ: *Trans Am Ophthalmol Soc* 1989;87:445–462.

nial mass (patients 2, 3, 4, and 6); while the other four may have had both MG and an intracranial mass (patients 1, 5, 7, and 8).

The clinical distinction between ocular myasthenia and pseudomyasthenia is not possible except by observation of certain neuro-ophthalmologic findings. No single test is infallible. However, strongly unilateral paresis, especially with pupillary disturbances and/or complaints of facial or ocular pains, optic nerve or trigeminal nerve involvement, or changes in cerebrospinal fluid are evidence of a cranial nerve lesion. Tests of optic nerve function might have resulted in an earlier diagnosis. Close observation of the patient is essential for a disease with a questionable diagnosis. Moorthy et al.[37] found that if the following changes occur, they are highly suggestive of, but not pathognomonic of, this disease:

1. Weakness and fatigue confined to the extraocular muscles, eyelids, and orbicularis oculi muscles are suggestive of MG. Variability of paresis, worsening on sustained effort and improving after rest, involvement of muscles innervated by more than one cranial nerve, especially if bilateral, and the absence of pupillary involvement are consistent with ocular myasthenia. Cogan's lid twitch sign, although highly suggestive of myasthenia, cannot be said to be absolutely diagnostic.[39]

2. Response to anticholinesterase agents—From a practical standpoint, it appears to be unwise to accept a diagnosis of MG on the basis of the response to these drugs. Seven of eight patients with intracranial masses showed a positive response to edrophonium, and four of five patients responded to oral anticholinesterase medication.

3. Repetitive nerve stimulation and single-fiber EMG are often helpful, although neither is entirely specific for MG. The finding of an elevated AChR ab titer is virtually diagnostic of MG. However, despite a serum antibody titer in a 40-year-old woman with a long history of myasthenic signs and marked respiratory distress, Tissot et al.[40] had certain diagnostic doubts concerning MG. The differential diagnosis of Bell's phenomenon is described by Miller et al.[41] The presence of the upward rolling of the eyes during forcible eye closure was seen in a 32-year-old woman with a myasthenic ophthalmoplegia who could not voluntarily elevate either eye above the horizontal line. The oculocephalic test (doll's head maneuver) also failed to overcome the eye muscle paresis. This finding of a preserved Bell's phenomenon means that attempting to close the eyes against resistance produces a stronger stimulus than other voluntary vertical eye movements. Therefore, an intact Bell's phenomenon together with a paresis of vertical eye movement is not pathognomonic for a supranuclear paralysis of upward gaze.

Therapy of Ocular Myasthenia

Surgery of the eye muscles is necessary in patients with long-standing paresis giving rise to incongruent and concomitant squints with individual muscle overaction or underaction. Although systemic therapy for myasthenic paresis controls motility disturbances in most patients, and spontaneous remission often occurs in rare cases, ocular morbidity may nevertheless cause chronic disability. Acheson and Elston[42] reported their experience of extraocular muscle surgery in five patients with stable MG for at least 2 years. The follow-up was 6 months to 6 years. In all five patients, a larger stable field of binocular single vision was achieved postoperatively. The treatment was a conventional recession and resection procedure (with additional Faden and adjustable sutures in certain operations).

Evoli et al.[11] reported on the results of therapy in 48 patients with ocular myasthenia: 19 patients (40%) responded to anticholinesterase drugs. Corticosteroids were effective in 14 of 18 patients (78%). Corticosteroids failed to bring about improvement in 4 patients with severe long-standing disease (marked bilateral ptosis and ophthalmoplegia in 3 patients, nearly complete monolateral ptosis in another patient). Twenty-two patients underwent thymectomy: a thymoma was found in 3 patients (13.6%), an involuted thymus in 11 (50%), and a hyperplasia of the thymus in 8 patients (36.4%).

EPIDEMIOLOGY

Ocular Myasthenia

Evoli et al.[11] diagnosed MG in 360 patients between 1968 and 1986. In 132 patients, the onset of the disease was strictly confined to the extraocular muscles. Generalization of the disease occurred in 84 of these patients (64%), mostly within a year of onset, while the remaining 48 patients (26 men, 22 women) continued with ocular myasthenia alone. Oosterhuis[34] examined 374 patients with MG (140 men, 234 women) from 1965 to 1984. Ocular myasthenia was found in 46 patients (12.3%). In the early onset group ($\leq$ 39 years of age), 6 men and 3 women were found, but in the late onset group ($\geq$ 40 years of age), 26 men and 11 women with ocular signs were counted. In an additional publication, Oosterhuis[43] presented the natural course of MG in a long-term follow-up study of 73 patients living in Amsterdam between 1926 and 1965. Of 35 cases with initial ocular signs, 11 cases remained purely ocular, 21 cases became generalized within 2 years, and in 3 cases, generalization occurred between 10 and 22 years after onset (Table 2).[44–47]

Oosterhuis[34] calculated that the incidence of MG is about four per 10^6, which implies that the average neurologist only sees one new patient in 3 years.

TABLE 2 (cont.).
Epidemiology of MG

Prevalence Rate	Incidence Rate per Yr per Million	Name and Number of Inhabitants of the Town/County	Time of Investigation	Number, Sex, Age of Patients	Female to Male	Thymectomy	Classification	Reference
125 per million	10.4 (including 2 patients with transient neonatal MG)	County of Viborg (Denmark): 230,760	Jan 1, 1973 to Dec 31, 1987	36 patients: 21 women (0–76 yr, average: 46.3), 15 men (4–75 yr, average: 50.7)	1.4 to 1	. . .	TMG: 2; type I: 8 (22%); type II: 19 (53%); type III: 5 (14%); type IV: 2 (5.5%); (Osserman and Genkins)	44
9.6 per 100,000		Counties of Hordaland 396,222; Sogn and Fjordane 106,049 (Norway)	Jan 1, 1984	48 patients: (mean age: 53 yr) (Jan 1, 1984), 32 women, 16 men	2.0 to 1	13 patients	Type I: 5 (10%); type IIA: 19 (40%); type IIB: 18 (38%); type III: 2 (4%); type IV: 4 (8%)	45
Analysis in various island areas: 7.5; 17.6; 31.4; 45.0 per million	Mean annual incidence: 2.5	Sardinia (Italy)	Jan 1, 1958 to Dec 31, 1986	110 patients: 80 women (73%) (mean age: 37.1, SD 18.1); 30 men (27%) (mean	2.7 to 1	58 patients (52.7%), histology of thymus: thymoma (16 patients,	Ocular: 45 patients (40.9%); bulbar signs: 20 patients (18.2%);	46

105.3 per million on Dec 31, 1987; 142.2 women, 61.9 men	Not investigated	Ferrara (Italy) 370,374 (192,827 women, 177,547 men)	1956–1988	age: 45.2, SD 16.6). Improvement after surgery: 38 patients (65.5%)	2.5 to 1	27.6%); hyperplasia (29 patients, 50%); normal (10 patients, 17.2%)	generalized signs: 15 (13.6%)	47
				39 patients (range: 13–78 yr, mean age: 47.1 yr); 28 women (mean age: 49.5, SD 17.4), 11 men (mean age: 47.8, SD 18.1)		28 patients (72%); 20 women, 8 men	Type I: 3 (8%); type II: 33 (84%); type III: 3 (8%); (Osserman and Genkins)	
53 per million	3.1 (women: 4.7; men: 1.5)	Amsterdam (Holland) 852,500 (443,700 women, 418,800 men)	1961–1965	58 patients (40 women, 18 men)	2.2 to 1	Not performed	. . .	43

GENERALIZED MG

Follow-up Studies in Patients With MG

A long-term follow-up of 73 patients with MG since 1926[43] showed that maximum severity of the disease occurred during the first 7 years after onset in 87%. Eighteen (29%) patients, 8 of whom had a thymoma, died in a myasthenic crisis. Death occurred in 13 patients within 3 years after onset, 3 in the sixth year of onset, and 2 patients (8 and 17 years after onset) in a crisis precipitated by an operation and an upper respiratory tract infection. At the end of the study (1985), 16 patients (22%) were in complete remission, 13 (18%) had improved considerably, 12 (16%) had improved moderately, 12 (16%) had remained unchanged, and 2 had deteriorated. The disease was classified (Osserman and Genkins) as ocular (11 patients), mild (14), moderate (24), severe with rapid progression (15), and severe with late progression (9). Thymomas were found in 14 patients (9 men, 5 women: 6 at surgery, 4 at autopsy, and 4 with radiologic investigation). In all patients with thymomas, MG was generalized.

Donaldson et al.[48] compared the course of the disease in patients with onset before 50 and at or after 50 years of age in 165 patients. A significantly greater percentage of older patients progressed to severe disease than did the younger group (36% of 55 patients compared with 18% of 110 patients). Seventy-one percent of patients under 50 were women, but only 29% of those over 50 were women. Thymoma was more common in the older population. A significantly greater percentage of older patients progressed to severe disease than in the younger group (36% compared with 18%). More of the younger than the older patients were in remission or were asymptomatic with medication.

Diagnosis of Generalized MG

Investigation of bulbar myasthenic signs: The ear, nose, and throat specialist or the phoniatrician may be the first to be consulted by patients with MG, because dysarthry, dysphagia, or dyspnea occur as initial signs in about 30% of those patients. Three characteristic case histories are given by Lamprecht.[49]

An electrophysiologic test like the acoustic stapedial reflex is not painful and does not require the cooperation of the patient. A unilateral acoustic stimulus causes a bilateral contraction of the stapedius, the smallest striated muscle in humans. In nine untreated patients with MG, the stapedial reflex amplitude was reduced to less than 10% of the initial amplitude following continuous stimulation for 120 seconds, whereas the maximum decay in normal subjects was only 50%.[50]

Differential Diagnosis of Fatigue Syndromes

Fatigue may be a normal consequence of intensive physical exertion or mental effort, or it may be symptomatic of a variety of specific illnesses.[51] Fatigue is peripheral in MG as well as in mitochondrial myopathies. In postviral fatigue syndrome, a muscle membrane disorder, probably arising from defective myogenic enzymes was postulated by Jamal and Hansen.[52] In ten patients with this syndrome, abnormal jitter values were found with single-fiber electromyography. Patients with upper motor neuron muscle weakenss due to multiple sclerosis showed greater fatiguability of the anterior tibial muscle, induced by repetitive electrical stimulation, than healthy subjects.[53] Investigation of the metabolic basis of human muscular fatigue and recovery was undertaken by Boska et al.[54] Changes in maximum voluntary contraction correlate best with $H_2PO_4^-$, suggesting that this metabolite is an important factor in human muscle fatigue. Moussavi et al.[55] showed in physiologic experiments that low-intensity exercise can produce long-standing depression of muscular force generation. Immunologic abnormalities in 100 patients who were suffering from chronic fatigue syndrome were found by Lloyd et al.[56] Changes in the cellular and humoral immune systems of these patients were documented. In a prospective study, patients with unexplained chronic postviral fatigue were investigated.[57] Patients with neuromuscular disease showed markedly less mental fatigue than patients with postviral fatigue or with affective disorders. The fatigue associated with postviral fatigue appeared central in origin, suggesting that it is not primarily a neuromuscular disease. Only some of the patients with neuromuscular diseases also suffered from psychiatric disorders. A 68-year-old woman with MG of 47 years' duration showed depressive episodes that developed following tapering off of prednisone.The depressive symptoms resolved after electroconvulsive therapy.[58]

Misdiagnosis

Patients with MG are too often misdiagnosed as having another disorder. A 38-year-old woman experienced progressive muscular weakness, dizziness, and dyspnea that was diagnosed at first as amyotrophic lateral sclerosis.[59] The disease was misdiagnosed for at least 4 months. The misdiagnosis was compounded by the misinterpretation of the first edrophonium test. A biopsy specimen taken from the vastus lateralis showed denervation with small group atrophy. The patient had moderate bilateral ptosis and ophthalmoplegia with weak orbicularis oculi muscles. After several days, a second edrophonium test was positive. The limb muscles had gained nearly normal power after treatment with anticholinesterase drugs, prednisone, and plasma exchange. Another patient, a 17-year-old woman with MG, developed muscle weakness, dysarthria, dysphagia, dyspnea, and bilateral ptosis. However, the nasal speech resulted in the first diagnosis of velopharyngeal incompetence. A third patient, an 18-year-old woman, had noted swelling of her eyes that required her to tilt her head backward to see. There was ptosis, worse at night, and she experienced occasional diplopia. A general physical examination revealed thyromegaly. The final diagnosis was MG and autoimmune thyroiditis.

In contrast to these three case histories, false-positive diagnoses are also made: In a 60-year-old woman with a 6-week history of progressive ptosis, blurred vision without diplopia, dysarthry, dysphagia for liquids, mild proximal weakness of the upper extremities, and an 11-kg weight loss, MG was suspected.[60] Ten milligrams of edrophonium chloride gave an equivocal result. No thymoma was present. The AChR ab assay was equivalent at 1 unit. The disease did not improve despite increasing doses of prednisone. Tongue fasciculations were seen. The patient then developed pneumonia requiring intubation. Following edrophonium administration, vital capacity improved transiently, but shortly after extubation, her respiratory status once again deteriorated. There was no further improvement despite therapy with prednisone, pyridostigmine, and many plasma exchanges. She developed distal weakness in all extremities and moderate wasting in the legs. Later, a left conjugate gaze paresis was noted in addition to the right gaze palsy. Fasciculations of the weak extremity muscles were seen on the hospital day 103. She died about 3 weeks later. The diagnosis of an unusual amyotrophic lateral sclerosis was made.

While a postive response to edrophonium chloride should usually be regarded as confirmatory for MG, the possibility of a false-positive test must be considered, especially in those patients with atypical physical findings. Dirr et al.[61] reported on the gradual onset of intermittent double vision in a 19-year-old woman who complained of general malaise after walking. Her symptoms were variable, often worse in the late afternoon. She could not abduct her left eye beyond the midline. After intravenous injection of 10 mg edrophonium, abduction of the left eye improved. However, pyridostigmine did not change the picture. Several weeks later, coarse nystagmus developed and magnetic resonance imaging revealed a large cystic lesion of the brain stem, a biopsy specimen of which demonstrated a low-grade astrocytoma.

DRUG-INDUCED MG

With the possible exception of D-penicillamine, "there are no drugs that are absolutely contraindicated in patients with MG."[62] However, numerous drugs are well known to interfere with neuromuscular transmission and will therefore make the muscular weakness of these patients worse. It is most desirable to avoid drugs that may adversely affect neuromuscular transmission. The emergency room physician should be cautious when prescribing drugs to patients with MG for conditions not related to MG[63] Nevertheless, in certain cases, these drugs must be used for the management of other illnesses, and thorough knowledge of their deleterious side effects can minimize their potential danger in such a situation. It is then necessary to use a drug with known side effects that has been shown to have the least effect on the neuromuscular junction.[62] For instance, from the group of aminoglycoside antibiotics, neomycin is known to be the most toxic, but tobramycin is the least dangerous antibiotic of this group to neuromuscular transmission.

Neuromuscular weakness is related to the dose of the drug. The serum levels are reversible in part with cholinesterase inhibitors. Aminoglycosides are generally considered to have the most potent effect on the neuromuscular junction, compared with other antibiotic subgroups.[63] Besides aminoglycosides, other antibiotics like polypeptides, penicillins, monobasic amino acid antibiotics, sulfonamides, and tetracyclines have been reported to cause transient worsening of myasthenic weakness.[62, 64] Chemotherapeutic agents like the fluoroquinolones, ciprofloxacin and norfloxacin, have been associated with exacerbation of MG.[65, 66] Two different types of drugs are known to interfere with neuromuscular transmission, those acting directly at the motor end plate and those with an immune mechanism, like D-penicillamine.[67] Among the cardiovascular drugs, β-blockers are known to cause serious side effects by potentiation of muscular weakness in MG. Propranolol is the β-blocker that most effectively impairs neuromuscular transmission, whereas atenolol has the least effect on neuromuscular transmission. Drugs used for the treatment of glaucoma, like timolol maleate or betaxolol, have been shown to cause an abrupt reduction of muscle strength in patients with MG. Steroid-induced exacerbation of MG can occur at the beginning of high-dose therapy. In 75% of cases, this worsening can be obviated by varying doses of cholinesterase inhibitors. With oropharyngeal weakness, plasma exchange can be used to prevent dangerous exacerbations.[62]

The cardiovascular drugs like quinine, quinidine, procainamide, and trimethaphan, and also calcium channel blockers and even β-blockers, have or may have serious side effects on patients with MG. Weakness of the muscles can be aggravated. On the other hand, drugs for the therapy of MG, such as anti-acetylcholinesterase inhibitors like pyridostigmine, can lead to a threatening bradycardia that may result in a ventricular tachyarrhythmia. A 78-year-old man with MG was treated with 180 mg pyridostigmine bromide a day. He developed an episode of angina pectoris with ventricular fibrillation.[68]

A direct effect of chloroquine on the neuromuscular junction was postulated in a 39-year-old man who developed double vision and generalized weakness 1 week after the onset of therapy with 300 mg of chloroquine a day.[69] This antimalarial drug was given to treat a presumed reticular erythematous mucinosis of the abdominal skin. The edrophonium chloride test gave a postitive result. Anti-AChR abs were absent. Five days after the last dose of chloroquine, myasthenic paresis had completely disappeared. With informed consent of the patient, a provocative test with chloroqine was reinstituted. About 1 week later, the patient again had ptosis, diplopia, and a generalized type of muscle weakness.

Treatment with the major tranquilizer clozapine has also resulted in myasthenic paresis in a 23-year-old patient.[70] Verapamil caused paresis of MG in a 72-year-old woman who also showed an increased anti-AChR ab titer.[71]

D-penicillamine (DPA) can induce MG. However, after discontinuation of the drug, the immunogenic effect is reversible and the clinical signs of MG disappear. Katz et al.[72] reported an ocular myasthenia due to DPA treatment for rheumatoid arthritis in a 68-year-old woman. Two weeks after she discontinued DPA, the ocular paresis cleared with no other treatment. However, Zakarian et al.[73] described persistent signs in a 60-year-old woman with arthritis treated with high-dose DPA for nearly 1 year. A bilateral facial paresis, together with dysphagia, mastication difficulties, and dysphonia, had developed and persisted. The edrophonium chloride test revealed a transient improvement of signs and DPA was discontinued. The anti-AChR abs showed a limiting value. Despite therapy with pyridostigmine and later with neostigmine, myasthenic paresis persisted. After a follow-up of 4 years, bilateral ptosis was also noticed for the first time.

DPA has been shown to induce anti-AChR abs. A 58-year-old man was treated with DPA for psoriatic arthritis. Four-and-a-half years later, ocular myasthenia developed. The patient had HLA DR1 antigen.[74] In 19 patients with DPA-induced MG, anti-AChR abs were compared to those from 204 patients with idiopathic MG. Antigenic specificities of the circulating antibodies were determined from the capacity of monoclonal antibodies to inhibit binding of the serum antibodies to the AChR against certain determinants on the AChR. It was shown that the antibody repertoire in the serum of idiopathic and DPA-induced MG is very similar. Antibodies to the main immunogenic region, which is located on the extracellular surface of the α subunit, were the predominant group.[75]

GENERAL ANESTHETICS IN PATIENTS WITH MG

Patients with MG are sensitive to the neuromuscular blocking effects of nondepolarizing muscle relaxants like vecuronium or d-tubocurarine or pancuronium. The duration of action of vecuronium is shorter than that of the others. A cumulative dose together with the infusion technique and integrated EMG monitoring of the first interosseous muscle were used to determine the potency of vecuronium in 10 patients with MG and in 20 healthy subjects under thiamylal, N_2O, O_2, and fentanyl anesthesia.[76] The patients with MG were approximately twice as sensitive to muscle relaxants than were the healthy subjects. A 74-year-old woman who was scheduled for gastrectomy received 1 mg of pancuronium immediately before induction of anesthesia to prevent succinylcholine fasciculation. Two minutes later, she became apneic and unresponsive. Postoperatively, a very high titer of AChR abs was found, and computed tomography demonstrated the presence of a thymoma. She did not show any muscle weakness. Seven months later, a thymectomy was performed. This time, pancuronium was examined in a dose-related manner with a neuromuscular transmission monitor. Small doses of pancuronium blocked neuromuscular transmission in a dose-dependent manner. Reversal of the neuromuscular blockade was achieved with neostigmine and atropine. The postoperative course was uneventful.[77]

A 28-month-old boy with a 1-year history of reactive airway disease developed severe generalized muscle weakness, which required ventilator support, after receiving muscle relaxants and steroids for 1 week.[78] Muscle relaxation with pancuronium bromide was stopped after 2 hours because of tachycardia and was replaced with vecuronium bromide. Ultrastructure of the neuromuscular junction of the intercostal muscles indicated terminal axon degeneration and atrophy with depletion of the secretory vesicles. The authors discuss the possibility that the reversible myasthenic syndrome represents neurotoxicity due to high doses of steroidal nondepolarizing blocking agents. Pancuronium and vecuronium are steroidal neuromuscular blocking agents that are structurally similar to corticosteroids.

A 30-year-old woman who had been treated years earlier with pyridostigmine, azathioprine, and steroids as well as with thymectomy was symptomless for several years without treatment. General anesthesia for elective gynecologic surgery was induced with thiopental and 7 mg vecuronium to produce neuromuscular blockade. The prolonged neuromuscular blockade in this patient was partly due to the potentiating effect of 1% enflurane.[79] Smith[80] in discussing this publication, proposed the administration of a more conservative dose of vecuronium for such a short elective procedure. Edrophonium and neostigmine were used as antagonists to atracurium, vecuronium, or pancuronium neuromuscular blockade.[81-83]

Patients with MG are more sensitive than healthy subjects to the neuromuscular depressant effects of isoflurane. Among halogenated anesthetic agents, isoflurane has been shown to suppress normal, healthy neuromuscular transmission more than halothane. However, in myasthenia, even halothane produces a significant depressant neuromuscular effect. Nilsson and Muller[84] showed that isoflurane produces approximately twice as strong a neuromuscular blocking effect as halothane in patients with MG. The occurrence of HLA-B8, together with anti-AChR abs, seems to predispose patients with MG to the neuromuscular depression produced by isoflurane. Rowbottom[85] studied the clinical and electromyographic effects of isoflurane in eight patients undergoing thymectomy. Isoflurane provided good intubating and operating conditions without the need for muscle relaxants in these patients. Recovery from anesthesia was rapid and associated with minimal weakness or respiratory depression.

Thoracic epidural anesthesia can be used as the primary anesthetic for transsternal thymectomy in patients with MG. It still seems prudent to avoid muscle relaxants in myasthenic patients with MG unless they are absolutely necessary. Burgess and Wilcosky[86] recommend further study of thoracic epidural anesthesia as a method of providing optimal operating conditions.

THERAPY

An overview of the therapeutic results in 374 patients with MG between 1965 and 1984 (follow-up, 3 to 22 years; mean, 12 years) was presented by Oosterhuis.[34]

Early onset MG without a thymoma (n=165) was mainly treated with thymectomy, late-onset MG without a thymoma (n=92) mainly with anticholinesterase or immunosuppressive agents (IS). Patients with ocular MG (n=46) were mainly treated with anticholinesterase agents. Therapy in patients with thymoma (n=71) consisted of thymectomy and/or IS. Myasthenic death occurred in 17 patients (5.2%), none of whom was treated with IS. Five patients died from the side effects of prednisone (diabetes, intestinal bleeding, urosepsis, tracheomalacia, and preexistent obesity), and 7 died from invasive thymoma or thymoma-associated myocarditis. Patients with thymomas were most severely affected: crises occurred in 51%, and the total death rate was 23%.

In a retrospective study of follow-up observations of 100 patients over 9 years, Emskötter et al.[87] found that the severity of myasthenic symptoms in the individual patient appeared to be determined within the first 3 years of the disease. Fifty percent of the cases were at least transiently improved with thymectomy. The favorable results with steroids or plasma exchange were confirmed. During the follow-up period of 9 years, a good prognosis was reported. In over 70% of the patients, a remission occurred or only minimal myasthenic signs were observed.

Drug Therapy

The kinetics of orally administered pyridostigmine were investigated in 18 patients with generalized MG.[88] Pyridostigmine plasma levels and decrement of neuromuscular transmission in the trapezius muscle on repetitive accessory nerve stimulation were repeatedly measured. Six patients were investigated two or three times at intervals of 2 weeks to 3 years, with a total of 27 investigations. Mean plasma pyridostigmine concentrations during the period of investigation varied widely among patients and did not correlate with the daily dose. The influence of concurrent medication with glucocorticoids was not apparent. Significant correlations between pyridostigmine concentrations and functional parameters were present in 3 of 11 patients in whom the plasma levels changed by at least 25 ng/mL during the investigation, and peak levels did not exceed 100 ng/mL. These findings provide an additional reason for avoiding high plasma concentrations. Patients exhibiting high plasma levels (above 100 ng/mL) showed cholinergic overstimulation as well as poor neuromuscular function.

High-Dose Immunoglobulin

The precise mode of action of immunoglobulin (Ig) is unknown at present. Postulated mechanisms underlying Ig effects in MG include: (1) competing with anti-AChR abs for binding to AChr; (2) preventing attachment of Fc receptor-positive inflammatory cells to the anti-AChR ab bound to the motor end plate; (3) decreasing synthesis of anti-AChR abs; and (4) exerting an anti-idiotypic effect.[89] Ig was given to 12 patients with MG. Improvement occurred in 11, beginning 3.6 ± 2.7 days after Ig was initiated, becoming maximal in 8.4 ± 4.6 days, and lasting 52 ± 37 days.[90]

A 7-year-old girl with ocular myasthenia who developed ptosis of the right eye at the age of 18 months was treated on alternate days with prednisolone combined with anticholinesterase agents. Treatment was initiated at the age of 2 years and 9 months. Despite a dosage increase to 30 mg, and later 55 mg on alternate days at the age of 7 years, she failed to make favorable progress. Therefore, at the age of 8 years, 300 mg/kg/day immunoglobulin (Ig) was given for 5 consecutive days. Improvement began on day 4, and all the symptoms disappeared within 14 days. Additional infusions of Ig after an interval of 2 weeks appeared to be effective. Ocular symptoms recurred 7 months after the initiation of Ig therapy, when she was receiving pyridostigmine bromide and prednisone. Despite an increase of the pyridostigmine dose, improvement of the symptoms was restricted. New Ig infusions were given five times every 2 or 3 days, with further improvement. Some months later, Ig infusions were discontinued and ocular symptoms gradually worsened again. There was no change after a new increase in the dose of prednisolone and pyridostigmine and another 5-g dose of immunoglobulin. The levels of AChR abs were not correlated with clinical improvement or aggravation.[91]

A 4-year-old girl with myasthenic ptosis, beginning in the left eye, was treated with anticholinesterase drugs, but responded poorly. After several months of therapy, ptosis had increased and amblyopia of the left eye was observed. She was therefore treated with human immunoglobulin intravenously (400 mg/kg/day for 5 days). The ptosis began to improve about 1 week after the immunoglobulin therapy began. Two weeks after the onset of this high-dose therapy, the right-sided ptosis disappeared for a whole day and the left-sided ptosis showed some improvement. Pyridostigmine chloride therapy was repeated. During the following months, additional doses of immunoglobulin were administered (7.5 g once every 2 or 3 months) with a total dose of 82.5 g in 1985. Subsequently, she was maintained in remission and the anti-AChR ab titer declined to normal. She remained in remission.[92]

Immunosuppressive Therapy

The mean peripheral blood lymphocyte count was decreased in 43 patients with MG. Significant lymphopenia was observed in 26 patients treated with prednisolone. In addition, B cells, T cells, CD4$^+$ cells, and their subsets decreased, while the proportions of CD8$^+$ cells were increased. After thymectomy in 23 patients, lymphocyte and B cell levels decreased.[93]

Prolonged corticosteroid therapy can have a negative effect on the bone. Bone mineral content was measured in 23 patients with MG who had been treated with an average dose of 50 mg fluocortolone every other day, continued for between 1 and 120 months. Measurements were obtained at the proximal and distal parts of the forearm. The results were compared with the bone mineral content values in age- and sex-matched control subjects. No signs of major bone loss were noticed in any of the patients with MG.[94] Donaldson et al.[48] stated in a retrospective review of 165 patients with MG that 62% receiving steroids developed complications of treatment. Obesity (40%), cataracts (19%), and infections (18%) were most common, while mental disturbances, hypertension, diabetes mellitus, and bone disease—including osteoporosis, aseptic necrosis of the femoral head, and pathologic fractures—were less frequently seen. Gastrointestinal disorders were rarely seen as a result of prednisone treatment (5%). Cataracts and infections were significantly more common in the older group of patients (> 50 years). Five patients developed one or more complications from azathioprine therapy (12% were treated with this medication): drug fever was seen in 2, granulocytopenia or anemia in 3, and hepatitis in 2 patients.

A new derivate of prednisolone Deflazacort, which is believed to have fewer side effects than other glucocorticoid drugs, was given to 14 patients with MG.[95]

Azathioprine

Twenty-seven patients with MG were treated with azathioprine (aza) in conjunction with pyridostigmine and prednisolone.[96] In four of these patients (14.8%), treatment was discontinued because of side effects (jaundice in one and abnormal liver function in another patient; portal hypertension after 3 years of treatment in a third, and recurrent upper respiratory infections after 4 years of treatment in a fourth). Aza treatment was associated with marked clinical improvement in all remaining 23 patients, resulting in reduction of the dose of pyridostigmine and prednisolone. The median duration of treatment was 7 years (range, 1 to 10 years). The median dose of aza was 100 mg daily (range, 75 to 200 mg). Clinical improvement was usually observed after 6 months. A 52-year-old man with MG and normal liver function developed clinical evidence of portal hypertension 3 years after starting treatment with aza. A liver biopsy specimen showed nodular regenerative hyperplasia.[97]

In a controlled study, aza has been used in two different groups of patients with MG.[98] In one group of 32 patients, aza without additional medication was given; in the second group of 57 patients, a combination of aza and steroids was administered. In both groups, positive outcomes were achieved (in 24 [75%] patients in the aza group and in 40 [70%] in the combination group). Aza treatment induced a reduction in the anti-AChR ab level, which was correlated with clinical improvement and greatly decreased the need for steroids. Severe toxicity was noted in 1 patient, who developed marked bone marrow depression. The most frequent side effects were nausea and abdominal discomfort. An increase in the transaminase level and gastric intolerance were additional side effects.

In a follow-up study of 20 patients with initially marked generalized MG, Michels et al.[99] observed stable clinical remission of these patients while receiving aza. However, 12 patients (60%) developed a relapse after discontinuation of aza, 8 patients within 3 to 11 months, and 4 patients within 27 to 70 months. Four of these 12 patients gained a new stable remission within 4 to 8 months when treated again, and aza could be discontinued a second time for periods of 8 to 62 months.

Cyclosporine

The most widely used of the more recent immunosuppressive agents is cyclosporine which has been proved successful in preventing the rejection of transplanted tissue. It acts chiefly on T lymphocytes through the interleukin-2 pathway. The result is the inhibition of helper T cells and cytotoxic cells. Drachman et al.[100] claim that cyclosporine will eventually find its place as an adjunct in the treatment of MG with other effective immunosuppressive drugs.

In 19 patients with MG (18 with a generalized MG, 1 with ocular MG), treatment with cyclosporine (5.6 ± 1.6 mg/kg/day over 11.6 ± 1.6 months) was undertaken. Previously, 4 patients had been unsuccessfully treated with aza, 1 with cyclophosphamide, 12 with steroids. Cyclosporine was beneficial in 14 patients with severe MG.[101]

Plasmapheresis

A distinct improvement after plasma exchange was seen in 36 of 43 patients (84%) with generalized MG.[87] A better result in therapy was obtained in patients with an acute deterioration of the disease and with oculo-facio-pharyngeal manifestation. MG with late onset improved in only 60% of the patients.

A 25-year-old man and a 42-year-old woman, both with severe generalized MG, were treated with plasma exchange in which citrate was used as the anticoagulant. After the plasma exchange was performed, muscle weakness worsened considerably and dyspnea increased. Edrophonium chloride produced no change in the condition in either patient,[102] although improvement occurred in one after the administration of calcium gluconate. In experimental autoimmune MG in rabbits and in rats, decremental muscle response to 3-Hz repetitive nerve stimulation worsened significantly after injection of the citrate anticoagulant. It follows that citrate can endanger the patient during and after plasmapheresis and should no longer be used.

A decrease in the mean serum concentration of C4, IgM, and anti-AChR abs of

IgG class after plasma exchange was the main finding in eight selected patients with MG during a 5-day trial.[103] All patients improved during the treatment, including two patients without detectable antibodies to AChR in the serum. The concentrations of IgG and IgA did not change significantly.

Recovery from global amnesia during plasma exchange in a 47-year-old woman was described by Aarli et al.[104] After 5 months of prednisone therapy, she contracted an acute infectious disease. During the first day of the illness, her memory gradually failed. She had no memory for the events of the 2 previous weeks. Memory for the previous 6 months was weak. During the 5 days of plasma exchange, the MG improved and her memory improved dramatically.

Thymectomy

Oosterhuis[34] examined 374 patients (140 men and 234 women) from 1965 to 1984. In early onset generalized MG ($\leq$ 39 years) without thymoma, thymectomy was performed on 136 patients, of whom 36% reached a complete remission without immunosuppressives (IS). In 21 patients who underwent thymectomy, IS also had to be given. Maximum improvement took place in the first half year after surgery, but in many patients complete remission was established only after 3 to 5 years. Late-onset generalized MG ($\geq$ 40 years) was seen in only 8 patients between 40 and 55 years of age. Thymomas were detected in 71 of 328 patients (21.6%) with generalized MG (12.6% of early onset, and 26% of late onset) and in none with pure ocular MG. Thymectomy was performed in 22 of 25 patients with early onset MG and a thymoma, and in 33 of 46 patients with late-onset MG and a thymoma. In 7 patients, remission occurred following surgery. In 20 patients, remission was the result of IS therapy. In most patients, thymectomy did not seem to have influenced MG favorably.

A prospective follow-up of 20 patients with MG after thymectomy showed that the anti-AChR ab titers changed in pari passu with the clinical state in 9 of 16 patients. The $CD4^+$ $CD8^+$ cell levels were also closely related to the clinical change within 1 year after surgery in 8 patients who had a preoperative elevation of the cell levels. This study suggests that the $CD4^+$ $CD8^+$ cell levels may serve as indicators for long-term prognosis of MG.[105]

Thymectomy in 32 children (aged from 3 to 15 years) was performed via a T-shaped sternotomy approach. In 27 patients, hyperplasia of the thymus, and in 5, a transition from hyperplasia to involution of thymus tissue was found. In the immediate postoperative stage, a myasthenic crisis occurred in 6 and a cholinergic crisis in 3 patients. Yudin et al.[106] reported that the late term result was favorable in 75% of their patients. Shkrob et al.[107] reported on the thymus operations on 43 of 51 patients with MG and emphasized the need for special care in the follow-up during the preoperative and postoperative period.

Mulder et al.[109] found abs in 43 of 76 patients (56.5%) who were treated with

TABLE 3.
Thymectomy

Number of Patients	Age (yr) at the Time of Surgery	Operative Technique	Mortality Rate	Clinical Remission (Osserman Classification)	Postoperative Improvement (Osserman Classification)	Reference
52	Mean age: 34 (range, 18 mo to 82 yr)	Radical transsternal thymectomy	1 postoperative death (respiratory insufficiency and sepsis in acute fulminating MG of Osserman stage III); 4 late deaths (8%) resulted from unrelated diseases (6 mo to 9 yr after surgery)	I: 2 (18%) in remission; IIA: 7 (27%) in remission; IIB, III, and IV: 5 (33%) in complete remission	I: 1 (9%) improved; IIA: 9 (35%) improved; IIB, III, and IV: 8 (53%) improved. 5 of 7 patients with thymomas improved (71.4%) 26 patients with thymic hyperplasia demonstrated a response rate of 72% Nineteen patients with normal or atrophic thymus demonstrated a response rate of 37%	108
84	0–20: 10 21–30: 17 31–40: 21 41–50: 17 51–70: 19	Median sternotomy after bilateral submammary skin incision	No operative deaths, 1 patient (4%) died 5 months after surgery from complications related to a recurrent myasthenic crisis	11 of 27 men (40.7%), 19 of 57 women (33.3%) I: no comment II: 12 (39%) III: 17 (37%) IV: no comment	Twelve of 27 men (44.4%), 25 of 57 women (43.8%) I: no comment II: 12 (39%) III: 18 (39%) IV: no comment	109

(Continued.)

TABLE 3   (cont.).

Number of Patients	Age (yr) at the Time of Surgery	Operative Technique	Mortality Rate	Clinical Remission (Osserman Classification)	Postoperative Improvement (Osserman Classification)	Reference
425	Between 8 and 67 <14 years: 40 (9.4%) 14–18: 62 (14.6%) 18–30:139 (32.7%) 30–50: 148 (34.8%) 50–60: 27 (6.4%) >60: 9 (2.1%)	Total longitudinal median sternotomy	Overall mortality: 3% Mortality in series (1): 7% series (2): (3.3%) series (3): 0.57% 5 out of 54 patients with thymoma died postoperatively (9.2%)	DSS: disability status scale 1972–1977: 2.75 1977–1982: 2.13 1982–1957: 2.10 30% of patients recovered sufficiently	40% of patients improved sufficiently	110
30	Between 16 and 73; mean, 39	Median sternotomy with a collar incision	No perioperative mortality	Eleven of 12 patients with symptoms for 2 years were in stage II and one was in stage III. All 12 patients were free from symptoms after surgery (stage I); of the 12 patients with symptoms for 3 years, 10 were in stage III preoperatively; 4 of	Ninety-seven percent improvement rate; three stage improvement in 1 patient (3.3%); two stage in 10 patients (33%); one stage in 18 patients (60%); 20 patients (67%) were asymptomatic; 6 patients (20%) required no medication	111

			these 10 became symptom free. 6 patients had had symptoms for 4 years; 5 of them were in stage IV, and only 1 of the 5 became asymptomatic after surgery	
142 thymomas	Between 8 mo and 73 yr; mean, 44±14	Surgery and postoperative radiation (30 Gy in 3 wk or 40 Gy in 4 wk with complete resection and over 50 Gy in 6 wk with incomplete resection)	Death by tumor occurred in 5 of 81 patients (6.2%) with MG, and in 18 of 61 patients (29.5%) without MG. Causes of death other than tumor were myasthenic crisis in 10 patients, pure red cell aplasia in 3 patients, and malignant fibrous histiocytoma pneumonia, and hepatitis; 1 patient each	No statistically significant differences in the survival rates of patients undergoing complete resection according to cell type (33 of 36 patients with lymphocyte predominant type—survival rate of 96% at 5 years— and 61 of 77 patients with mixed type—survival rate of 98% at 5 and 10 years)
				112

surgery (Table 3).[108-112] In 19 patients (44%), a remission occurred, and in 21 patients (49%), improvement occurred. In contrast, only 21 of the 33 patients (63.6%) in whom no antibody was detected benefited from surgery. Nine (27%) achieved remission and 12 (36.4%) patients showed improvement. Lennquist et al.[111] stated that, according to his observations on 30 patients, there was a tendency toward a higher success rate after surgery among patients younger than 30 years and also in those older than 60 years of age. Jaretzki and Wolff[113] recommended the en bloc transcervical-transsternal maximal thymectomy to ensure removal of all available thymus in all patients. The results of surgical-anatomic studies on 50 consecutive specimens demonstrated that gross and microscopic thymic tissue can frequently be found from the level of the hyoid bone to the diaphragm, and from hilum to hilum beyond the phrenic nerves. Anatomic studies have demonstrated that thymic tissue lay outside the two cervical lobes in 32% of the patients, and in the region of the aortopulmonary window in 24%.[114]

During this 34-year period, 114 operations on patients with thymoma were performed.[115] Repeat surgery for thymomas were necessary in 23 patients (20%) at intervals of 2 months to 17 years 10 months after the initial operation. Twelve patients had MG (52%), but it was a determinant for repeat surgery in only 2 patients.

REFERENCES

1. Finley JC, Pascuzzi RM: Rational therapy of myasthenia gravis. *Semin Neurol* 1990; 10:70–82.

2. Pachner AR: Myasthenia gravis. *Immunol Allergy Clin North Am* 1988; 8:277–293.

3. Newsom-Davis J: Autoimmunity in neuromuscular disease, in Raine CS (ed): *Advances in Neuroimmunology. Ann NY Acad Sci* 1988; 540:25–38.

4. Eymard B: Myasthénie auto-immune et syndrome myasthénique de Lambert-Eaton. *Ann Med Intern* 1989; 140:462–466.

5. Breucking E: Neurologische und neuromuskuläre Erkrankungen (Myasthenia gravis, M.Parkinson) und Cholinesterasemangel. *Anästh Intensivmed* 1989; 30:326–333.

6. Gajdos P: Traitement de la myasthénie. *Presse Med* 1989; 18:1732–1734.

7. Christadoss P: Immunogenetics of experimental autoimmune myasthenia gravis. *Crit Rev Immunol* 1989; 9:247–278.

8. Spencer RF, Porter JD: Structural organization of the extraocular muscles, in Büttner-Enever JA (ed): *Reviews of Oculomotor Research*, vol 2, *Neuroanatomy of the Oculomotor System*. Amsterdam, Elsevier, 1988, pp 33–79.

9. Porter JD, Burns LA, McMahon EJ: Denervation of primate extraocular muscle. A unique pattern of structural alterations. *Invest Ophthalmol Vis Sci* 1989; 30:1894–1908.

10. Iwasaki Y, Kinoshita M: Ocular myasthenia gravis associated with autoimmune hemolytic anemia and Hashimoto's thyroiditis. *Am J Ophthalmol* 1989; 107:90–91.

11. Evoli A, Tonali P, Bartoccioni E, et al: Ocular myasthenia: Diagnostic and therapeutic problems. *Acta Neurol Scand* 1988; 77:31–35.

12. Porter JD, Burns LA, May PJ: Morphological substrate for eyelid movements: Innervation and structure of primate levator palpebrae superioris and orbicularis oculi muscles. *J Comp Neurol* 1989; 287:64–81.

13. Walsh FB, Hoyt WF: *Clinical Neuro-Ophthalmology*, vol 1, ed 3. Baltimore, Williams & Wilkins Co, 1969, p 339.

14. Gangadhar DV, Johnson LN, Borchert M: Isolated weakness of the orbicularis oculi muscle from myasthenia gravis. *Neuro Ophthalmol* 1989; 9:327–329.

15. Chia LG: Facial weakness without ocular weakness in myasthenia gravis. *Muscle Nerve* 1988; 11:185–186.

16. Schmidt D: Ocular myasthenia, in Daroff RB, Neetens A (eds): Neurological Organization of Extra-Ocular Movement. *Bull Soc Belge Ophthalmol* 1989; 237:353–380.

17. Bartoccioni E, Scuderi F, Evoli A, et al: Ocular myasthenia gravis: Two different diseases. *Lancet* 1986; 1:1038.

18. Morel E, Vernet-der Garabedian B, Eymard B, et al: Binding and blocking antibodies to the human acetylcholine receptor: Are they selected in various myasthenia gravis forms? *Immunol Res* 1988; 7:212–217.

19. Tsujihata M, Yoshimura T, Satoh A, et al: Diagnostic significance of IgG, C3, and C9 at the limb muscle motor end-plate in minimal myasthenia gravis. *Neurology* 1989; 39:1359–1363.

20. Mossman S, Vincent A, Newsom-Davis J: Myasthenia gravis without acetylcholine-receptor antibody: A distinct disease entity. *Lancet* 1986; 1:116–118.

21. Hayashi M, Kida K, Yamada I, et al: Differences between ocular and generalized myasthenia gravis: Binding characteristics of anti-acetylcholine receptor antibody against bovine muscles. *J Neuroimmunol* 1989; 21:227–233.

22. Evoli A, Bartoccioni E, Batocchi AP, et al: Anti-ACh-R-negative myasthenia gravis: Clinical and immunological features. *Clin Invest Med* 1989; 12:104–109.

23. Winterkorn JMS, Odel JG, Behrens MM: Sleep test for myasthenia gravis. Presented at the VIIIth International Neuro-Ophthalmology Symposium, June 23–29, 1990, Winchester, England.

24. Oh SJ, Cho HK: Edrophonium responsiveness not necessarily diagnostic of myasthenia gravis. *Muscle Nerve* 1990; 13:187–191.

25. Phillips LH, Melnick PA: Diagnosis of myasthenia gravis in the 1990s. *Semin Neurol* 1990; 10:62–69.

26. Rodgin SG: Ocular and systemic myasthenia gravis. *Am Optom Assoc* 1990; 61:384–389.

27. Gilchrist JM, Sanders DB: Myasthenic u-shaped decrement in multifocal cervical radiculopathy. *Muscle Nerve* 1989; 12:64–66.

28. Scoppetta C, Casali C, D'Agostini S, et al: Repetitive stimulation in myasthenia gravis: Decrementing response revealed by anticholinesterase drugs. *Electroencephalogr Clin Neurophysiol* 1990; 75:122–124.

29. Emeryk B, Rowinska-Marcinska K, Nowak-Michalska T: Pseudoselectivity of the neuromuscular block in ocular myasthenia: A SFEMG study. *Electromyogr Clin Neurophysiol* 1990; 30:53–59.

30. Keesey JC: AAEE Minimonograph no. 33: Electrodiagnostic approach to defects of neuromuscular transmission. *Muscle Nerve* 1989; 12:613–626.

31. Trontelj JV, Khuraibet A, Mihelin M: The jitter in stimulated orbicularis oculi muscle: Technique and normal values. *J Neurol Neurosurg Psychiatry* 1988; 51:814–819.

32. Jabre JF, Chirico-Post J, Weiner M: Stimulation SFEMG in myasthenia gravis. *Muscle Nerve* 1989; 12:38–42.

33. Massey JM, Sanders DB, Howard JF: The effect of cholinesterase inhibitors on SFEMG in myasthenia gravis. *Muscle Nerve* 1989; 12:154–155.

34. Oosterhuis HJGH: Long-term effects of treatment in 374 patients with myasthenia gravis. *Monogr Allergy* 1988; 25:75–85.

35. Davis TL, Lavin PJM: Pseudo one-and-a-half syndrome with ocular myasthenia. *Neurology* 1989; 39:1553.

36. Shinton RA, Jamieson DG: Exercise induced diplopia as a presentation of midline cerebral tumour. *J Neurol Neurosurg Psychiatry* 1989; 52:916–917.

37. Moorthy G, Behrens MM, Drachman DB, et al: Ocular pseudomyasthenia or ocular myasthenia "plus": A warning to clinicians. *Neurology* 1989; 39:1150–1154.

38. Mindel JS, Charney JZ: Bilateral intracavernous carotid aneurysms presenting as pseudo-ocular myasthenia gravis. *Trans Am Ophthalmol Soc* 1989; 87:445–462.

39. Cogan DG: Myasthenia gravis. A review of the disease and a description of lid twitch as a characteristic sign. *Arch Ophthalmol* 1965; 74:217–221.

40. Tissot R, Roullet E, Mahieux F: Fatigabilité musculaire et accès de détresse respiratoire chez une femme de 40 ans. *Rev Neurol (Paris)* 1990; 146:61–66.

41. Miller NR, Griffin J, Cornblath D, et al: Intact Bell's phenomenon in a patient with myasthenia gravis and upward gaze paresis. *Arch Ophthalmol* 1989; 107:1117.

42. Acheson JF, Elston JS: Surgical management of strabismus in myasthenia gravis. Presented at the VIIIth International Neuro-Ophthalmology Symposium. June 23–29, 1990, Winchester, England.

43. Oosterhuis HJGH: The natural course of myasthenia gravis: A long term follow up study. *J Neurol Neuosurg Psychiatry* 1989; 52:1121–1127.

44. Sørensen TT, Holm EB: Myasthenia gravis in the county of Viborg, Denmark. *Eur Neurol* 1989; 29:177–179.

45. Thorlacius S, Aarli JA, Riise T, et al: Associated disorders in myasthenia gravis: Autoimmune diseases and their relation to thymectomy. *Acta Neurol Scand* 1989; 80:290–295.

46. Giagheddu M, Puggioni G, Sanna G, et al: Epidemiological study of myasthenia gravis in Sardinia, Italy (1958–1986). *Acta Neurol Scand* 1989; 79:326–333.

47. Tola MR, Granieri E, Paolino E, et al: Epidemiological study of myasthenia gravis in the province of Ferrara, Italy. *J Neurol* 1989; 236:388–390.

48. Donaldson DH, Ansher M, Horan S, et al: The relationship of age to outcome in myasthenia gravis. *Neurology* 1990; 40:786–790.

49. Lamprecht A: Dysarthrie, Dysphagie oder Dyspnoe als Grund der Erstvorstellung bei Myasthenia gravis pseudoparalytica und bei amyotropher Lateralsklerose. *Laryngolrhinootologie* 1990; 69:48–51.

50. Bischoff C, Klingelhöfer J, Conrad B: Decay and recovery of the stapedial reflex by prolonged stimulation in the diagnosis of myasthenia gravis. *J Neurol* 1989; 236:343–348.

51. Swartz MN: The chronic fatigue syndrome—one entity or many? *N Engl J Med* 1988; 319:1726–1728.

52. Jamal GA, Hansen S: Post-viral fatigue syndrome: Evidence for underlying organic disturbance in the muscle fibre. *Eur Neurol* 1989; 29:273–276.

53. Lenman AJR, Tulley FM, Vrbova G, et al: Muscle fatigue in some neurological disorders. *Muscle Nerve* 1989; 12:938–942.

54. Boska MD, Moussavi RS, Carson PJ, et al: The metabolic basis of recovery after fatiguing exercise of human muscle. *Neurology* 1990; 40:240–244.

55. Moussavi RS, Carson PJ, Boska MD, et al: Nonmetabolic fatigue in exercising human muscle. *Neurology* 1989; 39:1222–1226.

56. Lloyd AR, Wakefield D, Boughton CR, et al: Immunological abnormalities in the chronic fatigue syndrome. *Med J Aust* 1989; 151:122–124.

57. Wessely S, Powell R: Fatigue syndromes: A comparison of chronic "postviral" fatigue with neuromuscular and affective disorders. *J Neurol Neurosurg Psychiatry* 1989; 52:940–948.

58. Pande AC, Grunhaus LJ: ECT for depression in the presence of myasthenia gravis. *Convulsive Ther* 1990; 6:172–175.

59. Wheeler SD: Misdiagnosis of myasthenia gravis. *J Natl Med Assoc* 1987; 79:425–429.

60. Noseworthy JH, Rae-Grant AD, Brown WF: An unusual subacute progressive motor neuronopathy with myasthenia-like features. *Can J Neurol Sci* 1988; 15:304–309.

61. Dirr LY, Donofrio PD, Patton JF, et al: A false-positive edrophonium test in a patient with a brainstem glioma. *Neurology* 1989; 39:865–867.

62. Howard JF: Adverse drug effects on neuromuscular transmission. *Semin Neurol* 1990; 10:89–102.

63. Adams SL, Mathews J, Grammer LC: Drugs that may exacerbate myasthenia gravis. *Ann Emerg Med* 1984; 13:532–538.

64. Friedli WG: Diagnostische Aspekte der Myasthenie. *Schweiz Rundsch Med (Praxis)* 1989; 78:1037–1044.

65. Moore B, Safani M, Keesey J: Possible exacerbation of myasthenia gravis by ciprofloxacin. *Lancet* 1988; 1:882.

66. Rauser EH, Ariano RE, Anderson BA: Exacerbation of myasthenia gravis by norfloxacin. *DICP Ann Pharmacother* 1990; 24:207–208.

67. Lacomblez L, Warot D: Myasthénie et médicaments. *Therapie* 1990; 45:273–275.

68. Brachmann J: Kammerflimmern bei Myasthenia gravis. *Dtsch Med Wschr* 1988; 113:1575.

69. Robberecht W, Bednarik J, Bourgeois P, et al; Myasthenic syndrome caused by direct effect of chloroquine on neuromuscular junction. *Arch Neurol* 1989; 46:464–468.

70. Jiménez MD, Yusta A, Lesmes A, et al: Síndrome miasténico inducido por clozapina. *Rev Clin Espanol* 1990; 186:42–43.

71. Casado I, Nevado L, Dorrego FG: Miastenia asocjada con verapamil. *Rev Clin Espanol* 1989; 185:379–380.

72. Katz LJ, Lesser RL, Merikangas JR, et al: Ocular myasthenia gravis after D-penicillamine administration. *Br J Ophthalmol* 1989; 73:1015–1018.

73. Zakarian H, Viallet F, Acquaviva PC, et al: Syndrome myasthénique induit par la D-pénicillamine au cours de la polyarthrite rhumatoïde. Problèmes soulevés par une évolution autonomisée. *Sem Hôp Paris* 1989; 65:2052–2056.

74. Ferbert A: D-Penicillamin-induzierte okuläre Myasthenie bei Psoriasisarthritis. *Nervenarzt* 1989; 60:576–579.

75. Tzartos SJ, Morel E, Efthimiadis A, et al: Fine antigenic specificities of antibodies in sera from patients with D-penicillamine-induced myasthenia gravis. *Clin Exp Immunol* 1988; 74:80–86.

76. Eisenkraft JB, Book WJ, Papatestas AE: Sensitivity to vecuronium in myasthenia gravis: A dose-response study. *Can J Anaesth* 1990; 37:301–306.

77. Enoki T, Naito Y, Hirokawa Y, et al: Marked sensitivity to pancuronium in a patient without clinical manifestations of myasthenia gravis. *Anesth Analg* 1989; 69:840–842.

78. Benzing G, Iannaccone ST, Bove KE, et al: Prolonged myasthenic syndrome after one week of muscle relaxants. *Pediatr Neurol* 1990; 6:190–196.

79. Lumb AB, Calder I: "Cured" myasthenia gravis and neuromuscular blockade. *Anaesthesia* 1989; 44:828–830.

80. Smith DC: "Cured" myasthenia. *Anaesthesia* 1990; 45:252.

81. Donati F, Lahoud J, McCready D, et al: Neostigmine, pyridostigmine and edrophonium as antagonists of deep pancuronium blockade. *Can J Anaesth* 1987; 34:589–593.

82. Astley BA, Katz RL, Payne JP: Electrical and mechanical responses after neuromuscular blockade with vecuronium, and subsequent antagonism with neostigmine or edrophonium. *Br J Anaesth* 1987; 59:983–988.

83. Smith CE, Donati F, Bevan DR: Dose-response relationships for edrophonium and neostigmine as antagonists of atracurium and vecuronium neuromuscular blockade. *Anesthesiology* 1989; 71:37–43.

84. Nilsson E, Muller K: Neuromuscular effects of isoflurane in patients with myasthenia gravis. *Acta Anaesthesiol Scand* 1990; 34:126–131.

85. Rowbottom SJ: Isoflurane for thymectomy in myasthenia gravis. *Anaesth Intensive Care* 1989; 17:444–447.

86. Burgess FW, Wilcosky B: Thoracic epidural anesthesia for transsternal thymectomy in myasthenia gravis. *Anesth Analg* 1989; 69:529–531.

87. Emskötter TH, Lachenmayer L, Kunze K: Akut- und Langzeitverläufe bei Myasthenia gravis— Kriterien für den Einsatz immunmodulatorischer Massnahmen. *Akt Neurol* 1988; 15:130–133.

88. Breyer-Pfaff U, Schmezer A, Maier U, et al: Neuromuscular function and plasma drug levels in pyridostigmine treatment of myasthenia gravis. *J Neurol Neurosurg Psychiatry* 1990; 53:502–506.

89. Zweiman B: Theoretical mechanisms by which immunoglobulin therapy might benefit myasthenia gravis. *Clin Immunol Immunopathol* 1989; 53:83–91.

90. Arsura E: Experience with intravenous immunoglobulin in myasthenia gravis. *Clin Immunol Immunopathol* 1989; 53:170–179.

91. Sakano T, Hamasaki T, Shimizu H, et al: High-dose intravenous immunoglobulin for myasthenia gravis. *Hiroshima J Med Sci* 1988; 37:7–9.

92. Maruyama Y, Takeshita S, Sekine J, et al: High-dose immunoglobulin for juvenile myasthenia gravis. *Acta Paediatr Jpn* 1989; 31:544–548.

93. Shimizu H, Ichikawa Y, Yoshida M, et al: Lymphocyte subsets of the peripheral blood in myasthenia gravis determined by two-color flowcytometry. *Autoimmunity* 1990; 6:173–182.

94. Harmut M, Kusek V, Matulic-Bedenic I, et al: Bone mineral content in patients with myasthenia gravis treated with cortisone. *Arh Hig Rada Toksikol* 1988; 39:359–363.

95. Dubrovsky AL, De Rosa E, Cammarota A, et al: Deflazacort en el tratamiento de la miastenia gravis. *Prensa Med Argent* 1989; 76:150–154.

96. Fonseca V, Havard CWH: Long term treatment of myasthenia gravis with azathioprine. *Postgrad Med J* 1990; 66:102–105.

97. Fonseca V, Havard CWH: Portal hypertension secondary to azathioprine in myasthenia gravis. *Postgrad Med J* 1988; 64:950–952.

98. Mantegazza R, Antozzi C, Peluchetti D, et al: Azathioprine as a single drug or in combination with steroids in the treatment of myasthenia gravis. *J Neurol* 1988; 235:449–453.

99. Michels M, Hohlfeld R, Hartung HP, et al: Myasthenia gravis: Discontinuation of long-term azathioprine. *Ann Neurol* 1988; 24:798.

100. Drachman DB, McIntosh KR, De Silva S, et al: Strategies for the treatment of myasthenia gravis, in *Advances in Neuroimmunology*. *Ann NY Acad Sci* 1988; 540:176–186.

101. Goulon M, Elkharrat D, Gajdos PH: Traitement de la myasthénie grave par la ciclosporine. Etude ouverte de 12 mois. *Presse Med* 18:341–346.

102. Wirguin I, Brenner T, Shinar E, et al: Citrate-induced impairment of neuromuscular transmission in human and experimental autoimmune myasthenia gravis. *Ann Neurol* 1990; 27:328–330.

103. Thorlacius S, Mollnes TE, Garred P, et al: Plasma exchange in myasthenia gravis: Changes in serum complement and immunoglobulins. *Acta Neurol Scand* 1988; 78:221–227.

104. Aarli JA, Gilhus NE, Thorlacius S, et al: Recovery from global amnesia during plasma exchange in myasthenia gravis: Report of a case. *Acta Neurol Scand* 1989; 80:351–353.

105. Matsui M, Fukuyama H, Akiguchi I, et al: Circulating CD4$^+$CD8$^+$ cells in myasthenia gravis: Supplementary immunological parameter for long-term prognosis. *J Neurol* 1989; 236:329–335.

106. Yudin YB, Kogan OG, Prokopenko YD, et al: Surgical results of myasthenia in children. *Chirurgija (Moskva)* 1989; 11:72–75.

107. Shkrob OS, Vetshev PS, Ippolitov IK, et al: Surgical interventions for concurrent and concomitant diseases in patients with myasthenia. *Chirurgija (Moskva)* 1990; 2:5–9.

108. Hatton PD, Diehl JT, Daly BDT, et al: Transsternal radical thymectomy for myasthenia gravis: A 15-year review. *Ann Thorac Surg* 1989; 47:838–840.

109. Mulder DG, Graves M, Herrmann C: Thymectomy for myasthenia gravis: Recent observations and comparisons with past experience. *Ann Thorac Surg* 1989; 48:551–555.

110. Molnar J, Szobor A: Myasthenia gravis: Effect of thymectomy in 425 patients. A 15-year experience. *Eur J Cardiothorac Surg* 1990; 4:8–14.

111. Lennquist S, Andåker L, Lindvall B, et al: Combined cervicothoracic approach in thymectomy for myasthenia gravis. *Acta Chir Scand* 1990; 156:53–61.

112. Nakahara K, Ohno K, Hashimoto J, et al: Thymoma: Results with complete resection and adjuvant postoperative irradiation in 141 consecutive patients. *J Thorac Cardiovasc Surg* 1988; 95:1041–1047.

113. Jaretzki A, Wolff M: "Maximal" thymectomy for myasthenia gravis. *J Thorac Cardiovasc Surg* 1988; 96:711–716.

114. Jaretzki A: Thymectomy for myasthenia gravis. *Ann Thorac Surg* 1990; 49:686–688.

115. Kirschner PA: Reoperation for thymoma: Report of 23 cases. *Ann Thorac Surg* 1990; 49:550–555.

CHAPTER 16

Stroke

Jonathan D. Trobe, M.D.

Professor of Ophthalmology, Associate Professor of Neurology, W.K. Kellogg Eye Center, Departments of Ophthalmology and Neurology, University of Michigan Medical School, Ann Arbor, Michigan

The past 2 years continued a familiar trend in diagnosis and treatment of stroke. Epidemiologic studies, some very flawed because of the need to make tenuous presumptions about the pathogenesis of ischemic stroke, have nevertheless added helpful information about risk factors, prevalence, and natural history. Structural imaging, the principal diagnostic tool, keeps improving. Metabolic imaging is probably getting better too, but it is still too expensive and crude to aid the clinician. Treatment of acute ischemic stroke remains worthless; trials are in progress but enthusiasm is not high. Prevention of ischemic stroke with medical means (antiplatelet agents, anticoagulants) was reaffirmed as modestly effective. The ardor for carotid endarterectomy has cooled, even among surgeons, as the results of four multicenter trials are awaited. The only truly felicitous news came in the treatment of arteriovenous malformations: both the surgeons and the radiation therapists claim better results.

EPIDEMIOLOGY

The ability to subdivide stroke into different mechanistic subgroups is a critical step in improving both prevention and care.[1] Better imaging and pathologic corre-

Reprinted from *Current Neuro-ophthalmology®*, vol. 3.
Copyright 1991, Mosby–Year Book, Inc.

lation has taught us that the single category called ischemic stroke may result from many different conditions: proximal artery occlusion, artery-to-artery embolism, cardiogenic embolism, lipohyalinosis, hypotension, vasculitis, and small vessel thrombosis. Hemorrhagic stroke is now divided into parenchymatous hemorrhage and subarachnoid hemorrhage. The problem is that in life—when pathologic material is not available—these distinctions often remain presumptive. Recent reports revolve about that point.

Even after thorough clinical examination, computed tomography (CT), noninvasive vascular imaging, and cerebral angiography, 580 (40%) of 1,273 ischemic strokes entered in the Stroke Data Bank of the National Institutes of Neurological and Communicative Disorders and Stroke (NINCDS) were of undetermined cause.[2] It is instructive to review the criteria used for the ischemic strokes *when the cause was known:* (1) large artery occlusion: angiographic evidence of occlusion or >90% stenosis of the internal carotid artery or siphon, basilar artery, or major cerebral artery stem; (2) cardiac embolism: intracranial artery occlusion without prior transient ischemic attack (TIA) if associated with a likely cardiac source; (3) lacunar infarct: typical clinical lacunar syndrome together with a small, deep infarct on CT or a normal CT 1 week following the stroke; (4) artery-to-artery embolism: greater than 50% proximal artery stenosis, carotid artery ulceration, and a hemispheric surface infarct on CT; (5) other causes: evidence of arteritis, dissection, fibromuscular dysplasia, sickle cell anemia, migraine, or mycotic aneurysms.

To appreciate how fragile these criteria are, consider only the category of cardiac embolism. Ramirez-Lassepas et al.[3] and Hachinski et al.[4] point out what every neurologist has sensed, namely that the cardiac conditions most likely to cause cerebral emboli rarely exist in the absence of other arteriosclerotic risk factors. Cerebral angiography, a relatively dangerous procedure in the elderly stroke patient, is not always able to facilitate diagnosis of an embolic infarct,[5] and even necropsy findings may be inconclusive.[6] The lack of a gold standard for the diagnosis of cardiogenic stroke cannot be overlooked in interpreting studies of this topic. For example, Kittner et al.[7] found that three features were closely related to cardiogenic embolism: (1) systemic embolism; (2) abrupt onset; and (3) diminished level of consciousness. The traditional associations of rapid improvement, seizure at onset, deficit present on awakening, and prior ipsilateral TIA were not significantly related to cardiac embolism. But the authors were forced to define cardiogenic embolism as a probabilistic entity (low-, medium-, and high-risk groups), and draw their conclusions based on differences in the prevalence of each clinical feature within each of the various risk groups. The tortured and often circular reasoning in this paper is unfortunately typical of much of the research in this area of stroke.

It should be no surprise, then, that stroke data banks do not agree on criteria for defining stroke mechanisms and are generating slightly different relative prevalence figures.[8] Even the proportion of hemorrhagic strokes is not particularly consistent, for example, between NINCDS (26.6%)[2] and Lausanne (10.9%).[8] Differences could be partly explained by the fact that the Lausanne bank excluded subarachnoid hemorrhage. Also, patients in the NINCDS bank were drawn from a higher concentration of tertiary care centers, which attract the more serious hemorrhagic strokes.

The importance of accession factors in epidemiologic studies becomes even clearer if we compare the hospital-based stroke data bank figures to those of large community studies. The Oxfordshire Community Stroke Project in Great Britain is the most sophisticated study of its type.[9, 10] Over 4 years, many of the 675 patients with first-ever stroke had been evaluated with CT (80%), necropsy (37%), lumbar puncture, chest x-ray, standard blood trests, electrocardiography, echocardiography, and cardiologic examination. Ischemic stroke made up 81%, parenchymatous hemorrhage 10%, subarachnoid hemorrhage 5%, and undetermined cause 5%. These proportions are consistent with the results of other community studies, reminding us that the currently untreatable forms of stroke are preponderant.

Despite reports of progress in dealing with intracranial aneurysms and arteriovenous malformations, the 30-day mortality rate for hemorrhagic stroke continues to be very high. In the Oxfordshire Community Stroke Project, the 30-day mortality rate was 10% for infarct, 50% for parenchymatous hemorrhage, and 46% for subarachnoid hemorrhage.[10]

The Oxfordshire study has yielded other interesting information. In the initial report of 244 patients with their first stroke, major arteriosclerotic risk factors (hypertension, ischemic heart disease, TIA, peripheral vascular disease, cervical bruit, diabetes mellitus) were present in 60% of individuals at the time of the stroke. In 20%, major potential cardiac sources of emboli (atrial fibrillation, mitral stenosis or regurgitation, myocardial infarction within 6 weeks, deep vein thrombosis with patent foramen ovale) were identified. Only 4% had nonatheromatous, nonembolic conditions: migraine, arteritis, arterial trauma, autoimmune disease, thyroid cancer, major surgery. So, while our journals are filled with fascinating accounts of unusual causes of stroke, from a health planner's point of view, they are a pittance!

Health planners will certainly wish to take stock of the results of evaluating 163 consecutive patients with TIA in two public hospitals.[11] After a typical workup (which did not include noninvasive vascular imaging) estimated at a cost of $3,000 per patient, *treatment was altered in only two patients,* one who had lupus erythematosus and syphilis, the other who had had a recent myocardial infarction and whose echocardiogram showed a mural thrombus. The authors boldly recommend that we cast aside laboratory studies in favor of history and physical examination as sole criteria with which to exclude nonarteriosclerotic causes of TIA. Larger scale studies of this type, which are relatively inexpensive, should be welcomed—and funded—by insurers.

Returning to the Oxfordshire study, we find that although 20% had major cardiac sources of emboli, only 3% had cardiac lesions as the sole predisposing factor. This evidence is a further caution against implicating the heart as the source for 20% of strokes, as other investigators have done.[12]

Cerebral lacunes, those located deep within brain parenchyma in the domain of penetrating (rather than circumflex) vessels, have generally been ascribed to the effects of chronic hypertension on vascular endothelium (lipohyalinosis). But the drive to call more and more ischemic strokes cardioembolic has swept up cerebral lacunes as well.[13] Support for that position came from a preliminary report that found cerebral lacunes after experimentally induced emboli in normotensive rats.[14]

Two articles present indirect evidence against the theory that lacunar strokes are caused by cardiac emboli. Gandolfo et al.[15] have provided an impressive case-control study to show that hypertension is powerfully associated with lacunar stroke. Cigarette smoking and diabetes mellitus, both possibly associated with small vessel disease, were also considered precursors, but hyperlipidemia, high hematocrit, and atrial fibrillation—factors associated with large vessel or cardiac embolism—were not. The other important contribution came from Ringelstein et al.[16] who studied the CT stroke patterns in 60 patients with a reasonably secure diagnosis of cardiogenic embolism. None of the patients had a cerebral lacune (defined as a deep infarct on CT measuring < 2cm). However, 7 (12%) had striato-capsular infarctions measuring 2 cm or greater. Thus, as long as the imaging definition of a hemispheric lacune is restricted to a striatocapsular ovoid of 2 cm diameter or less, one can be reasonably confident that emboli have not caused it.

Defining the risk factors for stroke is confounded not only by the fact that there are several stroke mechanisms, but also by the fact that the risk factors themselves interact. Cigarette smoking has only recently been accepted on the short list of major risk factors because there have been many negative studies. A major metanalysis, or statistical reappraisal, of data from 32 reputable published studies found an overall relative stroke risk of 1.5 for cigarette smokers.[17] In a prospective case-control study of cigarette smoking and ischemic stroke among young adults aged 15 to 45 years, Love et al.[18] discovered that smokers were 1.6 times more likely to have stroke than nonsmokers. Stroke risk worsened both with the number of cigarettes smoked per day and number of years of smoking. This study has special importance because there were relatively few other risk factors in this age group.

In an Australian study[19] that attempted to measure the relationship of cigarette smoking to various stroke subgroups, the authors made an interesting observation: the relative risk was a gigantic 5.7 for noncardioembolic ischemic stroke, whereas it was not increased at all for cardioembolic stroke. Does this mean that cigarettes exert their effect primarily on blood vessels?

There is more new information on that point. The Framingham study[20] had shown that stroke risk fell significantly within 2 years of smoking cessation and to the level of nonsmokers within 5 years. Investigators suggested that cigarettes acted on thrombogenic circulatory factors such as fibrinogen[21] or prostacyclin.[22] But the previously cited Australian study[19] discovered that a significant relative risk was still present 10 years after cessation. In view of that finding, we must attach importance to another report[23] that demonstrated less cervical carotid artery atherosclerosis (as measured with B-mode ultrasound) in former than current smokers, and a preliminary report suggesting that cervical carotid atherosclerosis decreases with each passing year after cessation of smoking![24]

Reviewing the half-century evolution of epidemiologic concepts of cerebrovascular disease during his career as a distinguished clinician-scientist, Scheinberg[25] makes the following points:

1. The presumed decline in the frequency of stroke in the past decades may be an artifact of improved reporting in geographic areas, such as Rochester, Minnesota, where white Americans live.
2. Control of discretionary stroke risk factors, such as hypertension, smoking, and alcohol should command our attention. The role of diet and oral contraceptives needs further clarification.
3. The management of TIAs will probably have a negligible impact on the frequency of stroke because TIAs precede stroke in fewer than 10% of patients.

DIAGNOSIS

Improvements in stroke diagnosis rest primarily on imaging. Three areas occupy most efforts: (1) improved imaging of acute stroke; (2) better correlation of imaging with altered brain function; and (3) better prediction of future stroke.

In the depiction of acute ischemic stroke, magnetic resonance imaging (MRI) is superior to CT, especially when gadolinium enhancement is used.[26] Experimentally, MRI changes are seen within 30 minutes of infarction, even without gadolinium.[27] Cerebral blood flow imaging techniques, such as single photon emission CT (SPECT), may be more sensitive to the abnormal anatomy of fresh infarct within the first 48 hours than CT,[28] but they offer no special prognostic value and are no more sensitive than MRI (although they are less expensive).

There has been some debate about whether CT or MRI is more sensitive to subarachnoid bleeding. MRI does not demonstrate blood directly unless methemoglobin has been released from red blood cells, which takes several hours. So, whereas MRI can infer an intraparenchymal hemorrhage by demonstrating displacement of tissue, it would not depict fresh blood in the subarachnoid space, which normally has no mass effect. There has been a report on 30 patients in whom subarachnoid bleeding was estimated to be 8 hours to 5 days old that was demonstrated better with MRI than with CT![29] As an added bonus, in 14 (50%) patients, MRI showed the flow void corresponding to the ruptured aneurysm. The authors also point out that chronic brain hemorrhage is seen much better with MRI than with CT, because as electron density wanes, lingering paramagnetic substances alter the MRI signal. Despite this report, CT should remain the imaging study of choice for suspected intracranial (including subarachnoid) hemorrhage because it is quick, less easily degraded by patient motion, and excellent at showing acute extravascular blood.

MRI is so sensitive to arteriovenous malformations (AVMs) that the term cryptic AVM has been changed to angiographically occult AVM.[30] Some of these AVMs are also seen with CT, but MRI has added much greater specificity to their diagnosis. The typical MRI appearance of AVMs is a mixed intensity signal on T2-weighted images surrounded by signal void believed to represent hemosiderin from old bleeding.[31] These MRI characteristics serve to distinguish AVMs from gliomas or demyelinating plaques.

Metabolic imaging extends our understanding of disordered brain function within ischemic or potentially ischemic tissues. Two techniques are being used: MRI spectroscopy and positron emission tomography (PET). MRI spectroscopy facilitates precise topographic measurements of inorganic phosphates and lactic acid, indicators of ischemia. Its greatest utility thus far has been to measure the effects of thrombolysis on reversing ischemic damage in experimental stroke.[32] It is still a long way from clinical application. PET facilitates measurement of a broad range of metabolic changes, but its application has also been limited to experimental stroke because it is expensive and cumbersome.

There has been a flurry of articles purporting to show that cerebral blood flow imaging studies can pinpoint reduced cerebrovascular reserve in patients who will be at risk for stroke.[33] The rationale goes something like this: many patients have reduced cerebral blood flow because of stenotic vessels, but few have strokes. Perhaps those few who will have strokes can be identified by showing that the cerebral blood vessels are already completely vasodilated and extracting maximal oxygen. If the administration of acetazolamide or CO_2, which normally dilate cerebral vessels, does not result in increased cerebral blood flow, the patient is said to have reduced cerebrovascular reserve.[34] This finding has been used to justify revascularization procedures, but, as best as I can discover, no prospective studies have been conducted.

Are migraineurs at greater risk of complications of angiography than the general population? This dictum was not confirmed in a series of 149 angiographies performed on 142 migraineurs at one institution.[35]

MANAGEMENT

The non-surgical prevention of ischemic stroke consists of antiplatelet and anticoagulation therapy. Large-scale studies supported both kinds of treatment, but not impressively.

The Antiplatelet Trialists' Collaboration metanalyzed the statistical data on the more than 30 bonafide studies on aspirin in the prevention of stroke and death.[36] Aspirin came out as reducing stroke risk by 14% compared to placebo; however, the more dramatic effects of aspirin on preventing cardiac deaths may have skewed the result, as none of the individual studies except one showed a statistically significant preventive effect of aspirin on stroke. Even if aspirin is not incredibly effective in stroke prevention, its prophylactic use in doses of 325 mg/day was supported by the US Physicians' Health Study.[37] That study found that, among 22,000 American male physicians, there was no reduction in stroke, but a

47% reduction in nonfatal heart attacks, leading to premature termination of the study.

Two multicenter randomized studies concluded that ticlopidine, which acts on platelet membranes rather than prostaglandin pathways, was effective in stroke prevention. In the Ticlopidine Aspirin Stroke Study,[38] the 3-year rate for nonfatal stroke or death in 3,069 patients with recent TIA, stroke, or retinal ischemia was 17% for ticlopidine and 19% for aspirin. Although this was called a significant benefit from ticlopidine, it seemed to this reader to be a slim victory, especially considering that nausea, diarrhea, skin rash, and leukopenia occur in 1% to 5% of patients. The smaller Canadian-American Ticlopidine Study, which compared ticlopidine to placebo, produced comparable results.[39] The stampede to ticlopidine has not begun, and forecasts are dim.

Anticoagulation for nonvalvular (nonrheumatic) atrial fibrillation (NVAF) has been recommended because patients with untreated NVAF in the Framingham study, among others, were found to have a five times greater risk of stroke than age-matched control subjects and because strokes occurred within weeks of onset of atrial fibrillation.[40] A recently completed placebo-controlled trial[41] comparing warfarin to aspirin or placebo in 420 patients with chronic NVAF found two strokes in the anticoagulated group and 13 in the aspirin and placebo groups. The authors concluded that anticoagulation was indicated. They kept the prothrombin time below 1.5 times normal to avoid the hazards of bleeding.[42]

Surgical prevention of ischemic stroke consists of carotid endarterectomy, superficial temporal artery-middle cerebral artery anastomosis (extracranial-intracranial bypass, or EC/IC bypass), and angioplasty. There were no remarkable published developments in angioplasty. Endarterectomy is still being performed, but less so; it is the subject of four multicenter prospective studies. As for EC/IC bypass, since its send-up in the multicenter trial,[43] it has had a dwindling (but vocal) circle of devotees.[44]

Shivers about the dangers of carotid endarterectomy have evidently spread across the land, as the number of procedures dropped sharply from 107,000 in 1985 to 83,000 in 1986.[45] Apart from myocardial infarction—the principal source of morbidity from endarterectomy—a major problem has been middle cerebral artery stroke. Recent evidence suggests that this may result from perfusion breakthrough, since the desired postoperative increase in perfusion is not met with appropriate autoregulatory vasoconstriction and excess blood flow leads to a hemorrhagic infarct.[46]

With regard to the safety and efficacy of carotid endarterectomy, one series[47] documented a perioperative stroke/death rate of 1.7% and a late (beyond 30 days after surgery) risk of stroke of under 1% per year. A second series[48] found a late risk of 1.7% per year. Both series suggested that endarterectomy improves on the nonsurgical treatment, but the missing ingredient was a concurrent matched population and independent evaluation. In a companion editorial to the first study, Matchar[49] lists the cognitive traps that lead to treatments that are as likely to harm as help: (1) considering that the risks of surgery and the natural risk of late stroke are low, it is unlikely that any single surgeon will witness either event until many procedures are done, at which time the adverse event will be submerged by the favorable outcomes; (2) adverse postoperative events are apt to be dismissed as the result of peculiar high-risk patient factors and considered unlikely to bear on the next case; and (3) poor outcomes are generally judged as less regrettable when they follow aggressive intervention (the "college try") than when they occur out of benign neglect.

There are currently four multicenter carotid endarterectomy trials underway: two involving asymptomatic patients with carotid artery stenosis and two involving patients with carotid distribution TIA or stroke.[50] The earliest results may be expected in 1992. In the meantime, the following criteria for surgery were suggested[50]: surgical morbidity/mortality not to exceed 3% for asymptomatic patients; 5% for TIAs; and 7% for minor stroke. Each hospital is advised to perform a critical audit of surgeons performing this operation. This reviewer has yet to uncover such an audit or any serious attempt to conduct one.

Although the EC/IC bypass trial[43] convinced most people that the operation was not helpful in preventing stroke, it has been criticized for failing to evaluate a subgroup of patients who have chronically reduced cerebral perfusion. A study by Powers et al.[51] should still the critics. That study found no significant difference in the stroke rates between 29 EC/IC bypass cases and 21 unoperated cases that had PET evidence of reduced regional cerebral perfusion pressure.

The treatment of acute ischemic stroke remains a gigantic frustration. Based on successes in coronary ischemia, in experimental stroke, and in uncontrolled miniseries in patients,[52] four large trials of recombinant tissue plasminogen activator are underway. There is reason to be wary. Fatal brain edema occurred in the first two patients treated within 4 hours of stroke in one trial.[53] Hemodilution therapy, with starch or dextran, has been not just a disappointment, but a menace: a large trial was suspended because of excessive mortality.[54]

In the treatment of hemorrhagic stroke, including intraparenchymal and subarachnoid bleeding, the news was generally better.

The death rate of patients in whom the intracranial aneurysms ruptured and were treated at the Mayo Clinic declined from 57% in 1955 to 1964 to 42% in 1975 to 1984.[55] Perhaps that decline was caused by a dramatic shortening of the interval from hemorrhage to surgery (12 days to 2 days). In point of fact, an impressive randomized study from Helsinki of the effect of timing of aneurysm surgery on outcome showed slightly less morbidity and mortality in noncomatose patients who underwent surgery within 7 days of bleeding than in those operated on after that time.[56] Early (before 4 days) surgery is now standard to avoid the risks of rebleeding (peak, 7 to 10 days) and vasospasm (peak, 4 to 14 days).[57]

Has a solution arrived for the anguishing dilemma of whether or not to perform angiography in a patient with an isolated third cranial nerve palsy? Teasdale et al.[58] report that dynamic CT scanning (15 to 18 axial 3-mm sections with 1.5-mm overlap and intravenous nonionic contrast agent flowing in during image acquisition) demonstrated 10 of 10 aneurysms later verified with angiography. Aneurysms ranged in length from 7 to 15 mm; 9 of 10 were at the carotid-posterior communicating junction, 1 at the basilar-superior cerebellar artery junction, and none had caused subarachnoid hemorrhage. In the same study, dynamic CT incorrectly predicted aneurysms in only 4 of 62 normal angiograms (specificity, 94%). This paper, which is somewhat marred by a jumbled presentation, follows on two previous neuroradiologic studies[59, 60] that had shown that dynamic CT could depict intracranial aneurysms of only 8 mm length, but had cautioned that bone artifact in the region of the cranial base might obscure the third cranial nerve aneurysms. The authors assert that dynamic CT "is simple to perform . . . the risks are less than those of angiography, the examination takes less time, can be performed on an outpatient basis and is much cheaper . . . dynamic CT scanning should be the first radiological examination undertaken in patients presenting with a partial or complete third cranial nerve palsy in the absence of subarachnoid haemorrhage." They have a compelling case: others should now try to reproduce these results.

I was surprised to discover that berry aneurysms are no longer considered congenital lesions. According to Stehbens,[61] a respected authority, they should be considered "hemodynamically induced degenerative changes related to atherosclerosis associated with loss of the tensile strength and/or cohesive properties of the vessel wall." The turgid prose that enveloped this quote did not allow easy grasp of the argument, but the supportive bibliography is impressive.

Intracranial AVMs are the subject of a raft of papers dealing with natural history,[62, 63] treatment with extirpative surgery,[64-66] and treatment with radiation surgery.[67-71] The state of the art, as well summarized by Heros and Korosue[72, 73] and Ogilvy,[74] is this:

1. Untreated AVMs will bleed at a rate of 3% to 4% per year, slightly higher than the previously estimated 1% to 2%. If the AVM presents with hemorrhage, it will rebleed at a rate of 6% within the first 6 months, then settle into a rebleeding rate equal to that of previously unruptured AVMs. Neither the size and location of the lesion nor the age of the patient affect the rate of rebleeding. Angiographically occult AVMs rebleed at the same rate as angiographically manifest AVMs. However, venous angiomas, now imaged frequently as convexity linear signal voids with MRI, probably do not bleed, and should be left alone.

2. Mortality from an AVM hemorrhagic episode is 10%. Morbidity is 30%, a concept difficult to gauge quantitatively because headaches, dementia, and progressive neurologic deficits are attributed to AVMs with some controversy.

3. Surgical results have improved substantially in the past decade, largely because of greater microsurgical skill and preoperative embolization.[75] Although neurosurgeons are becoming bolder about attacking brain stem AVMs if they are close to the surface, opinion is shifting toward treatment with radiation surgery. Surgical treatment of large AVMs based in the cerebral cortex is now often preceded by staged embolization to avoid intraoperative and postoperative hemorrhage from normal perfusion breakthrough. Even with skilled embolization, the combined morbidity and mortality rate in a recent series[73] was 38%.

4. Radiation surgery for AVM is now available through proton beam, helium beam, cobalt-source focused gamma rays (gamma knife), and linear accelerator-source x-rays. These methods make use of stereotactic localization to deliver highly concentrated radiation. All modalities appear to produce comparable results: 75% to 80% complete obliteration of the AVM after 2 years with substantial improvement in headaches and seizures and no rebleeding after 2 years. There are three drawbacks: (a) rebleeding continues in the 2-year interval until the AVM is completely obliterated; (b) new neurologic deficits resulting from radiation necrosis occur in 3% to 10% of cases; and (c) lesions of 3.5 cm diameter or greater cannot be obliterated with radiation surgery.

5. Several issues in AVM treatment remain to be resolved. Is linear accelerator-source x-ray therapy, which is the most widely available and least expensive modality, equal to the more esoteric techniques? Can embolization reduce the nidus of large AVMs to bring them within range of radiation surgery? What is the optimal dose to obliterate the lesion yet not cause surrounding brain necrosis? Are there long-term risks of oncogenesis? Is extirpative surgery or radiation surgery the safest approach to small superficial lesions in eloquent cerebral cortex, basal ganglia, or brain stem?

CLINICAL ENTITIES

The interest in lupus anticoagulant and its association with neurologic disease has passed from a preoccupation to a virtual obsession.[76–78] Lupus anticoagulant (LA) is now considered only one of two important antiphospholipid antibodies (APLAb), anticardiolipin antibody (ACLA) being the other. As Levine and Welch[78] acknowledge, serious evidence for a cause and effect relationship between APLAb and stroke does not exist; at best, APLAb are markers for a higher stroke risk. Digre et al.[76] described six young patients who had amaurosis fugax and APLAb and no other risk factors. Some had elevated antinuclear antibody levels. The effect of anticoagulants and aspirin on the visual symptoms was unclear. In a retrospective review, Briley et al.[77] found that 25 of 80 patients with ACLA had encephalopathy, migraine-like headaches, amaurosis fugax, or ischemic optic neuropathy. Two patients improved after treatment with plasmapheresis or immunosuppression. They concluded that in patients with unexplained cerebral ischemia, establishing the presence of ACLA may have prognostic and therapeutic importance. On the basis of this sort of research, the ordering of APLAb titers has joined echocardiography for mitral valve prolapse as the most habit-forming medical maneuvers in young patients with stroke or TIA. Incidentally, Chancellor et al.[79] found that none of 66 young adults with ischemic stroke had APLAb.

When older patients complain of isolated transient bilateral blindness (lone bilateral blindness), are they at special risk of stroke? Dennis et al.[80] followed up 14 patients with this symptom for a mean of 2.4 years in the Oxfordshire Community

Stroke Project and found that 5 developed a first-ever stroke—a 16-fold increase in expected incidence. The patients ranged in age from 46 to 82 years and had the same stroke risk factor profile as patients with TIAs. They quite properly concluded that lone bilateral blindness in middle-aged or elderly individuals with vasculopathic attributes should be considered a posterior circulation TIA.

The clinical manifestations of hypotensive brain ischemia were superbly described by Howard et al.[81] Following cardiac surgery, documented hypotension, or pulmonary embolism, eight patients demonstrated a combination of three syndromes: (1) visual inattention, visual misreaching, disordered smooth pursuit, and absent voluntary saccades; (2) bibrachial distal weakness and disordered finger-tip position sense and two-point discrimination; and (3) transient cortical blindness giving way to dyslexia, dyscalculia, dysgraphia, and verbal and nonverbal memory loss. The deficits usually improved within days of onset, but some abnormalities persisted. CT scans showed abnormalities compatible with infarcts primarily in the posterior border zone (watershed) regions between the three circumflex cerebral arteries. Although the authors presumed that the bibrachial and saccadic features probably reflect slightly more anterior border zone ischemia, CT findings did not document that point. They also suggested that the vulnerable zone tends to be more anterior if hypotension occurs in a setting of hemodynamically significant carotid stenosis. To wit, a PET study[82] showed high cerebral blood volume relative to flow, a sign of vasodilatation in underperfused brain tissue, in the anterior border zone regions ipsilateral to severe carotid stenosis. In my opinion, these papers are describing important clinical phenomena that may be quite common after cardiothoracic procedures. By the time the patient recovers full consciousness in the intensive care unit, the findings may be hard to document. But as with other postoperative cognitive disturbances that are being discovered, they may have a lingering impact on the patient.

REFERENCES

1. Sterman AB, Furlan AJ, Pessin M, et al: Acute stroke therapy trials: An introduction to recurring design issues. *Stroke* 1987; 18:524–527.

2. Sacco RL, Ellenberg JH, Mohr JP, et al: Infarcts of undetermined cause: The NINCDS Stroke Data Bank. *Ann Neurol* 1989; 25:382–390.

3. Ramirez-Lassepas M, Cipolle RJ, Bjork RJ, et al; Can embolic stroke be diagnosed on the basis of neurological clinical criteria? *Arch Neurol* 1987; 44:87–89.

4. Hachinski VC, Rem JA, Boughner DR, et al: The common coincidence of carotid and cardiac lesions, in Stober T, Schimrigk K, Ganten D, et al (eds): *Central Nervous Control of the Heart.* Boston, Martinus Nijhoff, 1986, pp 215–220.

5. Gates PC, Barnett HJM, Silver MD: Cardiogenic stroke, in Barnett HJM, Mohr JP, Stein BM, et al (eds): *Stroke. Pathophysiology, Diagnosis, and Management.* New York, Churchill Livingston, 1986, pp 1085–1109.

6. Fisher CM, Adams RD: Observations on brain embolism with special reference to hemorrhagic infarction, in Furlan AS (ed): *The Heart and Stroke.* Berlin, Springer-Verlag, 1987, pp 17–36.

7. Kittner SJ, Sharkness MD, Price TR, et al: Infarcts with a cardiac source of embolism in the NINCDS Stroke Data Bank: Historical features. *Neurology* 1990: 40:281–284.

8. Bogousslavsky J, van Melle G, Regli F: The Lausanne Stroke Registry: Analysis of 1,000 consecutive patients with first stroke. *Stroke* 1988; 19:1083–1092.

9. Sandercock PA, Warlow CP, Jones LN, et al: Predisposing factors for cerebral infarction: The Oxfordshire community stroke project. *Br Med J* 1989; 298:75–80.

10. Bamford J, Sandercock P, Dennis M, et al: Infarction, intracerebral and subarachnoid haemorrhage. *J Neurol Neurosurg Psychiatry* 1990; 53:16–22.

11. Rolak LA, Gilmer W, Strittmatter WJ: Low yield in the diagnostic evaluation of transient ischemic attacks. *Neurology* 1990; 40:747–748.

12. Caplan LR, Hier DB, D'Cruz I: Cerebral embolism in the Michael Reese Stroke Registry. *Stroke* 1983; 14:530–536.

13. Miller V: Lacunar stroke. A reassessment. *Arch Neurol* 1983; 38:443–447.

14. Futrell N, Millikan C, Watson BD, et al: Lacunes following embolic stroke in normotensive rats. *Stroke* 1988; 19:13.

15. Gandolfo C, Caponnetto C, Del Sette M, et al: Risk factors in lacunar syndromes: A case control study. *Acta Neurol Scand* 1988; 77:22–26.

16. Ringelstein EB, Koschorke S, Holling A, et al: Computed tomographic pattern of proven embolic brain infarctions. *Ann Neurol* 1989; 26:759–765.

17. Shinton R, Beevers G: Meta-analysis of relation between cigarette smoking and stroke. *Br Med J* 1989; 298:75–79.

18. Love BB, Biller J, Jones MP, et al: Cigarette smoking. A risk factor for cerebral infarction in young adults. *Arch Neurol* 1990; 47:693–698.

19. Donnan GA, Adena MA, O'Malley HM, et al: Smoking as a risk factor for cerebral ischaemia. *Lancet* 1989; 2:643–647.

20. Wolf PA, D'Agostino RB, Kannel WB, et al: Cigarette smoking as risk factor for stroke. *JAMA* 1988; 259:1025–1029.

21. Wilkes HC, Kelleher C, Meade TW: Smoking and plasma fibrinogen. *Lancet* 1988; 1:307–308.

22. Nadler JL, Velasco JS, Horton R: Cigarette smoking inhibits prostacyclin formation. *Lancet* 1983; 1:1248–1250.

23. Tell GS, Howard G, McKinney WM, et al: Cigarette smoking cessation and extracranial carotid atherosclerosis. *JAMA* 1989; 261:1178–1180.

24. Homer D, Ingall TJ, Whisnant JP: The effect of smoking on carotid occlusive disease. *Neurology* 1988; 38:148.

25. Scheinberg P: Controversies in the management of cerebral vascular disease. *Neurology* 1988; 38:1609–1616.

26. Imakita S, Nishimura T, Yamada N, et al: Magnetic resonance imaging of cerebral infarction: Time course of gadolinium DTPA enhancement and CT comparison. *Neuroradiology* 1988; 30:372–378.

27. Berry I, Brant-Zawadzki M, Manele C: MRI study of a feline model of acute cerebral ischemia. *J Neuroradiol* 1988; 15:95–107.

28. Hayman LA, Taber KH, Jhingran SG, et al: Cerebral infarction: Diagnosis and assessment of prognosis by using 123IMP-SPECT and CT. *AJNR* 1989; 10:557–562.

29. Jenkins A, Hadley DM, Teasdale GM, et al: Magnetic resonance imaging of acute subarachnoid hemorrhage. *J Neurosurg* 1988; 68:731–736.

30. Ogilvy CS, Heros RC, Ojemann RG, et al: Angiographically occult arteriovenous malformations. *J Neurosurg* 1988; 69:350–355.

31. Smith HJ, Strother CM, Kikuchi Y, et al: MR imaging in the management of supratentorial intracranial AVMs. *AJNR* 1988; 9:225–235.

32. Lee BCP, Brock JM, Sibert A, et al: P31 spectroscopy and thrombolytic treatment of experimental cerebral infarct. *AJNR* 1989; 10:47–52.

33. Herold S, Brown MM, Frackowski RSJ, et al: Assessment of cerebral hemodynamic reserve—correlation between PET parameters and CO_2 reactivity measured by the intravenous xenon-133 injection technique. *J Neurol Neurosurg Psychiatry* 1988; 51:1045–1051.

34. Rogg J, Rutigliano M, Yonas H, et al; The acetazolamide challenge: Imaging techniques designed to evaluate cerebral blood flow reserve. *AJNR* 1989; 10:803–810.

35. Shuaib A, Hachinski VC: Migraine and the risks from angiography. *Arch Neurol* 1988; 45:911–912.

36. Antiplatelet Trialists' Collaboration: Secondary prevention of vascular disease by prolonged antiplatelet treatment. *Br Med J* 1988; 196:316–320.

37. Steering Committee of the Physicians' Health Study Research Group. Preliminary report: Findings from the aspirin component of the ongoing Physicians' Health Study. *N Engl J Med* 1988; 318:262–264.

38. Hass WK, Easton JD, Adams HP Jr, et al: A randomized trial comparing ticlopidine hydrochloride with aspirin for the prevention of stroke in high-risk patients. *N Engl J Med* 1989; 321:501–507.

39. Gent M, Blakely JA, Easton JD, et al: The Canadian American Ticlopidine Study (CATS) in thromboembolic stroke. *Lancet* 1989; 1:1215–1220.

40. Wolf PA, Dawber TR, Thomas HE, et al: Epidemiologic assessment of chronic atrial fibrillation and risk of stroke: The Framingham study. *Neurology* 1978; 28:973–977.

41. Boston Area Anticoagulation Trial for Atrial Fibrillation Investigators: The effect of low-dose warfarin on the risk of stroke in patients with nonrheumatic atrial fibrillation. *N Engl J Med* 1990; 323:1505–1511.

42. Petty GW, Lennihan I, Mohr JP, et al: Complications of long-term anticoagulation. *Ann Neurol* 1988; 23:570–574.

43. The EC/IC Bypass Study Group: Failure of extracranial-intracranial arterial bypass to reduce the risk of ischemic stroke: Results of an international randomized trial. *N Engl J Med* 1985; 313:1191–1200.

44. Bannister CM: Status of extracranial-intracranial anastomoses for cerebral ischaemia 2 years after the international bypass study (editorial). *Br J Neurosurg* 1988; 2:139–142.

45. Pokras R, Dyken ML: Dramatic changes in the performance of endarterectomy for diseases of the extracranial arteries of the head. *Stroke* 1988; 19:1289–1290.

46. Schroeder T, Sillesen H, Sorensen O, et al: Cerebral hyperperfusion following carotid endarterectomy. *J Neurosurg* 1987; 66:824–829.

47. Sundt TM, Whisnant JP, Houser OW, et al: Prospective study of the effectiveness and durability of carotid endarterectomy. *Mayo Clin Proc* 1990; 65:625–635.

48. Turner DA, Jay Tracy PAC, Haines SJ: Risk of late stroke and survival following carotid endarterectomy procedures for symptomatic patients. *J Neurosurg* 1990; 73:193–200.

49. Matchar DB: Decision making in the face of uncertainty: the case of carotid endarterectomy. *Mayo Clin Proc* 1990; 65:756–760.

50. Callow AD, Caplan LR, Correll JW, et al: Carotid endarterectomy: What is its current status? *Am J Med* 1988; 85:835–838.

51. Powers WJ, Grubb RL, Raichle ME: Clinical results of extracranial -intracranial bypass surgery in patients with hemodynamic cerebrovascular disease. *J Neurosurg* 1989; 70:61–67.

52. Mori E, Tabuchi M, Yoshida T, et al: Intracarotid urokinase with thromboembolic occlusion of the middle cerebral artery. *Stroke* 1988; 19:802–812.

53. Koudstall PJ, Stibbe J, Vermeulen M: Fatal ischaemic brain oedema after early thrombolysis with tissue plasminogen activator in early stroke. *Br Med J* 1988; 297:1571–1573.

54. The Hemodilution in Stroke Study Group: Hypervolemic hemodilution treatment of acute stroke: Results of a randomized multi-center trial using pentastarch. *Stroke* 1988; 20:317–323.

55. Ingall TJ, Whisnant JP, Wiebers DO, et al: Has there been a decline in subarachnoid hemorrhage mortality? *Stroke* 1989; 207:718–724.

56. Ohman J, Heiskanen O: Timing of operation for ruptured supratentorial aneurysms: A prospective randomized study. *J Neurosurg* 1989; 70:55–60.

57. Wiebers DO: Intracranial aneurysm, in Johnson RT (ed): *Current Therapy in Neurologic Disease,* vol 3. Philadelphia, BC Decker Inc, 1990, pp 192–194.

58. Teasdale E, Statham P, Straiton J, et al: Non-invasive radiologic investigation for oculomotor palsy. *J Neurol Neurosurg Psychiatry* 1990; 53:549–553.

59. Schmid U, Steiger H, Huber P: Accuracy of high resolution computed tomography in direct diagnosis of cerebral aneurysms. *Neuroradiology* 1987; 29:152–159.

60. Vonofakos D, Hacker H, Grau H: Direct visualisation of intracranial aneurysms by multiplane dynamic CT. *Am J Neuroradiol* 1983; 4:425–428.

61. Stehbens WE: Etiology of intracranial berry aneurysms. *J Neurosurg* 1989; 70:823–831.

62. Brown RD, Wiebers DO, Forbes G, et al: The natural history of unruptured intracranial arteriovenous malformations. *J Neurosurg* 1988; 68:352–357.

63. Heros RC, Korosue K, Diebold PM: Surgical excision of cerebral arteriovenous malformations: Late results. *Neurosurgery* 1990; 26:570–578.

64. Kashiwagi S, Van Loveren HR, Tew JM, et al: Diagnosis and treatment of vascular brainstem malformations. *J Neurosurg* 1990; 72:27–34.

65. Meyer FB, Sundt TM, Fode NC, et al: Cerebral aneurysms in childhood and adolescence. *J Neurosurg* 1989; 70:420–425.

66. Chyatte D: Vascular malformations of the brain stem. *J Neurosurg* 1989; 7:847–852.

67. Kemeny AA, Dias PS, Forseter DM: Results of stereotactic radiosurgery of arteriovenous malformations: An analysis of 52 cases. *J Neurol Neurosurg Psychiatry* 1989; 52:554–558.

68. Levy RP, Fabrikant JL, Frankel KA, et al; Stereotactic heavy-charged-particle Bragg Peak radiosurgery for the treatment of intracranial arteriovenous malformations in childhood and adolescence. *Neurosurgery* 1989; 24:841–852.

69. Loeffler JS, Alexander E, Siddon RL, et al: Stereotactic radiosurgery for intracranial arteriovenous malformations using a standard linear accelerator. *Int J Radiat Oncol Biol Phys* 1989; 17:673–677.

70. Betti OO, Munari C, Rosler R: Stereotactic radiosurgery with the linear accelerator: Treatment of arteriovenous malformations. *Neurosurgery* 1989; 24:311–321.

71. Steinberg GK, Fabrikant JL, Marks MP, et al: Stereotactic heavy-charged-particle Bragg-Peak radiation for intracranial arteriovenous malformations. *N Engl J Med* 1990; 323:96–101.

72. Heros RC, Korosue K: Radiation treatment of cerebral arteriovenous malformations (editorial). *N Engl J Med* 1990; 323:127–129.

73. Heros RC, Korosue K: Arteriovenous malformations of the brain. *Curr Opinion Neurol Neurosurg* 1990; 3:63–67.

74. Ogilvy CS: Radiation therapy for arteriovenous malformations: A review. *Neurosurgery* 1990; 26:725–735.

75. Adelt D, Bruckmann H, Krenkel W, et al: Combined neuroradiological and neurosurgical treatment of intracranial arteriovenous malformations. *J Neurol* 1988; 235:355–358.

76. Digre KB, Durcan FJ, Branch DW, et al: Amaurosis fugax associated with antiphospholipid antibodies. *Ann Neurol* 1989; 25:228–232.

77. Briley DP, Coull BM, Goodnight SH Jr: Neurological disease associated with antiphospholipid antibodies. *Ann Neurol* 1989; 25:221–227.

78. Levine SR, Welch KMA: Antiphospholipid antibodies. *Ann Neurol* 1989; 26:386–389.

79. Chancellor AM, Glasgow GL, Ockelford PA, et al: Etiology, prognosis, and hemostatic function after cerebral infarction in young adults. *Stroke* 1989; 20:477–482.

80. Dennis MS, Sandercock PAG, Bamford JM, et al: Lone bilateral blindness: A transient ischaemic attack. *Lancet* 1989; 1:185–188.

81. Howard R, Trend P, Ross Russell MD: Clinical features of ischemia in cerebral arterial border zones after periods of reduced cerebral blood flow. *Arch Neurol* 1987; 44:934–940.

82. Leblanc R, Yamamoto YR, Tyler JL et al: Borderzone ischemia. *Ann Neurol* 1987; 22:707–713.

CHAPTER 17

Migraine and Facial Pain

B. Todd Troost, M.D.

Professor and Chairman, Department of Neurology, Bowman Gray School of Medicine, Wake Forest University, Winston-Salem, North Carolina

Since the time of the last review,[1] several general reviews of migraine have appeared.[2-5] My contributions[2, 3] were similar except for minor modifications and new citations, such as a review of the neuro-ophthalmologic aspects of migraine, and I also included comments on other headache syndromes. Saper[4] reviews migraine, migraine variants, and related headaches and points out that an exact pathogenesis of migraine has yet to be found. It is his belief that the predilection to migraine-type headaches appears to be genetic, although migraine can be acquired or symptomatic following a number of physiologic assaults including head trauma, infection, and others. In this chapter, I will discuss some of the contributions made within the past 2 years to the understanding of migraine, its variants and treatment, as well as other types of facial pain.

When all has been said that can be, mystery still envelopes the mechanism of migraine. (W. Gowers, 1893).

PATHOPHYSIOLOGY

While it is true that the exact cause and mechanisms of migraine remain uncertain, many modern reviews are trying to integrate the two leading theories, that is, a primary vascular process vs. a primary neuronal process relating to spreading depression.[5] Welch[6] states that:

Migraine with aura, previously termed classical migraine, is now considered by most to be a disorder of central nervous system function. Indeed it is difficult to conceive that the stimulative followed by suppressive characteristics of the neurological symptoms and their spreading quality could be explained by anything other than a process of excitation and inhibition of central neurons. Patients with migraine plus aura may experience a state of central neuronal hyperexcitability which predisposes them to such a condition.

Welch then discusses two mechanisms for spreading depression, one based on the release of K^+ from neural tissue and the other on release of the excitatory amino acid glutamate. It is known that glutamate-induced spreading depression can be blocked by Mg^{2+}. Recently developed techniques of in vivo ^{31}P nuclear magnetic resonance (NMR) spectroscopy have enabled Dr. Welch and colleagues to measure intracellular Mg^{2+} in the brain tissue of patients with migraine. There was a decrease in intracellular Mg^{2+} in all patients compared to that in healthy subjects, and the change was even more significant during an attack.[7] He has also explored metabolic evidence for glutamate abnormality in patients with migraine by measurements in platelets.[8] He concludes that this neuronal hyperexcitability involved overaction of the excitatory amino acid glutamate. Stimuli that activate the migraine attack do so by evoking neuronal depolarization, slowing depolarization shifts, and spreading suppression of spontaneous neuronal activity possibly via glutamate and K^+-dependent mechanisms. A low level of Mg^{2+} in the brain, by promoting glutamate hyperactivity, neuronal hyperexcitability, and susceptibility ot glutamate-dependent spreading depression, may provide the link between the physiologic threshold for a migraine attack and the mechanisms of the attack itself.

Spierings[5] proposes the concept of the migraine process. With this concept, he is able to incorporate the phenomenon of spreading depression into Wolff's cerebral vascular constriction/dilatation model by considering them to be parallel. This as yet unspecified migraine process can explain the simultaneous occurrence of aura symptoms in headaches: headache without aura, and the occurrence of aura without headache.

Lance[9] proposes that monoamine centers in the midbrain are key to a suggested migraine process. The cortical projections from the locus ceruleus and nucleus raphe dorsalis affect cortical microcirculation by causing constriction, ischemia, and possible spreading depression. The periaqueductal gray matter responds to subsequent monoamine depletion by facilitating the perception of pain, commonly in a unilateral fashion. Glover and Sandler[10] find this an attractive model that possibly reconciles the vascular and neurogenic theories of migraine, while allowing 5-hydroxytryptamine (HT) receptors to play a major role. The midbrain centers are stimulated in some spontaneous cycle or by triggers such as stress or hormone fluctuations.

Seymour Solomon, the editor of *Headache Review,* suggests that there are two major questions about the pathophysiology of migraine and that they may not be interrelated.[11] What is the mechanism of the aura and what are the factors that cause pain? He points out that vasoconstriction causing ischemia, evoking the neurologic symptoms of the aura, and followed by compensatory vasodilation leading to the headache, has been the standard concept but it is too simplistic. The vasogenic mechanism proposed by Wolff and associates has given way to neurogenic concepts. The neurogenic rather than the vasogenic formulations of migraine are further supported by the work of Markowitz et al.[12] These authors report that plasma extravasation in the dura mater of the rat is neurogenically mediated and ergotamine preparations prevent such a reaction.[13] Solomon and associates also review arterial stenosis in migraine, discussing the concepts of vasospasm vs. arteriopathy.[14]

Two general reviews of pain have appeared in an issue of *Neurologic Clinics* devoted to pain: mechanisms and syndromes. The first[15] attempts to define a scientifically useful definition of pain: "Pain is an unpleasant sensory and emotional experience associated with actual or potential tissue damage, or described in terms of such damage." He then discusses the difficulties inherent in designing testable hypotheses about pain based on such a definition. Russell K. Portenoy, the guest editor of this issue of *Neurologic Clinics,* addresses the mechanisms of clinical pain.[15] He discusses a proposed taxonomy of chronic pain based on presumed pathophysiologic distinctions into categories of nociceptive, neuropathic, and psychogenic.

Fozard and Gray[16] discuss 5-HT$_{1C}$ receptor activation as a key step in the initiation of migraine. In June 1988, Brewerton[17] and his coworkers published a remarkable observation that *m*-chlorophenylpiperazine (*m*-CPP), a major metabolite of the antidepressant drug trazadone (Desyril) and a selective 5-HT$_1$ receptor agonist, can induce migraine-like headaches in humans. Other roles for 5-HT in the pathogenesis of migraine are reviewed and, putting all such evidence together,[16] they conclude that increased activation of 5-HT$_{1C}$ receptors may be a means to trigger migraine. If this were correct, a 5-HT$_{1C}$ receptor antagonist should be effective as a prophylactic agent in migraine as are methysergide and pizotifen. They conclude that the most plausible current scenario is that an inappropriate release or fluctuation in the activation of the 5-HT neurons of the brain stem, by activation of 5-HT$_{1C}$ receptors, would trigger the sterile inflammatory response around blood vessels, which has been claimed to play a role in the pathophysiology of acute migraine.

There appears to be an association between lupus anticoagulant, antiphospholipid antibodies, and migraine.[18] Hogan and colleagues reviewed the records of 15 patients referred for neurologic assessment who were found to have lupus anticoagulant or elevated anticardioplipin antibodies. A diagnosis of migraine, either as an acute or chronic problem, was made in 66% of these patients. Seven of the 15 patients had ischemic stroke and 2 patients had other thrombotic complications associated with lupus anticoagulant. Unfortunately, at this time, the prevalence of migraine in the population of patients with antiphospholipid antibodies is not known, but this work suggests a subgroup of patients with migraine and lupus anticoagulant who may have an increased susceptibility to stroke. Since some patients with migraine develop headache on exposure to bright sunlight, catecholamine responses to light in these patients were studied by Stoica and Enulescu.[19]

They found that increased light exposure increased norepinephrine excretion in healthy subjects, but in patients with migraine, exposure to high luminosity resulted in a depression of norepinephrine excretion and an augmentation of epinephrine excretion. Since propranolol reverses the pattern of this type of catecholamine response to photostimulation, this may be somehow related to the pathogenesis of the migraine attack.

Various studies on cerebral blood flow measured with a variety of techniques were made during this period of review. Robertson and colleagues[20] studied the effects of aging on cerebral blood flow in migraine. Cerebral blood flow was studied with the ^{133}Xe inhalation technique in 92 patients with migraine aged 19 to 35 years and compared them with 49 control subjects aged 22 to 80 years. Cerebral blood flow declined with age in both groups but at a slower rate in patients with migraine. The difference was most pronounced in classic migraine. The results suggested that differences exist in cerebral vascular resistance tone in patients with migraine, which may contribute to the threshold for migraine attack and result in differing age-related changes in blood flow. Delayed hyperemia following hypoperfusion in classic migraine was studied with ^{133}Xe inhalation and single photon emission computed tomography (SPECT).[21] Initially reduced regional cerebral blood flow persisting up to 3 hours was observed in the hemisphere appropriate to the focal neurologic deficit and hyperperfusion was noted later in the same region. Delayed hyperemia asymmetry often persisted beyond the duration of the clinical headache, and it was postulated that the tardive regional hyperperfusion was a consequence of previous focal arterial vasoconstriction. These observations promoted a series of letters[22, 23] discussing the implications and providing criticisms of the study that were later reviewed by the authors.[24]

Finally, with a relatively new technique, transcranial Doppler ultrasound (TCD), Thomas et al.[25] studied 10 patients with migraine and compared them to healthy control subjects without headaches. Patients with migraine during headache-free intervals demonstrated excessive cerebrovascular activity to CO_2, evidenced by an increase in middle cerebral artery blood flow velocity. Differences between the two study groups revealed no significant decrease in middle cerebral artery blood flow velocity with hypocapnia. However, the differences between middle cerebral artery blood flow velocity during hyperventilation and CO_2 inhalation were significantly different between patients with migraine and control subjects. This study presented observations with TCD that may allow differentiation of vascular from nonvascular headache. The authors conclude that TCD is a safe, rapid, and economical method to study the hemodynamic changes that occur in patients with vascular headaches and may improve diagnosis in a patient with complicated headache, as well as provide a means of monitoring response to therapy. Two papers appeared evaluating the use of TCD in common and classic migraine.[26, 27] During attacks, patients with common migraine exhibited reduction of flow velocities associated with an increase of pulse wave amplitude. Vascular bruits that were heard during the headache-free interval often disappeared. The authors propose that these changes represent caliper fluctuations of the large arteries, suggesting vasodilitation during attacks of common migraine and vasoconstriction during attacks of classic migraine.

Kobari[28] studied cortical and subcortical hyperperfusion during migraine and cluster headache with xenon computed tomography (CT). In spontaneously occurring headache in patients with common or classic migraine, local cerebral blood flow values for cerebral cortex and subcortical gray and white matter were diffusely increased by 20% to 40%, with the exception of the occipital lobes.

Different neuroimaging techniques such as brain mapping[29] and magnetic resonance imaging (MRI) have also been used in migraine.[30] In the MRI study, 19 of 74 patients had multiple foci of bright signal in the brain on T2-weighted MRI. Of note, none of these parenchymal abnormalities were detected on CT scans. Drake and colleagues[31] studied visual and auditory evoked potentials with migraine.

Regarding the pathophysiology of migraine and its relationship to hormone changes in women, it had been suggested that migraine frequently decreases during pregnancy; however, a recent report[32] described nine patients in whom migraine attacks began during pregnancy.

COMMON MIGRAINE

Most current headache classifications derive from the Ad Hoc Committee on Classification of Headache (*Arch Neurol* 1962; 6:173–176). Now there is a new classification of headache.[33] As indicated by the individuals who chaired the committees, it is believed that this classification and diagnostic criteria for headache are very important issues. The new headache classification has been discussed by Daroff.[34] It is modeled somewhat after the *Diagnostic and Statistical Manual of Mental Disorders* (DSM-III) containing a hierarchial constructed and operational diagnostic criteria for all headache disorders. Diagnoses can be made simply at the one- or two-digit levels, but when indicated in specialized centers or for research purposes, four-digit level diagnoses are possible. While a new classification may seem quite complex at first, the new classification will lead to substantive advances in the scientific underpinnings of the mechanisms and, therefore, the therapy of headaches.[34] For the edification of those dealing with migraine, the entire migraine classification is reproduced as follows:

1. Migraine
   1.1 Migraine without aura
   1.2 Migraine with aura
       1.2.1 Migraine with typical aura
       1.2.2 Migraine with prolonged aura
       1.2.3 Familial hemiplegic migraine
       1.2.4 Basilar migraine
       1.2.5 Migraine aura without headache
       1.2.6 Migraine with acute onset aura

1.3 Ophthalmoplegic migraine
1.4 Retinal migraine
1.5 Childhood periodic syndromes that may be precursors to or associated with
   migraine
   1.5.1 Benign paroxysmal vertigo of childhood
   1.5.2 Alternating hemiplegia of childhood
1.6 Complications of migraine
   1.6.1 Status migrainous
   1.6.2 Migrainous infarction
1.7 Migrainous disorder not fulfilling above criteria

One can see that it would be difficult to simply diagnose common migraine with this classification, but indeed the rubric common migraine is too broad to apply to most of these patients. Tension headache, known as muscle contraction headache by many, is a separate category, but of course many believe that there may be a continuum between common migraine and muscle contraction headache as discussed in our prior review.[1]

CLASSIC MIGRAINE

A major review appeared concerning the visual disturbances of migraine.[35] The review describes the visual alterations associated with migraine syndromes of particular interest to ophthalmologist and neuro-ophthalmologist: acephalic, ocular, and ophthalmoplegic. Several current theories of migraine pathophysiology were also discussed. Migrainous episodes are pointed out to be extremely common and must be differentiated from neurologic dysfunction due to ischemia, inflammation, seizure, and compression. This is an excellent review containing both historical aspects and an algorithm for diagnosis and listing of therapy which will be reviewed in the appropriate sections of this chapter. The following description of classic migraine is presented: Classic migraine occurs when visual or sensory motor disturbances precede or, more rarely, accompany the headache. Men and women are affected equally. Visual symptoms include positive and negative scotomata. Scintillating positive scotoma is the most frequent disturbance, occurring in 79% of patients with classic migraine. They are usually of a hemianoptic nature and last less than 1 hour. The positive scotoma may appear as sparkles, flashes of colors, or heat waves. The typical build-up and march of the scintillating scotoma is strongly suggestive of classic migraine, but occurs in only 10% of patients with migraine.

OPHTHALMOPLEGIC MIGRAINE

Hupp et al.,[35] in their review of the visual disturbance of migraine, include a section on ophthalmoplegic migraine. As pointed out, this relatively uncommon condition has been reported to occur in 2% to 17% of patients with migraine. Ophthalmoplegic migraine is much more common in children. Indeed, the onset of migraine after the second decade of life makes the diagnosis highly suspect. The authors indicate that the differential diagnosis of ophthalmoplegic migraine must include parasellar causes of painful ophthalmoplegia, including aneurysm, pituitary apoplexy, diabetic ophthalmoplegia, and the Tolosa-Hunt syndrome. The pathophysiologic mechanisms of ophthalmoplegic migraine are unknown but more theories suggest either a compressive or ischemic lesion of the involved ocular motor nerve. Different theories for the causation of ophthalmoplegic migraine are reviewed.

In a survey to attempt to define the incidence and characteristics of ophthalmoplegic migraine, charts from patients admitted over a 10-year period to the departments of neurology, neurosurgery, ophthalmology, and pediatrics serving a population of over 600,000 inhabitants in Copenhagen County, Denmark, were surveyed.[36] An initial 4 cases of ophthalmoplegic migraine were found (for an annual incidence of 0.7 per million inhabitants), but another 4 cases were added during their review. Only 2 of the 8 cases fulfilled the entire criteria for pain and associated symptoms required for migraine without aura (common migraine). In contrast, the clinical characteristics of the attack were said to be typical of the Tolosa-Hunt syndrome. The authors came to a conclusion with which I disagree; that is, when headaches were typical they were diagnosed as ophthalmoplegic migraine, whereas the proper diagnosis of the Tolosa-Hunt syndrome was made in 9 patients with migraine. On reviewing the actual case histories, every one of the 8 patients satisfy my criteria for ophthalmoplegic migraine. Recurrent episodes of third cranial nerve palsy or sixth cranial nerve palsy (2 of their cases had sixth cranial nerve palsy) often beginning in childhood with accompanying headache which disappeared spontaneously occurred; all patients had normal imaging studies, normal erythrocyte sedimentation rate, and 2 had normal arteriograms. In 1 patient who had 50 attacks over a 10-year period beginning at age 10 years and a family history of migraine, the authors concluded, incorrectly, that the most likely possibility was a retro-orbital inflammatory reaction. I continue to believe that the Tolosa-Hunt syndrome should be diagnosed only on the basis of excluding all other possibilities and it is likely that MRI will be the procedure of choice, particularly with high-resolution views of the orbit and cavernous sinus region.

RETINAL MIGRAINE

I am happy that the newest classification of headache reserves a separate category for retinal migraine.[33] Hupp et al.[35] unfortunately call this "ocular migraine," by which they mean transient monocular visual loss, but this is confusing to the uninitiated because classic migraine with its visual auras is thought of by some as visual or ocular migraine as well. Nonetheless, the review gives excellent coverage to the monocular visual disturbances of migraine, citing my recently republished definition[3]: A transient or permanent monocular visual disturbance accompanying a migraine attack or occurring in a person with a strong history of migrainous episodes. Anterior visual pathway migraine may be preferable but is cumbersome. As pointed out by Hupp et al.,[35] manifestations of retinal migraine that have been reported include ischemic optic neuropathy, central, and branch retinal artery occlusion, retinal pigmentary changes, central retinal vein occlusion, central serous retinopathy, vitreous hemorrhage, retinal hemorrhage with or without optic disc edema, and transient monocular visual loss. They gave an excellent review and excellent citations for all previous reported cases. Transient monocular visual loss is the most frequent clinical presentation of retinal migraine, usually occurring in young adults less than 40 years old. There is often a history of common or classic migraine or, more rarely, cluster headache. After repeated attacks, or occasionally with single spells, the patient may be left with a permanent visual field defect. Duration of the visual loss ranges from seconds to hours, with most cases lasting less than 30 minutes. However, long-lasting amaurotic spells with recovery are most likely due to migraine, with one report of recovery of vision after 7½ hours of amaurosis. As these authors point out, headache is an inconstant accompaniment of ocular migraine. However, headache rarely occurs with embolic amaurosis fugax. The authors admonition that the rarity of ocular migraine as a cause of transient monocular visual loss should make it a diagnosis of exclusion. This was highlighted by a recent case of mine[37] in which a young medical student had episodes of amaurosis fugax, occasionally accompanied by headache, and was considered to have retinal migraine. He turned out to have a large pituitary tumor!

Newman et al.[38] reported bilateral central retinal artery occlusions, disk drusen, and migraine. Central retinal artery occlusion occurred in a patient in the left eye at the age of 25 years when she was noted to have biltaeral intrapapillary drusen. Extensive investigation failed to establish the presence of any systemic disease or vasculopathy. Eight years later, she had a central retinal artery occlusion in the right eye. The authors discuss the possible association with retinal migraine as the patient's history was noteworthy for frequent headaches, the character of which changed to a form suggestive of classic migraine. In this patient, the combination of bilateral drusen and migraine might have contributed to the occurrence of bilateral sequential central retinal artery occlusions.[38]

CEREBRAL MIGRAINE

As in the past, I am using the term cerebral migraine to refer to all cerebral symptoms of migraine whether transient or permanent, Migraine stroke is a topic of review by Welch and Levine.[39] They review the diagnosis of migraine-related stroke and provide illustrative case histories. The Headache Classification Committee category of migrainous cerebral infarction[34] is amplified and further categorized with strictly defined diagnostic criteria. True migraine-induced stroke is revealed as only one of a number of migraine-related stroke syndromes. This manuscript reviews general concepts of the pathogenesis of migraine and typical and atypical cases and certainly provides some unusual cases that defy classification. Intracerebral hemorrhage in cases of migraine, retinal migraine, and ophthalmoplegic migraine are also reviewed. In considering the pathogenesis of migraine-induced stroke, the major categories considered are coagulation factors, hemodynamic factors, and neuronal factors. They cite their previous reviews of ten cases of migraine associated with lupus anticoagulant and also cite platelet hyperaggregability as a possible risk factor. Considering hemodynamic factors, they conclude that low flow in major intracerebral vessels may be due to increased downstream resistance and not, necessarily, to vasospasm.[40]

Migraine with vasospasm and delayed intracerebral hemorrhage was also reported by Cole and Aubie.[41] Three women with well-documented migraine associated with intracerebral hemorrhage were described. In each case, migraine headaches began during adulthood. Unusually severe and protracted headache heralded the onset of fixed neurologic deficits associated with lobar intracerebral hemorrhage. Striking carotid artery tenderness was characteristic. Except for a history of migraine, no cause for intracerebral hemorrhage could be established. Extensive spasm of the extracranial or intracranial arteries was demonstrated on arteriography. These authors believe that vasospasm associated with severe migraine attacks may result in ischemia of intracranial vessel walls, leading to necrosis, and subsequent vessel rupture when perfusion pressure is restored. The use of cocaine can also cause intracranial hemorrhage, and migraine-like headache associated with cocaine use has also recently been described.[42] The finding of such headache in the authors' minds expands the range of neurologic complications of cocaine use and is believed to be consistent with the potential role of serotonin in the development of migraine. In the subjects described, the desire to avoid the cocaine-induced headache eventually became part of the resolve to stop drug use. Vascular headache has also been described as a presenting symptom of multiple sclerosis.[43]

Differentiating new onset, severe migraine from intracranial hemorrhage may, on occasion, be a major problem, particularly if CT scans and spinal fluid examinations are normal in the presence of initial subarachnoid hemorrhage. Saper[44] reviews thunderclap headache and discusses other recent reports.[45, 46] Harling and associates[45] performed a prospective study of 49 patients presenting to the regional neurosurgeon unit with sudden onset of severe headache suggestive of subarachnoid hemorrhge. Thirty-five of the 49 patients had cerebrospinal fluid (CSF) and/or CT documentation of actual hemorrhage caused by aneurysm. Fourteen of the 49 patients had normal results on the CT and CSF studies. Eight of these 14 patients underwent arteriography, which was normal in all cases. All 14 of the patients with normal results on CT and lumber puncture (LP) who did not appear to have hemorrhage (including the 6 who did not undergo angiography) were followed up for 18 to 30 months after the acute attack. None of the patients suffered from hemorrhage during this time. Those authors reported that all patients in the series had described their attacks as "the worst I have ever experienced." The headache was precipitated by exercise, weight lifting, or sexual intercourse in 10 of the 35 patients with confirmed subarachnoid hemorrhage and in 3 of the 14 benign cases. Neck stiffness was present in 28 of the patients with subarachnoid hemorrhage and in 8 of the benign group. It should be emphasized, as it was by the authors, that it was not possible to categorize the patients into the hemorrhage or non-hemorrhage group on clinical grounds. Saper reviews the implications of these papers[44] and suggests that, nonetheless, the weight of current clinical opinion suggests that arteriography is not recommended in most incidences when CT and LP studies, performed soon after the event, return normal results. Saper also has reviewed more chronic headache syndromes including some with cerebral symptoms.[47]

BASILAR ARTERY MIGRAINE

McDonald reported the case of a 40-year-old woman with a 24-year history of basilar artery migraine.[48] She was admitted to the hospital after suffering a large cerebellar infarction causing hydrocephalus and deep stupor during an attack of migraine. Fortunately, the patient recovered after ventricular shunting and removal of the infarct. MRI studies in basilar artery migraine were performed in 18 patients with nonepileptiform basilar artery migraine.[49] In a few subjects, mild enlargement of the cortical sulci and increased signal intensity of white matter on T2-weighted images were present. Twelve of the patients also underwent CT of the head: 6 had abnormalities on MRI not detected with CT, but this finding did not modify the preexisting diagnosis or influence clinical management. The authors conclude that MRI is a useful but limited complementary diagnostic tool in cases of basilar artery migraine. Three patients with a history of migraine and coital cephalalgia associated with signs of vertebrobasilar deficiency were described.[50] The authors postulated that the ischemic disturbances were triggered by hemodynamic changes during orgasm.

CLUSTER HEADACHE

The underlying mechanism of cluster headache and its autonomic features are described as a "mystery surrounding an enigma."[51] Pupillometric studies were performed in eight patients with chronic paroxysmal hemicrania and in control subjects during basal conditions and after the instillation of tyramine, hydroxyamphetamine, and phenylephrine.[52] In patients with chronic paroxysmal hemicrania, the pupils on both symptomatic and nonsymptomatic sides were smaller in the basal state than in control subjects; this was particularly true on the symptomatic side. Mydriatic responses were similar on both the symptomatic and nonsymptomatic sides.

The same authors studied patients with cluster headache by testing forehead sweating patterns and found only minor differences when compared with patients who had brain stem lesions causing a typical Horner's syndrome. Patients who had typical reactions of definite evaporimetric asymmetries also had typical pupillometric patterns for a sympathetically denervated eye.[53] Further pupillary responsiveness in cluster headache was studied with infrared pupillometry, which defined an impairment of pupillary response to light and to nociceptive stimulation on the symptomatic side.[54] The variations and pupil diameter were induced by dark-light adaptation, light reflex, and electric stimulation of the sural nerve in patients with episodic and chronic cluster headache. More autonomic disturbances in cluster headache were described by Drummond.[55] Thirty patients were studied both during attacks and during headache-free periods. Ocular sympathetic function was impaired on the symptomatic side between cluster attacks and especially during cluster headache. Heat loss was greatest from the orbital region on the symptomatic side in association with ocular sympathetic dysfunction and with lacrimation, but the latter only during attacks.

Cluster minibouts were described as brief episodes of cluster headache lasting just 1 to 2 weeks.[56]

Raskin believes that the traditional designation of cluster headache as a vascular headache disorder is probably inaccurate.[57] He believes that the vascular alterations that occur appear to be epiphenomenal, as they are in migraine, resulting from a primary central nervous system dysfunction. He points out that it has been confirmed that patients with postganglionic lesions display no mydriasis in response to hydroxyamphetamine, patients with more proximal lesions demonstrate full mydriasis, and patients with cluster headache respond with *partial* mydriasis, again inconsistent with a postganglionic lesion. Since patients with Horner's syndrome in whom the lesion is distal to the bifurcation of a common carotid artery have sweat impairment restricted to the medial aspect of the forehead and lateral nose, other studies of facial sweating in patients with cluster headache have found impairment in the cheek as well as in the forehead. He points out that the results of conjunctival phenylephrine, a direct-acting receptor agonist, have been inconclusive, since first-order neuronal lesions cannot be distinguished from third-order neuronal injuiries. All the studies are consistent with a central nervous system origin for the Horner's syndrome that attends cluster headache, and inconsistent with a lesion of the pericarotid sympathetic plexus.[57] Ekbom has reviewed the terminology of cluster headache and suggests that certain phraseology be used to describe the periodicity such as the following: (1) attack or cluster headache attack; (2) cluster period; (3) remission.[58]

Substance P-like immunoreactivity was measured in iris, choroid, and retina obtained postmortem.[59] The possible functional involvement of iris substance P was studied in 22 patients with episodic cluster headache by using the anticholinesterase agent echothiophate iodide (EI), which also induces an atropine-resistant miosis, putatively due to release of substance P from trigeminal sensory neurons. In patients with cluster headache, EI eyedrops instilled into both eyes provoked a prolonged miosis with a more marked response in the pupil of the symptomatic eye. The authors propose that the hyperfunction of substance P-containing neurons may coexist with the previously documented sympathetic hypofunction in the innervation of the symptomatic pupil of cluster headache.[59] Cluster headache in women is rare but was the subject of a study of 82 women.[60] The clinical features of headache and the physiologic events related to reproductive life were compared with those of various control groups. No remarkable differences in clinical features between men and women were found. Unlike other forms of primary headache, the course of cluster headache did not seem to be modified by menstruation, pregnancy, or puerperium. The data also seemed to confirm a hypofertility trend, mostly after the onset of cluster headache, a fact that has been previously noted by other authors.

TRIGEMINAL NEURALGIA

An excellent review article concerning trigeminal neuralgia and related disorders appeared in a collection discussing pain. As Fromm states: "Because the oro-facial region has one of the densest and richest nerve supplies in the body, it is not surprising that the face and mouth are particularly sensitive to pain and that patients afflicted with oro-facial pain often come to feel that they are being subjected to the tortures of the damned."[61] He reviews the clinical characteristics of classical tic, how one arrives at a diagnosis in the 1990s, evidence concerning the pathogenesis of trigeminal neuralgia, and experimental data favoring both peripheral and central mechanisms in the etiology and pathogenesis of trigeminal neuralgia.

Microvascular cross compression was the subject of two reviews. First, Bederson and Wilson[62] evaluate their results from microvascular decompression and partial sensory rhizotomy in 252 cases. Patients with distortion of the fifth cranial nerve root caused by extrinsic vascular compression underwent microvascular decompression, those with no compression underwent partial sensory rhizotomy, and those with vascular contact but no distortion of the nerve root underwent decompression and rhizotomy. An excellent (75%) or good (8%) clinical outcome was achieved in 208 patients: 13 patients (5%) experienced little or no pain relief. Thirty-one patients (12%) suffered recurrent trigeminal neuralgia with an average of 1.9 pain-free years after operation; recurrence continued at a rate of approximately 2% per year thereafter. These authors conclude that vascular decompression may cause dysfunction of the trigeminal system in tic douloureux, but in patients who remain untreated for a long period, an intrinsic abnormality develops that may perpetuate pain even after microvascular decompression. They recommend posterior fossa exploration as the procedure of choice for patients with trigeminal neuralgia who are surgical candidates. Taking another tack, Adams[63] presents an alternative view and hypothesis believing that the evidence used to support the hypothesis of microvascular compression is insufficient and unconvincing. He believes that the basis of microvascular decompression could be trauma of the nerve during operative dissection and decompression. He believes that the concept of microvascular compression might be more convincing if microvascular decompression could be shown to cure a condition such as spasmodic torticollis, which cannot be remedied by damage to or section of the same cranial nerve or nerves.[63]

Most authors currently recommend medical therapy to be initiated with baclofen, which is believed to be less toxic than carbamazepine.[61] Another drug, pimozide, has been compared with carbamazepine in a double-blind crossover trial in 48 patients with trigeminal neuralgia who were refractory to medical therapy.[64] All of the patients treated with pimozide improved, while only 56% of patients treated with carbamazepine were relieved of their pain. The central and peripheral mechanisms that may underlie pimozide-induced improvement were discussed.

OTHER FACIAL PAIN

Temporomandibular joint dysfunction is considered controversial both as a cause of a variety of facial pains and in its therapy. Most agree that obvious organic disease of the temporomandibular joint causes pain, but pain is often attributed to dysfunction rather than disease of the joint. Most physicians and dentists will concede that psychologic factors are important in such patients, but many believe that psychological factors are predominant.[65] Controlled studies have been performed only in recent years. Ylitalo and associates compared the functional defects of the masticatory system in patients predisposed to temporomandibular joint (TMJ) disease because of rheumatoid arthritis with a control group of asymptomatic subjects.[66] There were no significant differences in the symptoms of TMJ dysfunction between the two groups. Roberts et al. evaluated the tenderness of masculatory muscles in patients undergoing arthrography for TMJ pain and dysfunction.[67] Tenderness was greater in patients with normal arthograms than in those with abnormalities. Solomon[65] concludes that while controlled studies are narrowing the concept of TMJ and myofascial pain dysfunction, it appears that the diagnosis is being made (probably mistakenly) with increasing frequency.

Post–lumbar puncture headache was reviewed in relation to body posture.[68] Three hundred neurologic inpatients were studied and evaluated for the significance of body posture after lumbar puncture. Immediate mobilization was compared with bed rest for 6 hours (3 hours prone followed by 3 hours supine posture). Contrary to the widely held belief, his investigation did not show significant differences between recumbent and ambulatory patients as to the frequency of post–lumbar puncture headache. Headache associated with nausea was significantly more frequent in the recumbent than in the ambulatory patients. Thus, these authors recommend immediate mobilization after lumbar puncture.

Cervicogenic headache was evaluated based on computer-generated measurements of cervical spine mobility in 15 patients.[69] The term cervicogenic only reflects the localization of the pain, without specifying a certain anatomic structure as the source of pain. Unfortunately, the statistical analysis is suspect in the study because multiple t tests were done on all the data presented and only certain joints showed a significant difference between control subjects and patients with headache. Multivariant statistics should have been used in this study.

Pathologic studies were performed on one case of the Tolosa-Hunt syndrome.[70] This was an unusual patient who died at age 73 years after developing pain and joint swelling at age 19. He underwent earlier biopsies of involved organs, which showed granulomatosis arteritis. At autopsy, multiple organs were found to have evidence of a systemic vasculitis, leading the authors to conclude that the Tolosa-Hunt syndrome may be only one manifestation of a chronic systemic vasculitis in some cases.

Atypical facial pain was described in a 72-year-old woman who was found to have ectasia of the basilar artery that responded dramatically to baclofen.[71] Chronic electrical stimulation after electrode implantation in the gasserian ganglion led to good results in two cases with chronic atypical pain due to deafferentation caused by prior surgery and trauma.[72] These authors conclude that such stimulation, used after failed medical therapy, was not as useful as thalamic stimulation, which could be used for the paint of herpes zoster or postherpetic neuralgia, even though that was not the condition being discussed. Watson, however, provided an extensive review of postherpetic neuralgia.[73] He reviews the origin, definition, natural history, pathogenesis, as well as prevention of postherpetic neuralgia. Therapeutic endeavors including medical and surgical approaches are also reviewed. Of interest to many is the use of topical capsaicin, which is the pungent principal of hot paprika or chile peppers. As Watson points out, capsaicin selectively stimulates and then blocks unmyelinated sensory afferent fibers from skin and mucous membranes. He suggests the following guidelines for the use of topical capsaicin:

1. It must be used four to five times daily (if used less, it may not effectively deplete substance P).
2. It should be used for 4 weeks (patients may not get relief for 2 or 3 weeks).

3. Patients should be seen regularly to encourage persistence and deal with capsaicin-burning.

4. If burning occurs, it may be tolerated by the prior application of 5% lidocaine ointment, covering a small area of skin initially, and by regular analgesics.

5. Hands should be washed after use to avoid eye exposure by inadvertent contact, and the ointment should be kept above the eyebrow and away from the eye if used for ophthalmic nerve involvement.[73]

He concludes that postherpetic pain persisting 1 month or longer occurs in only a small percentage of all patients with herpes zoster and, in most patients, it tends to diminish with time. The incidence is, however, directly related to age, meaning that any therapeutic claim for prophylaxis or treatment must be evaluated with these observations in mind.

THERAPY

A number of review articles on migraine or headache in general include sections on therapy.[3, 4, 9, 74] Saper[4] believes that there should be some general treatment considerations as follows:

A global recognition of the patient's life, emotional needs, and physiological vulnerabilities is essential. The traditional focus of physicians on symptoms must make way for an emphasis on the individual primarily and the symptom secondarily. The successful preventive as well as symptomatic treatment of migraine requires patience and innovativeness. Therapy in all cases must be modelled to meet individual differences in general health, psychological make-up, headache pattern, and patient compliance.

He believes that migraine can be treated in nonpharmacologic and pharmacologic ways. The pharmacologic treatment can be either symptomatic (rescue, abortive) or preventive. Nonpharmacologic treatment emphasizes a variety of different interventions, including biofeedback and stress management training, and avoidance of provoking influences ranging from dietary considerations to changing sleep time and awakening time. He believes, as do I, that linkage of certain foods to the onset of headache has not been satisfactorily established, but anecdotally, it is believed that many patients will regularly or periodically be sensitive to certain food components, including tyramine, monosodium glutamate, and many other additives and food products. Thereafter, the overall pharmacologic approach to the therapy of migraine is well reviewed.

The three calcium channel antagonists are verapamil (Isopin, Calan), diltiazem (Cardizem), and nifedipine (Procardia). Verapamil is usually administered beginning at 80 mg two to three times a day and is increased to approximately 160 mg three to four times per day. The starting dose of diltiazem is 30 mg two or three times a day and is increased to 90 mg three times per day if tolerated. Nifedipine may be initiated at 10 mg three times a day and increased to 60 to 90 mg three times a day. He points out that calcium antagonists are of special benefit in patients who suffer from migraine and simultaneous vasoconstrictive tendencies such as Raynaud's phenomenon/disease and asthma. β-Blocking agents aggravate these conditions.[4] He suggests as treatment for chronic daily headache a combination of tricyclic antidepressants and blocking agents but stresses concern for analgesic overuse and abuse. Beckett[74] reviews the contemporary management of migraine, emphasizing the nonsteroidal antiinflammatory drugs for abortive therapy of migraine.

In reviewing the search for the ideal headache drug, Lance[9] reviews ideas of pathogenesis as well as the inheritance of the migraine syndromes. Fromm[75] reviews the clinical pharmacology of drugs used to treat head and face pain. He reviews the indications, dosing regiments, and potential side effects of drugs used in the treatment of trigeminal and glossopharyngeal neuralgia, postherpetic neuralgia, temporal arteritis, and migraine based on their clinical pharmacology. Humphrey et al.[76] review advances in serotonin receptor pharmacology, discussing various antimigraine drugs that are currently under development. Peroutka[77] also reviews the pharmacology of current antimigraine drugs. The major finding of his analysis is that acute migraine agents such as the ergots and sumatriptan share a high affinity for 5-HT_{1D} receptors. This receptor appears to be present in certain intracranial blood vessels. It is also found in nerve terminals where it inhibits the release of 5-HT and other neurotransmitters. Theoretically, 5-HT_{1D} receptor agonists may acutely inhibit the release of vasoactive and/or pain-inducing substances in the perivascular space. Conceivably, drugs acting at this receptor would stop the progression of this perivascular process. In contrast, a number of prophylactic antimigraine drugs share a relatively affinity for 5-HT_2 receptors in human brain. Although this receptor is also found in certain blood vessels, it is present throughout the nervous system. The receptor appears to mediate neuronal depolarization at the cellular level. No hypothesis, at present, readily explains the effectiveness of prophylactic antimigraine drugs based on this receptor however.

Other reports describe studies with flunarizine, a calcium antagonist.[78–80] Sorge studies the use of flunarizine in a double-blind, placebo-controlled, crossover study in childhood migraine.[78] The main side effects were daytime sedation and weight gain. They conclude that flunarizine is an effective drug in the treatment of childhood migraine. Piccini[79] believed that flunarizine may interfere with dopaminergic systems. In a related article. Facchinetti and coauthors believe that opioid control of the hypothalamus-pituitary-adrenal axis cyclically fails in menstrual migraine.[81] This may relate to the difficulty in providing prophylaxis for migraine sufferers when the headache is directly linked to the menstrual cycle. No difference in the monthly frequency of attacks was found in one study of nifedipine in the prophylaxis of classic migraine.[82] Valproate is now being used by some for migraine prophylaxis.[83] In this study, an open trial, valproate therapy (600 mg twice a day) was evaluated in 22 patients with severe migraine who were resistant to previous prophylactic therapy. Despite a positive effect in their study, the authors conclude that these results must be confirmed with a controlled clinical trial. Incidental note is also taken of a second article detailing the use of pimozide for the therapy of severe trigeminal neuralgia.[84] Blanchard and colleagues[85] described the use of thermal biofeedback combined with cognitive therapy in the treatment of vascular headache. Raskin also provides a conceptual overview of how antimigraine drugs work.[86]

TEMPORAL ARTERITIS

Paice[87] reviews problems in the diagnosis, investigation, and therapy of giant cell arteritis. She points out that difficulties arise when the presenting feature is an unusual one, such as cough or claudication, and the physician, not suspecting giant cell arteritis, fails to ellicit other signs or symtpoms that would point to the correct diagnosis. Equally difficult are those cases in which the presenting features are classic, such as headache or sudden blindness, but the patient denies any associated symptoms to confirm the suspicion. This is made more difficult, of course, by those patients who have normal erythrocyte sedimentation rates (ESR).[88] Paice points out that values of less than 30 mm/hour (Westergren) were found in 22.5% of some untreated patients with clinical evidence of polymyalgia rheumatica or giant cell arteritis. It is also pointed out that the height of the ESR is not a predictor for the severity of the disease.

The mainstay of treatment for temporal arteritis is corticosteroid therapy, but there is still controversy over the optimum dose and duration of treatment. Delecoeuillerie et al.[89] reviewed the case notes of 132 patients with pure polymyalgia rheumatica and of 78 who had clinical evidence of giant cell arteritis. The authors conclude that high doses of steroids (above 12 mg of prednisolone per day) are of no value in polymyalgia rheumatica and the value of high-dose methylprednisolone (above 20 mg per day) for giant cell arteritis is doubtful. The flaws in the study were that it was retrospective and there was no randomization of the starting dose. Alternative therapies when complications ensue or even when high steroid therapies are ineffective include azathioprine, dapsone, methotrexate, and cyclosporine.[87] An unusual patient who presented with a lateral medullary syndrome and ipsilateral hemiplegia caused by giant cell arteritis was described.[90]

While it is true that stroke and blindness are the most common neurologic manifestations of temporal arteritis, there are a number of other neurologic and neuroophthalmologic manifestations. Reich and colleagues[91] reviewed the neurologic manifestations of temporal arteritis, including less well-recognized neuro-ophthalmologic features such as ophthalmoplegia, ischemic ophthalmopathy, and pupillary abnormalities.

Hayreh[92] reviews anterior ischemic optic neuropathy (AION) and the differentiation of arteritic from nonarteritic type and their management. As he reports, he has studied the subject of AION clinically and experimentally over the past 20 years. This important article deals particularly with three aspects of AION: (a) the differentiation of arteritic from nonarteritic AION; (b) management of arteritic AION and giant cell arteritis; and (c) currently prevalent misconceptions about AION. Eight factors are used to differentiate arteritic from nonarteritic AION: (1) systemic symptoms; (2) visual symptoms; (3) high ESR and C-reactive protein (CRP); (4) early massive visual loss; (5) chalky-white optic disk swelling; (6) AION associated with cilio retinal artery occlusion; (7) massive choroidal nonfilling of the choroid on fluorescein fundus angiography; and (8) temporal artery biopsy. He strongly emphasizes that temporal artery biopsy must be performed in every patient having a high index of suspicion of giant cell arteritis or of arteritic AION. Interestingly enough, he and his colleagues have found much less fluctuation in CRP than in ESR. He states, "In our experience, combined information from CRP and ESR is very useful in the diagnosis and evaluation of patients with giant cell arteritis and in their follow-up on systemic corticosteroids."

As far as therapy goes, Hayreh[92] believes strongly that when there is a reasonable index of suspicion for giant cell arteritis, with or without visual loss, that the patient be started immediately on systemic corticosteroids even before the temporal artery biopsy is performed. If a patient presents with no visual symptoms or visual loss, they start with at least 80 mg of oral prednisone daily, or even up to 120 mg, depending on the severity of systemic symptoms, ESR, and CRP. He does report, however, that they give megadose corticosteroid therapy intravenously to start with on an emergency basis when a patient with symptoms of giant cell arteritis has any one of the following ocular signs or symptoms: (1) visual symptoms (particularly amaurosis fugax); (2) a complete loss of vision in one eye; or (3) early evidence of second eye involvement (amaurosis fugax, visual field defect, optic disk edema, cilioretinal artery occlusion, or sluggish circulation in the central retinal artery). Their megadose therapy consists of giving usually three to four doses of the equivalent of 1 g of prednisone slowly by intravenous drip, every 6 to 8 hours. This is followed by 120 mg of prednisone orally daily.

He concludes with a review of misconceptions about AION:

1. AION is exclusively a disease of the elderly: "We have found that AION is a disease of all ages and no age is immune from it."

2. Eyes with AION must be blind or almost blind: "In our studies in nonarteritic AION, 41% of the eyes had 6/12 or better visual acuity. Even in arteritic AION the visual acuity was 6/12 or better in 26%."

3. AION always has pale optic disk edema: "Only about half of the eyes with arteritic AION really showed pale edema of the disk from the very start."

4. Asymptomatic optic disk edema is not seen in AION: "My studies have shown conclusively that asymptomatic optic disk edema may precede the visual loss in AION."

5. Neural ischemia is an all or none phenomenon.

6. AION is an early complication of hypertensive arterial disease. This miscon-

ception is based on a report by Elenberger and his theory was based on a retrospective review of records of only 18 cases of nonarteritic AION!: "Our prospective, detailed studies on about 525 patients of nonarteritic AION lend no support at all to this view."

7. Nonarteritic AION patients with systemic hypertension have an increased risk of cerebrovascular accidents and myocardial infarction: "From a prospective follow-up of about 525 patients in our clinic up to 15 years, I have so far detected no support for this view."

REFERENCES

1. Troost BT, McCormick GM: Migraine and facial pain, in Lessell S, vanDalen JTW (eds): *Current Neuro-Ophthalmology*. Chicago, Year Book Medical Publishers, 1989, pp 307–330.

2. Troost BT: Migraine and other headaches, in Tasman W, Jaeger EA (eds): *Duane's Clinical Ophthalmology*. Philadelphia, JB Lippincott, 1989, pp 1–29.

3. Troost BT: Migraine and other headaches, in Glaser JS (ed): *Neuro-Ophthalmology, ed 2*. Philadelphia, JB Lippincott, 1990, pp 487–517.

4. Saper JR: Migraine, migraine variants, and related headaches. *Otolaryngol Clin North Am* 1989; 22:1115–1130.

5. Spierings EL: Recent advances in the understanding of migraine. *Headache* 1988; 28:655–658.

6. Welch KMA. Migraine as a state of central neuronal excitability. *Headache Rev* 1990; 3:3–6.

7. Ramadan NM, Halvorson H, Vande-Lind A, et al: Low brain magnesium in migraine. *Headache* 1989; 29:590–593.

8. D'andrea G, Canazi AR, Joseph R, et al: Platelet excitatory amino acids in migraine. *Cephalalgia* 1989; 9:3–5.

9. Lance JW: A concept of migraine and the search for the ideal headache drug. *Headache* 1990; 30:17–23.

10. Glover V, Sandler M: Can the vascular and neurogenic theories of migraine finally be reconciled?. *Trends Pharmacol Sci* 1989; 10:1–3.

11. Solomon S: Mechanisms of migraine headache. *Headache Rev* 1990; 3:1.

12. Markowitz S, Saito K, Moskowitz MA: Migraine. *Cephalalgia* 1988; 8:83–91.

13. Markowitz S, Saito K, Moskowitz MA: Neurogenically medicated plasma extravasation in dura mater: Effect of ergot alkaloids. A possible mechanism of action in vascular headache. *Cephalalgia* 1988; 8:83–91.

14. Solomon S, Lipton RB, Harris PY: Arterial stenosis in migraine: Spasm or arteriopathy?. *Headache* 1990; 30:52–61.

15. Portenoy RK: Mechanisms of clinical pain, in Portenoy RK (ed): *Neurologic Clinics*, vol 7. *Pain: Mechanisms and Syndromes*. Philadelphia, WB Saunders, 1989, p 205.

16. Fozard JR: 5-HT 1c receptor activation: A key step in initiation of migraine?. *Trends Pharmacol Sci* 1989; 10:307–309.

17. Brewerton TD, Murphy DL, Mueller EA, et al: Induction of migrainelike headaches by the serotonin agonist m-chlorophenylpiperazine. *Clin Pharmacol Ther* 1988; 43:605–609.

18. Hogan MJ, Brunet DG, Ford PM, et al: Lupus anticoagulant, antiphospholipid antibodies and migraine. *Can J Neurol Sci* 1988; 15:420–425.

19. Stoica E, Enulescu O: Catecholamine response to light in migraine. *Cephalalgia* 1988; 8:31–36.

20. Robertson WM, Welch KMA, Levine SR, et al: The effects of aging on cerebral blood flow in migraine. *Neurology* 1989; 39:947–951.

21. Andersen AR, Friberg L, Skyhoj O, et al: Delayed hyperemia following hypoperfusion in classic migraine. *Arch Neurol* 1988; 45:154–159.

22. Vijayan N: Regional cerebral blood flow in classic migraine. *Arch Neurol* 1989; 46:605.

23. Spierings ELH, Graham JR: Cerebral hypoperfusion followed by hyperperfusion in classic migraine. *Arch Neurol* 1989; 46:605–606.

24. Andersen AR, Olesen J, Olsen TS, et al; In reply. *Arch Neurol* 1989; 46:606.

25. Thomas TD, Harpold GJ, Troost BT: Cerebrovascular reactivity in migraineurs as measured by transcranial Doppler. *Cephalalgia* 1990; 10:95–99.

26. Thie A, Fuhlendorf A, Spitzer K, et al: Transcranial Doppler evaluation of common and classic migraine. Part I. Ultrasonic features during the headache-free period. *Headache* 1990; 30:201–208.

27. Thie A, Fuhlendorf A, Spitzer K, et al: Transcranial Doppler evaluation of common and classic migraine. Part II. Ultrasonic features during attacks. *Headache* 1990; 30:209–215.

28. Kobari M, Myers JS, Ichijo M, et al: Cortical and subcortical hyperfusion during migraine and cluster headache measured by the Xe CT-CBF. *Neuroradiology* 1990; 32:4–11.

29. Hughes JR, Robbins LD: Brain mapping in migraine. *Clin Electroencephalogr* 1990; 21:14–24.

30. Kuhn MJ, Shekar PC: A comparative study of magnetic resonance imaging and computed tomography in the evaluation of migraine. *Comput Med Imaging Graphics* 1990; 14:149–152.

31. Drake ME, Pakalnis A, Hietter SA, et al; Visual and auditory evoked potentials in migraine. *Electromyogr Clin Neurophysiol* 1990; 30:77–81.

32. Chancellor AM, Wroe SJ, Cull RE: Migraine occurring for the first time in pregnancy. *Headache* 1990; 30:224–227.

33. Headache Classification Committee of the International Headache Society. Classification and diagnostic criteria for headache disorders, cranial neuralgias, and facial pain. *Cephalalgia* 1988; 8:12–72.

34. Daroff RB: New headache classification. *Surg Neurol* 1989; 31:112.

35. Hupp SL, Kline LB, Corbett JJ: Visual disturbance of migraine. *Surv Ophthalmol* 1989; 33:221–236.

36. Hansen SL, Borelli-Moller L, Strange P, et al: Ophthalmoplegic migraine: Diagnostic criteria, incidence of hospitalization and possible etiology. *Acta Neurol Scand* 1990; 81:54–60.

37. Dirr LY, Janton FJ, Troost BT: Non-benign amaurosis fugax in a medical student. *Neurology* 1990; 40:349.

38. Newman NJ, Lessell S, Brandt M: Bilateral central retinal artery occlusions, disk drusen, and migraine. *Am J Ophthalmol* 1989; 107:236–240.

39. Welch KMA, Levine SR: Migraine-related stroke in the context of the international headache society classification of head pain. *Arch Neurol* 1990; 47:458–462.

40. Moen M, Levine SR, Newman DS, et al: Bilateral posterior cerebral artery strokes in a young migraine sufferer. *Stroke* 1988; 19:525–528.

41. Cole AJ, Auble M: Migraine with vasospasm and delayed intracerebral hemorrhage. *Arch Neurol* 1990; 47:53–56.

42. Satel SL, Gawin FH: Migrainelike headache and cocaine use. *JAMA* 1989; 261:2995–2996.

43. Freedman MS, Gray TA: Vascular headache: A presenting symptom of multiple sclerosis. *Can J Neurol Sci* 1989; 16:63–66.

44. Saper JR: The thunderclap headache. *Headache Rev* 1989; 2:3–4.

45. Harling DW, Peatfield RC, Van Hille PT. Thunderclap headache: Is it migraine? *Cephalalgia* 1989; 9:87–90.

46. Wijdicks EFM. Long-term follow-up with 71 patients with thunderclap headache mimicking subarachnoid hemorrhage. *Lancet* 1988; 2:68–69.

47. Saper JR: Chronic headache syndromes, in Portenoy RK (ed): *Neurologic Clinics,* vol 7, *Pain: Mechanisms and Syndromes*. Philadelphia, WB Saunders, 1989, p 387.

48. McDonald JV: Basilar artery migraine. *J Neurosurg* 1990; 72:289–291.

49. Jacome DE, Laborgne J: MRI studies in basilar artery migraine. *Headache* 1990; 30:88–90.

50. Martinez JM, Roig C, Arboix A: Complicated coital cephalalgia. Three cases with benign evolution. *Cephalalgia* 1988; 8:265–268.

51. Solomon S: Cluster headaches. *Headache Rev* 1990; 3:1.

52. DeSouza CD, Salvesen R, Sand T, et al: Chronic paroxysmal hemicrania. XIII. The pupilllometric pattern. *Cehpalalgia* 1988; 8:219–226.

53. Salvesen R, deSouza CD, Sand T, et al: Cluster headache: Forehead sweating pattern during heating and pilocarpine tests. Variation as a function of time. *Cephalalgia* 1988; 8:245–253.

54. Micieli G, Magri M, Sandrini G, et al: Pupil responsiveness in cluster headache: A dynamic TV pupillometric evaluation. *Cephalalgia* 1988; 8:193–201.

55. Drummond PD: Autonomic disturbances in cluster headaches. *Brain* 1988; 111:1199–1209.

56. Sjaastad O, deSouza CD, Fragoso YD, et al: Cluster headache: On the significance of so-called minibouts. *Cephalalgia* 1988; 8:285–291.

57. Raskin NH: Cluster headache: Localization. *Headache* 1989; 29:579–580.

58. Ekbom K: Some remarks on the terminology of cluster headache. *Cephalalgia* 1988; 8:59–60.

59. Fanciullacci M, Pietrini U, Geppetti P, et al: Substance P in the human iris: Possible involvement in echothiophate-induced miosis in cluster headache. *Cephalalgia* 1988; 8:49–53.

60. Manzoni GC, Micieli G, Granella F, et al: Cluster headache in women: Clinical findings and relationship with reproductive life. *Cephalalgia* 1988; 8:37–44.

61. Fromm GH: Trigeminal neuralgia and related disorders, in Portenoy RK (ed): *Neurologic Clinics*, vol 7, *Pain: Mechanisms and Syndromes*. Philadelphia, WB Saunders, 1989, p 305.

62. Bederson JB, Wilson CB: Evaluation of microvascular decompression and partial sensory rhizotomy in 252 cases of trigeminal neuralgia. *J Neurosrug* 1989; 71:359–367.

63. Adams CBT, Chir M: Microvascular compression: An alternative view and hypothesis. *J Neurosurg* 1989; 57:1–12.

64. Lechin F, van der Dijs B, Lechin ME, et al: Pimozide therapy for trigeminal neuralgia. *Arch Neurol* 1989; 46:960–963.

65. Solomon S: Temporomandibular joint dysfunction. *Headache* 1989; 2:1.

66. Ettala Ylitalo UM, Syrjanen S, Halonen P: Functional disturbances of the masticatory system related to temporomandibular joint involvement by rheumatoid arthritis. *J Oral Rehabil* 1987; 14:415–427.

67. Roberts CA, Tallents RH, Katzberg RW, et al: Comparison of arthrographic findings of temporomandibular joint with palpation of the muscles of mastication. *Oral Surg Oral Med Oral Pathol* 1987; 64:275–277.

68. Vilming ST, Schrader H, Monstad I: Post-lumbar-puncture headache: The significance of body posture. *Cephalalgia* 1988; 8:75–78.

69. Pfaffenrath V, Dandekar R, Mayer ETH, et al: Cervicogenic headache: Results of computer-based measurements of cervical spine mobility in 15 patients. *Cephalalgia* 1988; 8:45–48.

70. Hannerz J: Pathoanatomic studies in a case of Tolosa-Hunt. *Cephalalgia* 1988; 8:25–30.

71. Martins IP, Ferro JM: Atypical facial pain, ectasia of the basilar artery, and baclofen: A case report. *Headache* 1989; 29:581–583.

72. Probst C: Treatment of atypical post-traumatic and postoperative facial neuralgia by chronic stimulation. Apropos of 2 cases, with review of the literature. *Neurochirurgie* 1988; 34:106–109.

73. Watson CPN: Postherpetic neuralgia, in Portenoy RK (ed): *Neurologic Clinics*, vol 7, *Pain: Mechanisms and Syndromes*. Philadelphia, WB Saunders, 1989, p 231.

74. Beckett BE: Contemporary management of migraine, part 1. *Am Pharm* 1990; 30:51–56.

75. Fromm GH: Clinical pharmacology of drugs used to treat head and face pain. *Neurol Clin* 1990; 8:143–151.

76. Humphrey PPA, Feniuk W, Perren MJ: Anti-migraine drugs in development: Advances in serotonin receptor pharmacology. *Headache* 1990; 29:12–16.

77. Peroutka SJ: The pharmacology of current anti-migraine drugs. *Headache* 1990; 30:5–11.

78. Sorge F, DeSimone R, Marano E, et al: Flunarizine in prophylaxis of childhood migraine. *Cephalalgia* 1988; 8:1–6.

79. Piccini P, Nuti A, Paoletti AM, et al: Possible involvement of dopaminergic mechanisms in the antimigraine action of flunarizine. *Cephalalgia* 1990; 10:3–8.

80. Centonze V, Magrone D, Vino M, et al: Flunarizine in migraine prophylaxis: efficacy and tolerability of 5 mg and 10 mg dose levels. *Cephalalgia* 1990; 10:17–24.

81. Facchinetti F, Martignoni E, Fioroni L, et al: Opioid control of the hypothalamus-pituitary-adrenal axis cyclically fails in menstrual migraine. *Cephalalgia* 1990; 10:51–56.

82. McArthur JC, Marek K, Pestronk A, et al: Nifedipine in the prophylaxis of classic migraine: A crossover, double-masked, placebo-controlled study of headache frequency and side effects. *Neurology* 1989; 39:284–286.

83. Srensen KV: Valproate: A new drug in migraine prophylaxis. *Acta Neurol Scand* 1988; 78:346–348.

84. Lechin F, van der Dijs B, Amat J, et al: Definite and sustained improvement with primozide of two patients with severe trigeminal neuralgia. *J Med* 1988; 19:243–256.

85. Blanchard EB, Appelbaum KA, Radnitz CL, et al: A controlled evaluation of thermal biofeedback and thermal biofeedback combined with cognitive therapy in the treatment of vascular headache. *J Consult Clin Psychol* 1990; 58:216–224.

86. Raskin N: Conclusions. *Headache* 1990; 29:24–28.

87. Paice E: Giant cell arteritis: Difficult decisions in diagnosis, investigation and treatment. *Postgrad Med J* 1989; 65:743–747.

88. Grodum E, Petersen HA: Temporal arteritis with normal erythrocyte sedimentation rate. *J Intern Med* 1990; 227:279–280.

89. Delecoeullerie G, Joly P, Cohen A, et al; Polymyalgia rheumatica and temporal arteritis: A retrospective analysis of prognostic features and different corticosteroid regimens. *Ann Rheum Dis* 1988; 47:733–739.

90. Collado A, Santamaria J, Ribalta T, et al: Giant-cell arteritis presenting with ipsilateral hemiplegia and lateral medullary syndrome. *Eur Neurol* 1989; 29:266–268.

91. Reich KA, Giansiracusa DF, Strongwater SL: Neurologic manifestations of giant cell arteritis. *Am J Med* 1990; 89:67–72.

92. Hayreh SS: Anterior ischaemic optic neuropathy. *Eye* 1990; 4:25–41.

PART SEVEN

DIAGNOSTIC METHODS

CHAPTER 18

The Visual Field

Michael Wall, M.D.

Associate Professor of Neurology, University of Iowa College of Medicine, Iowa City, Iowa

This chapter is a review of selected articles about the visual field. Perimetric studies in neuro-ophthalmologic and related disorders are summarized. Automated perimetry is the sensory visual system probe used for most of these studies and advances in this area are covered.

ISCHEMIC OPTIC NEUROPATHY

Traustason et al. reported a series of 47 eyes of 37 patients with ischemic optic neuropathy studied with automated perimetry.[1] They found a statistically significant altitudinal pattern of loss in 55% of patients; the spared hemifields routinely showed some loss of sensitivity. Most of the remainder (visual field without altitudinal characteristics) had diffuse visual field loss. This diffuse type of loss was more typical of patients with diabetes mellitus. This pattern difference was statistically significant. Twenty-eight examinations were performed of the visual field from 30 degrees to 60 degrees from fixation. The visual field defect characteristics were altered from that of the central 30-degree field in only one patient.

Kline reported six patients with nonarteritic ischemic optic neuropathy with progression over a 6-week period. He suggests this type of progression may not be uncommon.[2]

OPTIC NEURITIS

With threshold automated perimetry, generalized depression of the visual field has been found in resolved optic neuritis (idiopathic or secondary to multiple sclerosis).[3] This is likely from a combination of the classic cecocentral scotoma described with Goldmann perimetry and the arcuate nerve fiber bundle defects reported with tangent screen examination.

With automated static threshold testing, there is statokinetic dissociation in optic neuritis (Wedemeyer et al.).[4] This probably accounts for the increased sensitivity of static compared with kinetic stimuli for detection of visual loss in optic neuritis.

Berninger and Heider found paracentral scotomas with automated perimetry in the uninvolved eye in 9 of 16 cases tested; in all, the localized defects resolved with improvement in the involved eye.[5] Purvin and colleagues have reported a case of varicella optic neuritis with incomplete visual resolution.[6]

ENLARGEMENT OF THE BLIND SPOT

Corbett and colleagues have shown that with papilledema much of the blind spot enlargement is due to the peripapillary retina being regionally hyperopic; using plus lenses they refracted away much of the blind spot enlargement in five of six patients.[7] This contrasts with previous theories that attributed blind spot enlargement in papilledema to mechanical disruption of peripapillary retinal fibers or to the Stiles-Crawford effect.

Fletcher reported seven patients with the syndrome of monocular blind spot enlargement (big blind spot syndrome) without optic disk edema.[8] The scotomas in these cases were absolute, measuring 15 to 20 degrees in diameter with steep margins. They extended to within 5 to 10 degrees of fixation. Positive visual symptoms in the region of the scotoma were common (five of seven cases). Other visual functions including Snellen acuity, color, and pupillary responses were normal except for photostress recovery time that was prolonged. Ophthalmoscopy was characteristically normal. Multifocal electroretinography showed loss of retinal wave forms in the region surrounding the optic disk in two patients. The cause of this disorder is unknown.

Hamed and colleagues[9] and Dodwell et al.[10] reported an association of the big blind spot syndrome with or without disk edema and the multiple evanescent white dot syndrome (MEWDS).

Gass reviews the evidence that the idiopathic big blind spot syndrome as described by Fletcher is likely a part of the multiple evanescent white dot syndrome.[11] He notes that besides marked blind spot enlargement, patients with MEWDS may develop central and paracentral scotomas and photopsia. Faintly visible white spots at the level of the pigment epithelium in the midperipheral fundus are commonly noted; the spots may only last a few weeks. He states that the characteristic cineangiographic picture is of a wreath-like arrangement of tiny hyperfluorescent spots in the peripapillary and midperipheral fundi in the acute phase. He believes the disorder is an acute inflammatory disorder affecting primarily the pigment epithelium and outer retina.

PSEUDOTUMOR CEREBRI (IDIOPATHIC INTRACRANIAL HYPERTENSION)

Fifty patients with idiopathic intracranial hypertension were prospectively evaluated with Goldmann perimetry and automated perimetry performed on the same day.[12] Ninety-six percent of the patients had visual loss determined with Goldmann perimetry using an Armaly-Drance glaucoma strategy; 92% had visual field defects on threshold automated perimetry. In other words, in idiopathic intracranial hypertension, visual field loss was the rule. The most common visual field defects besides blind spot enlargement were glaucoma-like: nasal step defects, nasal depressions, and a generalized depression of the visual field; Bjerrum scotomas and cecocentral defects were less common. In this study, the major risk factor for visual field loss was recent weight gain.

Gittinger and Asdourian point out that not all visual loss of idiopathic intracranial hypertension is from the associated optic neuropathy. They report three patients with mottled macular pigmentation. Choroidal folds and macular stars were also observed. They suggest that the pigmentary changes are the result of macular edema.[13]

Visual loss in idiopathic intracranial hypertension often improves with treatment. A study of the right eyes of 19 patients with a decrease in papilledema grade had automated visual fields of the initial and final examinations compared. There was generalized loss, most pronounced on the nasal side of the field, on the initial examination. This was followed by generalized improvement, least in the central and inferior paracentral areas.[14]

Kashii and coauthors remind us that arteriovenous malformations can cause intracranial hypertension and patients can develop papilledema with resultant blindness if treatment is not instituted.[15]

OPTIC CHIASM

Ambuhl and colleagues studied 40 patients with pituitary tumor with automated perimetry (Octopus program 32).[16] Thirty-four patients had suprasellar extension of the tumor compressing the optic chiasm. Most of these patients showed symmetric visual field damage, most pronounced in the upper temporal quadrant. Following surgery, they noticed most of the recovery was in the central portion of the tested field; in the temporal quadrants, it was less. Three months postoperatively, the greatest recovery was in the lower temporal quadrant, less so in the upper temporal quandrant. The authors conclude that nerve fibers affected last by chiasmal compression show the most recovery and are the first fibers to recover. They did not find further recovery in the 7 patients they tested at 1 year (compared to the 3-month examination).

Purvin and colleageus report a case of a 13-year-old boy with chiasmal neuritis as a complication of Epstein-Barr virus infection. A junctional scotoma was present.[17]

Repka et al. studied the visual outcome after surgical removal of craniopharyngiomas in 30 patients. Twenty percent of eyes had normal visual field examinations at the time of presentation; 48% of eyes had field examinations that were normal in the immediate postoperative period. There was a slight decrease (44% normal) at long-term follow-up.[18]

HOMONYMOUS HEMIANOPIA

Messing and Ganshirt reported on the long-term follow-up of 37 patients with homonymous hemianopia.[19] Recovery was usually maximal by 6 months. They found the increase in visual field area after 3 years to be 6.5% in quadrantanopsia, 15.7% in hemianopia, and 36.7% in cortical blindness. They found the best recovery in occipital pole lesions. Etiology surprisingly did not appear to influence recovery (hemorrhage vs. infarction). Recovery usually took the form of fingerlike extensions in the periphery of the involved quadrants. They attributed this phenomenon to the effect of the cortical magnification factor.

Grossman and colleagues report a case of homonymous sector field defect following ischemic infarction (branch of the calcarine artery) of the occipital cortex.[20] The T2-weighted magnetic resonance imaging study documented a corresponding mid-occipital high-signal-intensity lesion along the calcarine fissure. The lesion did not involve the lateral geniculate nucleus. Previous case reports of horizontal sector hemianopia have shown the mechanism to be posterior lateral choroidal artery infarction causing lesions of the lateral geniculate nucleus; this unusual form of hemianopia has also been reported with lesions of the optic radiations.

Kölmel found that of 230 patients with homonymous visual field defects of central origin, 3 had homonymous paracentral scotomas.[21] All 3 defects were highly congruent. All complained of photophobia and difficulty reading. They note these lesions are usually from trauma, ischemia, or hypoxia.

Soza et al. report a case of bilateral homonymous hemianopia with sparing of the central 10 degrees of vision following subdural hematoma.[22] They attribute the visual field defect to posterior cerebral artery occlusion from uncal herniation.

MIGRAINE

Lewis and colleagues found 35% of 60 patients with migraine had visual field loss with automated static perimetry (Humphrey perimetry, program 30–2).[23] The incidence of visual loss was greater with increasing age and duration of the condition. The most common defect was a generalized depression (abnormal mean deviation). Homonymous defects were present in 3 (5%). The authors did not exclude patients with diabetes mellitus or hypertension. They retested 10 patients; in some, the defects were replicated. Since there is an appreciable learning effect with automated perimetry, this high incidence might not persist if repeat testing was done on all patients.

MISCELLANEOUS DISEASES

Enoch and associates have reported peripheral temporal step defects in patients with Gilles de la Tourette's syndrome.[24] The anatomic basis for this finding is unclear.

Lakhanpal and Selhorst remind us that bilateral altitudinal visual field defects can occur with occipital infarction.[25] They concluded the mechanism of this visual field defect when due to occipital lobe infarction is either from bilateral parieto-occipital watershed infarction from systemic hypotension or bilateral embolization of paired superior branches of the calcarine arteries.

FUNCTIONAL VISUAL LOSS

Smith and Baker assessed automated static perimetry in 15 consecutive patients who had functional visual loss.[26] Their most common finding was a severe peripheral depression (12 of 15 patients). They found tunnel or spiral type isopters with tangent screen evaluation in these patients. Four patients showed sector or hemianopic defects. The patterns of abnormality were not distinguishable from organic loss, and none of the visual field reliability indices were useful for determining functionality. They conclude that automated perimetry is unable to facilitate differentiation of functional from organic visual field loss.

AUTOMATED PERIMETRY

Automated perimetry has emerged as a powerful technique to detect damage to the sensory visual system. This is especially true concerning quantitation of visual field defects. However, besides the observation that patients with neurologic disease may have difficulty in performing a reliable automated visual field examination, some questions remain better answered with manual perimetry. For example, determining the presence of a hemianopia may be best found on the tangent screen or Goldmann perimeter. The use of these manual techniques allows more test points along either side of the vertical midline and multiple rechecking of clinically important test points.

Although manual perimetry excels at determining the presence of a hemianopia, automated perimetry is superior for demonstrating the visual loss of optic neuropathies and quantitating visual loss. However, the occurrence of various artifacts has emerged as an obstacle in the performance of automated perimetry that is overcome only with a highly trained technician and careful selection of patients.

Artifact in Automated Perimetry

Artifact in automated perimetry is a prime example of Murphy's law: if an artifact can occur, it will occur. Therefore, it is best when interpreting a disturbed visual field to ask the question, What artifact could have caused this?, before concluding damage to the sensory visual system has occurred.

Zalta has reported the presence of lens rim artifact in 10% of his cases.[27] He used a Humphrey 30–2 program that tested in the central 30 degrees. Visual loss usually took the form of a combination of absolute and relative defects involving the temporal quadrant either alone or in combination with another quadrant. Risk factors for lens rim artifact were older age, high hyperopic correction, and location-specific involvement attributed by the author to perimeter design.

Heuer and colleagues studied artifacts from improper refraction (refraction scotomas and depressions).[28] The depression of sensitivity was of similar magnitude at all eccentricities within the central 25 degrees and ranged from a 1.4 dB depression with a +1.00 D sphere error to a 7.6 dB depression with a +6.00 D error.

Lindenmuth et al. studied the effects of pupillary constriction (2% pilocarpine) on automated perimetry results. They showed the mean defect increased by an average of .67 dB in visual fields of constricted pupils compared with baseline fields.[29] In a later study, these authors showed the effects of pupillary dilation. Tropicamide 1% instillation produced a worsening of the mean defect by 0.83 dB compared with the baseline field.[30]

Meyer and coworkers studied the effects of blepharoptosis on the superior visual field.[31] They used a series of contact lenses with the superior portion of the lens made opaque to simulate eyelid ptosis. They found a progressive decrease in the superior visual field at the 90-degree vertical meridian that was proportional to the degree of simulated ptosis. Within the range of their study, each 1 mm increase in simulated eyelid ptosis corresponded to about 8 degrees of loss of the superior visual field.

PROBLEMS WITH THE GRAY SCALE

Zalta has shown visual field defects may be hidden by gray scale interpolation.[32] Two hundred ninety visual fields from 67 eyes of 51 patients were analyzed. In 2.4% of visual fields and 10.4% of eyes with well-established early glaucoma, he found a normal gray scale display despite an arcuate scotoma on the pattern deviation display. This report highlighted the utility of the Humphrey Statpac probability plot software.

RELIABILITY INDICES

Before analysis of any automated visual field, one should decide whether the field is reliable. This determination is based on the number of fixation losses, false-positive and false-negative responses, and the short-term fluctuation (intratest variability).

Katz and Sommer evaluated fixation losses, false-positive rates, and false-negative rates with the Humphrey Field Analyzer in patients with glaucoma and in healthy subjects.[33] They found 45% of patients with glaucoma and 30% of healthy subjects were unreliable based on the manufacturer's recommended reliability criteria (fixation losses >20%, false-positive or false-negative responses >33%). Fixation losses alone accounted for 41% of rejections of patients and for 67% of rejections of healthy subjects. Fixation losses can occur either from actual poor fixation effort or from small degrees of head tilt. In patients, the other common reason for rejection was false-negative results alone (44%).[33] The Humphrey perimeter determines false-positive results with a stimulus one log unit (10 dB) brighter than one previously seen. Because of the large magnitude of variability with a decrease in threshold sensitivity, reliable patients may have many false-positive responses. In other words, the slope of the frequency of seeing curve in disease may be shallow, so a stimulus one log unit brighter may actually not be seen by reliable subjects. The strategy of the Octopus perimeter is superior, using its brightest available stimulus to determine false-positive results.

The frequency of abnormalities of the reliability indices may depend on various factors such as patient selection and technique of the perimetrist, as Nelson-Quigg and coauthors have reported much lower rates of rejection than Katz and Sommer. These authors found the following rejection rates exceeding the manufacturer's recommended criteria in healthy subjects and patients with glaucoma to be: false-positive results, <1%; false-negative results, <1%; and fixation losses 19% to 30%.[34]

The last visual field index used as a reliability criteria is the short-term (root mean square, R.M.S.) fluctuation. This standard deviation-like value is an index of the variability of ten retested points. It becomes elevated with disease because of the increase in variability associated with a decrease in sensitivity. In addition,

Haefliger and Flammer have reported an increase in the short-term fluctuation in the region surrounding the physiologic blind spot.[35] Slight shifts in head position (tilt) can increase variability at the edge of a visual field defect.

Keltner and the Optic Neuritis Study Group recommend another approach to the problem of unacceptable rates of abnormal reliability indices—improved quality control.[36] They have shown dramatic improvement in reliability parameters with proper visual field testing technique.

ADVANCES IN STATISTICAL ANALYSIS

An important advance in automated perimetry has been the use of pointwise probability maps (Heijl et al.).[37, 38] Using a large data base of visual fields of healthy subjects, they determined confidence intervals at various probability levels. The test point results of an unknown visual field are compared to the normative data confidence intervals and the probability that the test point is normal is determined. The values are age-corrected and weighted for central location. That is, since variability increases with eccentricity, there is less variability closer to fixation and, therefore, confidence limits are narrower. Abnormal values are then mapped. These perimetric probability maps, therefore, show visual field results in terms of the frequency with which the measured findings are seen in a normal population. The authors emphasize that simple rules of thumb, like a depression of 5 dB, represents an abnormality lack precision. Heijl and Åsman have shown this type of analysis performed well in separating glaucomatous and healthy eyes.[37]

Another important paper by Heijl and colleagues studied the variability of the static perimetric threshold values across the central visual field.[39] The authors randomly selected 210 subjects between the age of 20 and 80 years with government population computers in Malmö, Sweden. Six patients followed in the Malmö General Hospital Eye Department were excluded, and the remaining subjects were invited for a free eye examination; 140 subjects accepted. Of these 140, 17 or 8% of those tested had visual field defects that were reproducible or explicable by ocular status or history. Eight subjects were either unable or unwilling to undergo the automated visual field test. This study represents the best approximation to date of the frequency of visual field defects in the general population using threshold automated perimetry. The study also showed that the variability of the measured threshold values was highly dependent on eccentricity with higher variability with increasing eccentricity. The authors suggest this may arise from the decrease in receptive field density with increasing eccentricity, leading to an increase in the signal-to-noise ratio and increased variability. There was a linear loss of sensitivity with advancing age.

Several studies have evaluated the effect of perimetric experience in healthy subjects[40] and in disease.[41, 42] There are three different patterns of learning. In some subjects, there is little if any learning effect. In others, the learning effect is primarily between the first and second visual fields. In some, there is a gradual learning effect over many visual fields. When present, the effect is about 1 to 2 dB on the mean sensitivity. Learning effects are more prominent peripherally than centrally. This explains the finding of a constricted field in some healthy subjects that improves with experience with the test. The effect may be decreased in patients previously subjected to manual perimetry. Obviously, these findings need to be considered when therapeutic decisions are made following the first visual field. A single automated visual field may be an inadequate basis for comparison.

Heijl and colleagues have also studied test-retest variability of disturbed (glaucomatous) visual fields.[43] Large degrees of intertest variability were found in this study, especially in areas of low sensitivity. In fact, test points with loss of 8 to 18 dB had a 95% prediction interval that included the full measurement spectrum of the perimeter! The authors caution that no conclusions should be drawn from threshold variations at a single test point when only two tests are compared. The intertest variability decreased when comparisons were based on the averages of several tests. This data on point-by-point variation of threshold value on retesting serves as the basis for the pointwise change analysis for the Humphrey software.

The important finding of this study is that the pointwise intertest variability increases with decreasing sensitivity of the test point.[43] This finding has major implications. Since variability increases with decreasing sensitivity, areas of visual loss (the area of greatest clinical importance) have the highest variability and are therefore the most difficult areas to tell whether change is occurring. This finding also suggests the most likely reason variability increases with eccentricity is sensitivity decreases with increasing eccentricity. Also, in this study, the authors elucidate important factors for determining change in glaucomatous visual fields: (1) comparisons should be based on more than two tests; (2) points with normal sensitivity show less random variability than disturbed points; and (3) variation in shallow defects increases with eccentricity.

INTERPRETATION OF AUTOMATED VISUAL FIELDS

Werner et al. compared the results of six experienced clinicians to six statistical models to determine progression of visual loss in glaucomatous fields.[44] The human observers agreed in only 15 of the 30 subjects. Five of the six statistical models agreed on 22 of the 30 subjects. Werner points out that there is no validated technique for detecting progressive visual field loss. He attributes this to the high variability present in abnormal fields, difficulties for human observers in analyzing large amounts of numeric data, and problems with the various types of statistical analyses presently used.

The location-dependent and threshold-sensitivity–dependent variability along with problems inherent in the gray scale make it difficult to decide if a visual field is normal. The probability maps of the Statpac software of the Humphrey Field

Analyzer make this interpretation easier (see previous section). Many clinicians now are primarily using probability maps and only secondarily using the raw numerical data and gray scale printouts.

Until major advances in statistical analysis are available, a combination of factors will remain important for proper clinical interpretation.[45] History, other examination findings, and the presence of abnormal test points in a clinically suspicious area are obviously important. Also, knowledge of the motivation of the patient and the likelihood of the presence of artifacts will remain necessary for deciding whether a visual field defect is present and whether change has occurred.

STATOKINETIC DISSOCIATION

Wedemeyer et al. have studied statokinetic dissociation in healthy subjects and in patients with resolved optic neuritis.[4] They did not find differences in stimulus detection for velocities between 1 and 8 degrees per second for either patients or healthy subjects. Both groups, though, showed a higher sensitivity for moving targets compared to stationary ones (statokinetic dissociation). Normal observers showed a minimal amount of statokinetic dissociation; patients with resolved optic neuritis had a three and a half times larger effect than normal. They hypothesize these results are due to a greater loss of X type than Y type retinal ganglion cell function in optic neuritis.

Yabuki and associates compared the results of kinetic and static perimetry in 162 eyes of 102 cases distributed among optic nerve lesions, chiasmal lesions, and retrochiasmal lesions.[46] Only 2 patients, both with optic nerve disorders, had more of a defect to kinetic perimetry than static perimetry. Twenty percent of eyes had more visual loss with static perimetry than kinetic perimetry. These findings agree with those of Riddoch that the presence of the phenomena suggests there will be some recovery of visual function.

NEW TYPES OF PERIMETRY

Color-Contrast Perimetry

Hart et al. have developed color-contrast perimetry using blue targets on an isoluminant yellow background.[47, 48] The stimuli were designed so that the contrast between target and background was from color, not luminance. Hart has used both kinetic and static color-contrast testing.[47] The kinetic strategy gave similar results to manual kinetic Goldmann perimetry, although the defect borders were less well defined. The static strategy was found to be more sensitive for glaucomatous damage (greater defect extent), but appeared no more sensitive than conventional (luminance increment) perimetry for finding the presence of glaucomatous visual field defects. The authors attribute this in part to the smaller dynamic range of blue/yellow visual field function in later stages of the disease.

High Pass Resolution Perimetry (Ring Perimetry)

Frisén has developed a new type of perimetry using high pass resolution targets.[49-52] These are doughnut-shaped targets that have been spatially high pass filtered. This leaves only the high spatial frequencies and produces a target that has the characteristic that its resolution and detection thresholds come at approximately the same time (vanishing optotypes). This leads to a steep frequency of seeing curve with a resultant easy stimulus discrimination criterion for the subject. This property should promote low variability. The method thresholds visual field test loci by targets changing in size rather than luminance. This is the likely reason that there is uniform variability across the visual field (unlike the increase in variability with increasing eccentricity with conventional automated perimetry). The perimeter is ergonomically designed, and many feedback devices are used. For example, following each legal response, the device presents a black square target to provide immediate visual confirmation of test location. Illegal responses call various messages. A constantly changing fixation mark and a message to "look here" decrease monotony. A message also prompts poor fixators to "look here" at the fixation target.

In a comparison study in patients with psuedotumor cerebri, the sensitivity and specificity of this perimeter were similar to that of the Humphrey perimeter.[53] Wanger and Persson found elevated mean thresholds or significant interocular differences with the ring test in 14 of 21 patients with elevated intraocular pressure. Differential light sensitivity automated perimetry was not abnormal with similar criteria.[54]

Dannheim and coworkers compared the ring test and automated perimetry (G1 program of Octopus perimeter) in 116 eyes of 63 patients with glaucoma, low tension glaucoma, and ocular hypertension. They found excellent correlation between the two tests for mean sensitivity of the entire field ($r = .91$) and each quadrant ($r = .9$).[55] Dannheim and Roggenbuck compared the ring test and automated perimetry (Octopus program 32) in 36 patients with chiasmal lesions. They found a good correlation of loss of quadrant sensitivity when they compared the scores to those in adjacent normal quadrants. They note that the program 32 examination took at least twice as long to administer as the ring test.[56] The ring test has many features of an excellent testing device: high sensitivity and specificity, low variability,[57] feedback procedures, and patient-friendly ergonomics.

Oculokinetic Perimetry

Nagata and Kani have developed a perimetric test in which the patient's response was to look at targets that reach threshold.[58] The next target in the sequence is presented relative to detection of the preceding target. This perimeter might be especially useful for certain groups of neuro-ophthalmologic patients and children.

Noise Field Campimetry

Aulhorn has reported a new perimetric method following the observation of one of her patients who described a scotoma when looking at a television screen filled with static.[59] She has developed a campimeter with a background of small black-and-white random dots flickering at high frequency similar to the "snow" of a television screen after the end of transmission. Interestingly, the blind spot and hemianopic defects are either incompletely seen or not perceived at all. The perimeter does appear to be sensitive for optic neuropathies. After detection of a scotoma, the perimeter can then present traditional static or kinetic perimetric targets in the disturbed area. It is a rapid screening test for patients with optic neuropathies.

Pattern Discrimination Perimetry

In this method, the subject is asked to detect a patch of nonrandom or coherent dots embedded in a background of dynamic random dots. Drum has reported that in patients with ocular hypertension or glaucoma, pattern discrimination results are abnormal in areas of the visual field that are normal with differential light sensitivity automated perimetry.[60]

Automated Pupil Perimetry

Kardon and colleagues have developed objective measurement of the visual field by quantifying the pupillary light reflex.[61] They presented stimuli with a modified Humphrey Field Analyzer and determined visual threshold responses with a computer-based infrared pupillometer. The authors demonstrated visual field defects that corresponded to those of conventional automated perimetry in patients with pre-geniculate lesions.

It is hoped that maturation of these new methods will provide enhanced sensitivity and specificity, reduce variability, and give an ergonomically effective, less time-consuming quantitation of the visual field.

REFERENCES

1. Traustason OI, Feldon SE, Leemaster JE, et al: Anterior ischemic optic neuropathy: Classification of field defects by Octopus automated static perimetry. *Graefes Arch Clin Exp Ophthalmol* 1988; 226:206–212.

2. Kline LB: Progression of visual defects in ischemic optic neuropathy. *Am J Ophthalmol* 1988; 106:199–203.

3. Wall M: Loss of P retinal ganglion cell function in resolved optic neuritis. *Neurology* 1990; 40:649–652.

4. Wedemeyer L, Johnson CA, Keltner JL: Statokinetic dissociation in optic nerve disease, in Heijl A (ed): *Proceedings of the Eighth International Perimetric Society Meeting,* Kugler, 1989, pp 9–14.

5. Berninger TA, Heider W: Electrophysiology and perimetry in acute retrobulbar neuritis. *Doc Ophthalmol* 1989; 71:293–305.

6. Purvin V, Hrisomalos N, Dunn D: Varicella optic neuritis. *Neurology* 1988; 38:501–503.

7. Corbett JJ, Jacobson DM, Mauer RC, et al: Enlargement of the blind spot caused by papilledema. *Am J Ophthalmol* 1988; 105:261–265.

8. Fletcher WA, Imes RK, Goodman D, et al: Acute idiopathic blind spot enlargement. A big blind spot syndrome without optic disc edema. *Arch Ophthalmol* 1988; 106:44–49.

9. Hamed LM, Glaser JS, Gass JD, et al: Protracted enlargement of the blind spot in multiple evanescent white dot syndrome. *Arch Ophthalmol* 1989; 107:194–198.

10. Dodwell DG, Jampol LM, Rosenberg M, et al: Optic nerve involvement associated wtih the multiple evanescent white dot syndrome. *Ophthalmology* 1990; 97:862–868.

11. Gass JDM: Retinal causes of the big blind spot syndrome. *J Clin Neuro-ophthalmol* 1989; 9:144–145.

12. Wall M: Idiopathic intracranial hypertension (pseudotumor cerebri): A prospective study of 50 patients. *Brain* 1991; 114:155–180.

13. Gittinger JW, Asdourian GK: Macular abnormalities in papilledema from pseudotumor cerebri. *Ophthalmology* 1989; 96:192–194.

14. Wall M: Sensory visual testing in idiopathic intracranial hypertension: Measures sensitive to change. *Neurology* 1990; 40:1859–1864.

15. Kashii S, Solomon SK, Moser FG, et al: Progressive visual field defects in patients with intracranial arteriovenous malformations. *Am J Ophthalmol* 1990; 109:556–562.

16. Ambuhl J, Mattle H, Sciler R: Visual fields in patients with pituitary tumors, in Heijl A (ed): *Proceedings of the Eighth International Perimetric Society Meeting,* Kugler, 1989, p 127.

17. Purvin V, Herr GJ, De Myer W: Chiasmal neuritis as a complication of Epstein-Barr virus infection. *Arch Neurol* 1988; 45:458–460.

18. Repka MX, Miller NR, Miller M: Visual outcome after surgical removal of craniopharyngiomas. *Ophthalmology* 1989; 96:195–199.

19. Messing B, Gansirt H: follow-up of visual field defects with vascular damage of the geniculostriate visual pathway. *Neuro-ophthalmology* 1987; 7:231–242.

20. Grossman M, Galetta SL, Nichols CW, et al: Horizontal homonymous sectoral field defect after ischemic infarction of the occipital cortex. *Am J Ophthalmol* 1990; 109:234–236.

21. Kölmel HW: Homonymous paracentral scotomas. *J Neurol* 1987; 235:22–25.

22. Soza M, Tagle P, Kirkham T, et al: Bilateral homonymous hemianopia with sparing of central vision after subdural hematoma. *J Neurol Sci* 1987; 14:153–155.

23. Lewis RA, Vijayan N, Watson C, et al: Visual field loss in migraine. *Ophthalmology* 1989; 96:321–326.

24. Enoch JM, Itzhaki A, Lakshminarayanan V, et al: Visual field defects detected in patients with Gilles de la Tourette syndrome: Preliminary report. *Int Ophthalmol* 1989; 13:331–344.

25. Lakhanpal A, Selhorst JB: Bilateral altitudinal visual fields. *Ann Ophthalmol* 1990; 22:112–117.

26. Smith TJ, Baker RS: Perimetric findings in functional disorders using automated techniques. *Ophthalmology* 1987; 94:1562–1566.

27. Zalta AH: Lens rim artifact in automated threshold perimetry. *Ophthalmology* 1989; 96:1302–1311.

28. Heuer DK, Anderson DR, Feuer WJ, et al: The influence of refraction accuracy on automated perimetric threshold measurements. *Ophthalmology* 1987; 94:1550–1553.

29. Lindenmuth KA, Skuta GL, Rabbani R, et al: Effects of pupillary constriction on automated perimetry in normal eyes. *Ophthalmology* 1989; 96:1298–1301.

30. Lindenmuth KA, Skuta GL, Rabbani R, et al: Effects of pupillary dilation on automated perimetry in normal patients. *Ophthalmology* 1990; 97:367–370.

31. Meyer DR, Linberg JV, Powell SR, et al: Quantitating the superior visual field loss associated with ptosis. *Arch Ophthalmol* 1989; 107:840–843.

32. Zalta AH: Normal gray scale displays in the presence of arcuate scotomas in automated threshold perimetry. *Ann Ophthalmol* 1990; 22:87–91.

33. Katz J, Sommer A: Reliability indexes of automated perimetric tests. *Arch Ophthalmol* 1988; 106:1252–1254.

34. Nelson-Quigg JM, Twelker JD, Johnson CJ: Response properties of normal observers and patients during automated perimetry. *Arch Ophthalmol* 1989; 107:1612–1615.

35. Haefliger IO, Flammer J: Increase of the short-term fluctuation of the differential light threshold around a physiologic scotoma. *Am J Ophthalmol* 1989; 107:417–420.

36. The Optic Neuritis Study Group: Visual Field Reading Center. Optic Neuritis Treatment Trial. *Invest Ophthalmol Vis Sci* 1990; 31:609.

37. Heijl A, Åsman P: A clinical study of perimetric probability maps. *Arch Ophthalmol* 1989; 107:199–203.

38. Heijl A, Lindgren G, Olsson J, et al: Visual field interpretation with empiric probability maps. *Arch Ophthalmol* 1989; 107:204–208.

39. Heijl A, Lindgren G, Olsson J: Normal variability of static perimetric threshold values across the central visual field. *Arch Ophthalmol* 1987; 105:1544–1549.

40. Heijl A, Lindgren G, Olsson J: The effect of perimetric experience in normal subjects. *Arch Ophthalmol* 1989; 107:81–86.

41. Werner EB, Adelson A, Krupin T: Effect of patient experience on the results of automated perimetry in clinically stable glaucoma patients. *Ophthalmology* 1988; 95:764–767.

42. Werner EB, Krupin T, Adelson A, et al: Effect of patient experience on the results of automated perimetry in glaucoma suspect patients. *Ophthalmology* 1990; 97:44–48.

43. Heijl A, Lindgren A, Lindgren G: Test-retest variability in glaucomatous visual fields. *Am J Ophthalmol* 1989; 108:130–135.

44. Werner EB, Adelson A, Krupin T: Effect of patient experience on the results of automated perimetry in clinically stable glaucoma patients. *Ophthalmology* 1988; 95:764–767.

45. Anderson DR: Interpreting automated perimetry. *Am J Ophthalmol* 1989; 108:189–190.

46. Yabuki K, Sakai M, Suzumura H, et al: A comparison of kinetic and static perimetry for lesions in

the visual pathway, in Heijl A (ed): *Proceedings of the Eighth International Perimetric Society Meeting,* Kugler, 1989, pp 15–19.

47. Hart WM Jr: Blue/yellow color-contrast perimetry compared to conventional kinetic perimetry in patients with established glaucomatous visual field defects, in Heijl A (ed): *Proceedings of the Eighth International Perimetric Society Meeting,* Kugler, 1989, pp 23–30.

48. Hart WM Jr, Silverman SE, Trick GL, et al: Glaucomatous visual field damage. Luminance and color-contrast sensitivities. *Invest Ophthalmol Vis Sci* 1990; 31:359–367.

49. Frisén L: High-pass resolution targets in peripheral vision. *Ophthalmology* 1987; 94:1104–1108.

50. Frisén L: A computer graphics visual field screener using high-pass spatial frequency resolution targets and multiple feedback devices. *Doc Ophthalmol Proc Ser* 1987; 42:441–446.

51. Frisén L: Computerized perimetry: Possibilities for individual adaptation and feedback. *Doc Ophthalmol* 1988; 69:3–9.

52. Frisén L: Acuity perimetry: Estimation of neural channels. *Int Ophthalmol* 1988; 12:169–174.

53. Conway MC, Wall M, Allely R: Specificity and sensitivity of perimetry comparing high-pass resolution, Humphrey automated and Goldmann techniques in pseudotumor cerebri patients and normals. *Invest Ophthalmol Vis Sci* 1989; 30:245.

54. Wanger P, Persson HE: Pattern-reversal electroretinograms and high-pass resolution perimetry in suspected or early glaucoma. *Ophthalmology* 1987; 94:1098–1103.

55. Dannheim F, Abramo F, Verlohr D: Comparison of automated conventional and spatial resolution perimetry in glaucoma. Perimetry Update 1988/89, in Heijl A (ed): *Proceedings of the Eighth International Perimetric Society Meeting,* Kugler, 1989, pp 377–382.

56. Dannheim F, Roggenbuck C: Comparison of automated conventional and spatial resolution perimetry in chiasmal lesions. Perimetry Update 1988/89, in Heijl A (ed): *Proceedings of the Eighth International Perimetric Society Meeting, 1989, pp 383–392.*

57. Douglas GR, Drance SM, Mikelberg FS, et al: Variability of the Frisén ring perimeter. Perimetry Update 1988/89, in Heijl A (ed): *Proceedings of the Eighth International Perimetric Society Meeting,* Kugler, 1989, pp 197–198.

58. Nagata S, Kani K: A new perimetry based on eye movement, in Heijl A (ed): *Proceedings of the Eighth International Perimetric Society Meeting,* Kugler, 1989, pp 337–340.

59. Aulhorn E, Kost G: Noise field campimetry. A new perimetric method (snow campimetry), in Heijl A (ed): *Proceedings of the Eighth International Perimetric Society Meeting, 1989, pp 331–336.*

60. Drum B, Breton M, Massof R, et al: Pattern discrimination perimetry. A new concept in visual field testing. *Doc Ophthalmol Proc Ser* 1987; 49:433–440.

61. Kardon R, Haupert C, Thompson HS: Automated pupil perimetry. *Invest Ophthalmol Vis Sci* 1990; 31:504.

CHAPTER 19

The Visual Evoked Potential in Clinical Neuro-Ophthalmology

Wim I. M. Verhagen, M.D., Ph.D.
Department of Neurology and Clinical Neurophysiology, Canisius Wilhelmina Hospital, Nijmegen, The Netherlands

Robert Jan Schimsheimer, M.D., Ph.D.
Erasmus Univerity, Academic Hospital Dijkzigt, Department of Clinical Neurophysiology, Rotterdam, The Netherlands

The visual evoked potential (VEP) is one of the most frequently used diagnostic investigations in clinical neuro-ophthalmology. This chapter presents recent articles that are of clinical importance.

METHODS AND AGE EFFECTS

The effects of reference electrode site, stimulus mode, and check size on pattern electroretinography (PERG) have been thoroughly investigated by Tan et al.[1] They paid special attention to the issue of recording from the occluded eye while stimulating the nonoccluded eye. With transient pattern stimulation, they concluded that this was not the case for the clinically significant P50, irrespective of the placement of the reference electrode. However, for the N95, there was an apparent crosscontamination due to widespread VEP P100 activity (ear reference electrode) or VEP N100 activity (midfrontal reference electrode). An ipsilateral temple reference electrode reduces this problem. Their conclusions were confirmed by the results in a patient who had a marked monoclular delay of a normal amplitude P100.

Shih et al. compared the site of two reference electrodes for the pattern visual evoked potential (PVEP) recording: the vertex vs. the linked mastoid processes. The diagnostic yield from the two montages was similar, although the linked mastoid reference provided a greater number of inadequate recordings due to a smaller P100 and increased contamination by muscle artifact. Nevertheless, there was an abnormal P100 in five patients with the linked mastoid reference, which was missed in the Cz (vertex) reference. Furthermore, the linked mastoid references may also be helpful in clarifying aberrant or ambiguous waveforms.[2]

During the past decade, several authors tried to measure visual acuity with visual evoked potentials. However, their methods did not always offer adequate and reliable clinical application. De Keyser et al. described a more precise stimulus method by decreasing the contrast level to 14% with a large variety of pattern sizes and a frequency of 1 Hz.[3] With this method, the authors were able to determine the visual acuity with VEP rapidly enough (maximally 20 minutes for both eyes) and accurately enough (up to 1/10) to be clinically useful. The accuracy was proven at lower and higher visual levels and was independent of patient cooperation. As long as the subject continues watching the screen, measurement is possible. Flexibility of the applied stimulus enlarges its applicability to children. Forty-two patients with ophthalmologic and neuro-ophthalmologic diseases were successfully investigated. This method appears to be a reliable tool for the objective assessment of visual acuity.

Pryds et al. studied flash evoked cortical potentials in 33 preterm infants with gestational ages of 27 to 33 weeks.[4] In all infants, responses were evoked during the first 12 hours after birth. Flash stimuli were delivered at the beginning of an interburst interval on the electroencephalogram, and recordings were performed with the eyes closed. The VEP latency decreased during the first hours of life with a magnitude of 6 ms per degree Celcius increase in core temperature. There was a significant negative influence of gestational age on VEP latency and amplitude, but there was no association between head circumference and latency. They also investigated the effect of background illumination and flash intensity on the VEP. Reducing flash intensity from 155 cd to 39 cd did not alter the VEP latency or amplitude. Also, a variation of background illumination below 200 lux did not cause VEP changes.

Harding et al. obtained PVEPs in ten premature babies born between 32 to 35 weeks.[5] All the infants underwent recording on at least two separate occasions between 32 and 46 weeks, the initial recording at or before 37 weeks. Pattern reversal stimulation was produced by a small, hand-held television monitor at 20 cm from the eye. The black-and-white checks subtended a visual angle of 2 degrees; the contrast was 78%. The results were compared with conventional flash VEP stimulation. The PVEP showed a major positive component around 280 ms. There was a negative correlation between the latency of this component and the gestational age. The flash VEPs in the same babies often showed an initial negative component, which was not seen in the PVEP. A very striking feature of this study is that the correlation with gestational age for the flash VEP negative component is less than it is for the pattern reversal positive component. Maturation factors such as myelination, synaptogenesis, and organization of the lateral geniculate nucleus might explain this feature.

MULTIPLE SCLEROSIS

The diagnosis of multiple sclerosis (MS) is still based primarily on clinical criteria, but an increasing number of laboratory tests and imaging methods are available to confirm the clinical diagnosis. The PVEP is still a powerful test for detecting white matter lesions. Several studies compared different investigations on sensitivity.

Sola et al. studied 41 patients with MS (possible, probable, and definite). They found that magnetic resonance imaging (MRI) and detection of cerebrospinal fluid (CSF) oligoclonal bands were the most sensitive techniques in demonstrating MS (positive in 88%), while the PVEP and helper suppressor T-cell ratio were altered in 54% and 46% of the patients with probable MS, respectively. The PVEP was abnormal in 67% of the patients with definite MS.[6] Rossini et al. reported a study of 41 patients with MS and found abnormalities on MRI in 78%, CSF immunology in 64%, and PVEP in 70%. Evoked potentials (VEP, somatosensory evoked potential [SSEP], and brainstem auditory evoked potential [BAEP]) were abnormal in 90%, while altered evoked potentials and normal MRI images were found in 22% of cases; defective CSF or MRI findings with normal evoked potentials were found in 7%.[7] Müller et al. found significant correlations between CSF immunoglobulin content, MRI parameters, and the sum of VEP latencies of both eyes in patients with definite but not in probable MS. This is in line with recent evidence indicating a close pathogenetic correlation between CSF immunoglobulins and the severity of demyelination.[8]

Rigolet et al. found no difference in sensitivity between PVEP and MRI testing in patients with MS.[9] Guérit and Argiles studied 65 patients with definite MS and found that the sensitivities of MRI, CSF immunoglobulins, and multimodality evoked potentials did not differ significantly from each other; the highest sensitivity was obtained with SSEPs (84.6%), but the "hit rate" increased 9.2% when PVEP was combined with SSEP.[10] Looking at the patients with definite MS, similar results can be found in other studies.[6, 7, 10–13] Pattern reversal visual evoked potentials proved to be much more sensitive than testing long loop electrocutaneous reflexes.[14]

Differences in sensitivity might be largely explained by criteria used for patient incorporation and sometimes the stimuli used in the tests. Incorporation in studies of patients with possible and/or probable MS includes patients that do not suffer from MS. MRI and PVEP were as frequently abnormal in patients with probable MS who ultimately were shown to have MS.[13] It is clear however that using high and low spatial frequencies in PVEP testing results in a higher detection rate.[10] Finally, PVEP is relatively inexpensive and widely available.

Hyperventilation might cause a significant reduction in P100 latency in MS.[15] This change appeared to be specific for demyelination, for it was not found in other types of pathologic conditions in the anterior visual pathways.[16]

MacFadyen et al. studied the retinal nerve fiber layer, neuroretinal rim area, and PVEP in 57 patients with MS; the yield of optic nerve abnormalities increased from 68% (VEP alone) to 90% in the definite and probable group.[17] This confirms that not only demyelination, but also extensive axonal loss commonly occurs in the optic nerve of patients with MS. The photopic electroretinogram in patients with MS and demyelinating optic neuritis showed a reduced amplitude of the b wave of all affected eyes, probably as a result of damage to the Müller's fibers.[18]

Visual evoked potentials have been used in follow-up studies of patients with MS during therapy. A double-blind, randomized trial of ACTH vs. dexamethasone vs. methylprednisolone did not show significant alterations of CSF or VEP or other evoked potentials.[19] The same was found in a double-blind, placebo-controlled trial with α-interferon and transfer factor.[20] Intrathecal and systemic corticosteroid therapy did not significantly alter PVEP latencies.[21]

ANTERIOR VISUAL PATHWAY LESIONS

It is well known that PVEP examination is an accurate method for the detection of anterior visual pathway compression by pituitary tumors.[22] None of 34 patients with a nonfunctioning chromophobe adenoma, tested by Holder and Bullock, had a completely normal PVEP and flash visual evoked potential (FVEP). Visual dysfunction was the main presenting symptom in 29 of the 34 patients. Thirty patients had binocular abnormalities, and only 4 eyes showed a normal PVEP. Sixteen eyes had an abnormality over the ipsilateral hemisphere, but it was significantly worse over the contralateral hemisphere. Seven eyes showed only contralateral abnormalities. These results are indicative of optic chiasm dysfunction. There was a very good correlation between the presence of a visual field defect and PVEP abnormalities, but a poor correlation with visual acuity.[23]

Mahaptra and Bathia prospectively analyzed 45 patients with post-traumatic unilateral blindness; CT scans were normal in all, and an optic canal fracture was seen in only one patient. Ninety percent of the patients with a positive (normal or disturbed) PVEP at the first test had complete or partial visual recovery. The authors state that repetitive testing is important in predicting the outcome because 20% of the patients with an initial absent PVEP showed visual improvement.[24]

Kaufman et al. reported a prospective long-term study of PERG and PVEP recordings of 63 eyes with four different types of optic neuropathy (optic neuritis, compressive and hereditary optic atrophy, and traumatic atrophy). They found that PVEP latency was usually abnormal in acute or chronic lesions, while PERG was usually normal in acute optic neuropathy. They also stress the importance of the use of different check sizes. The PERG correlated closely with failure of visual recovery.[25]

It is well known for many years that retinal as well as optic nerve disease may cause PVEP delay.[26] Holder studied PERG in 67 patients with a delayed PVEP due to a dysfunction distal to the optic nerve. In all cases, the mean positive P50 component was disturbed, showing especially an amplitude decrease or a diminished interocular P50 amplitude ratio. Only one patient had a marked P50 delay with no associated amplitude changes. No patient had an abnormality confined to the N95 component.[27] As previously mentioned, in optic nerve disease the PERG abnormality is usually confined to the N95 component, probably reflecting retrograde degeneration to the retinal ganglion cells.[26, 28] Therefore, PERG can facilitate the distinction between macular and optic nerve disease, which both cause PVEP abnormalities.

A foveal electroretinogram (ERG) can be obtained from the macular region in response to light modulation, provided that the surrounding retina is light-adapted to minimize the effects of stray light. Bagolini et al. have recently developed a new technique for the foveal ERG recording. Simultaneous foveal and parafoceal electroretinograms were recorded in 26 patients affected by central hereditary chorioretinal diseases (Stargardt's disease, cone dystrophy, vitelliform degeneration, pattern dystrophy) and in 14 age-matched control subjects. The mean foveal ERG amplitude was significantly lower in affected patients than in the control subjects. However, the b-wave implicit time showed no difference compared with that in the control group. The mean value of the amplitude ratio of foveal and parafoceal ERG was significantly reduced as compared with the control mean in Stargardt's disease and cone dystrophy only. In 46 of 52 affected eyes, at least one of the electrophysiologic parameters was abnormal. The authors suggest that simultaneous foveal and parafoveal ERG recording may be a sensitive technique in hereditary degenerations of the central retina.[29]

POLYNEUROPATHY

Chronic Inflammatory Demyelinating Polyradiculopathy

Gigli et al. described delayed P100 latencies in 4 of 6 patients with chronic inflammatory demyelinating polyradiculopathy (CIDP); only 1 patient presented with bilateral optic atrophy.[30] Thomas et al. found prolonged latencies of PVEP on one or both sides in all 6 of their patients; 2 patients had clinical visual disturbances and one other patient had a pale optic disk. MRI images of 5 patients showed periventricular, central white matter, brain stem, and cerebellum lesions that were indistinguishable from those observed in patients with MS.[31] In a study of 18 patients, 9 had a prolonged P100 latency. Of these 9 patients with disturbed PVEPs, 5 had abnormal MRI studies, the other 4 patients had neither clinical nor MRI signs of central nervous system demyelination.[32] Ohtake et al. found a delayed P100 in PVEP testing in 2 of 12 tested patients with CIDP. One patient had nystagmus without visual complaints, the other had optic neuritis. Both patients also had MRI abnormalities suggesting demyelination.[33] It is therefore clear that in CIDP, central nervous system demyelination may also be present and clinically manifest.

Diabetic Polyneuropathy

Collier et al. studied PVEP in 19 patients with diabetes mellitus and a mild peripheral neuropathy; they found a small but insignificant delay while Yaltkaya et al. found a significant latency prolongation in the P100 and N140 components in their study of 25 patients.[34, 35] Comparing the group on mean duration of the disease and ocular findings, one should expect Collier et al. to find more disturbances than Yaltkaya et al. The differences between the studies might therefore be explained by the stimulation method used.

Charcot-Marie-Tooth Disease

Cosi et al. investigated 13 patients with hereditary motor and sensory neuropathy (HMSN) type I and 5 with HMSN type II; all cases showed normal PVEP P100 latencies while P100 amplitudes were reduced in 44% of cases.[36] However, it is impossible to derive which patients the data are from; and the authors state that these patients probably belong to a subset which is a borderline between HMSN and the hereditary ataxias. Three of the 9 patients with HMSN type I described by Triantafyllou et al. showed abnormal PVEPs; in 2, the P100 latency was prolonged bilaterally, while in the third patient the interocular latency difference was abnormal. The visual system showed no clinical abnormalities.[37] These reports confirm earlier studies on cranial nerve involvement, especially in HMSN type I.

MISCELLANEOUS DISORDERS

Parkinson's Disease

It is well known that PERG and PVEP may be abnormal in Parkinson's disease.[38-41] The PVEP 100 and PERG are delayed, and the amplitude of the PVEP decreased. The PVEP abnormalities depend on pattern element size and spatial frequency as well as contrast level, with high frequencies being more involved in the early stage.[40-43] The retinal dopamine content is decreased in patients with Parkinson's disease compared to that in age-matched control subjects.[44] Levodopa treatment diminishes PVEP abnormalities.[45, 46] Gottlob et al. studied the effect of levodopa on PVEP and PERG in control subjects with different luminance levels and check sizes. At lower luminance levels, a significant decrease in PERG and PVEP latencies was found; for PVEPs, the latency changes occurred only at small check sizes (less than 100 minutes of arc). At a low luminance level, the retina might show a reduced dopamine release, resulting in a more pronounced levodopa effect.[47]

Migraine

Drake et al. found no significant differences in PVEP amplitude and latency in 50 patients with common migraine compared to control subjects, although the latencies and amplitudes were slightly higher in the patients with migraine.[48] Nyrrke et al. saw transient asymmetries of the amplitude spectrum of steady-state PVEPs in classic migraine. There was unilateral amplitude attenuation in 55% of their patients during the headache-free interval during serial recordings in at least one record, especially with high frequency stimulation (18 to 22 Hz). Treatment with metoprolol compared to placebo did not significantly affect the asymmetry.[49] In migraine, Diener et al. found larger amplitudes and increased latencies with transient and steady-state checkerboard stimulation. During migraine prophylaxis with metoprolol and propranolol, there was no significant difference in VEP amplitude and latency between responders and nonresponders. Both groups showed a significant amplitude reduction compared to the baseline recording, and the amplitude was restored to the level of the control group. VEP latencies were unchanged. It is still unclear how the drug effect is explained because it can be caused by purely retinal effect, purely cortical effect, or both.[50]

Alzheimer's Disease

Katz et al. studied six patients with Alzheimer's disease.[51] They found that the mean amplitude of the PERG P50 was significantly lower than that in the control group. They found no differences in flash ERG amplitude or latencies in flash ERG and PERG. PVEP was undisturbed, but the FVEP showed clear changes in waveforms in the patients with Alzheimer's disease; the major positive P2 component was prolonged in the flash VEP.[51-55] The PERG findings can be explained by the axon depletion in the optic nerve and degeneration of retinal ganglion cells in patients with Alzheimer's disease.[56] This is also in line with findings in other optic nerve lesions (see elsewhere).

Myotonic Dystrophy

The visual system is frequently involved in myotonic dystrophy (MD). PVEP P100 latency was significantly increased compared to the control group in a study of 60 patients by Ganes and Kerty. The mean ERG a-b amplitude was lower and latencies of a and b waves were prolonged. The VEP was abnormal in 50% of the patients, the ERG in 25%, probably due to the fact that skin electrodes were used instead of corneal electrodes.[57, 58] There was no consistent correlation between abnormal ERGs and VEPs.

Amyotrophic Lateral Sclerosis

In contrast to somatosensory evoked potentials, pattern reversal visual evoked potentials were normal in 27 patients with amyotrophic lateral sclerosis. This is in line with what could be derived from the study of Matheson et al., although they did mention abnormalities.[59, 60]

Friedreich's Ataxia

Abnormal PVEPs were recorded in 58% of the patients with Friedreich's ataxia studied by Kostić et al. Amplitudes were decreased and latencies prolonged, but this was not regular finding. This is in line with earlier studies, but these authors also detected a P100 latency increase in 6 of 18 examined siblings. It might be that these siblings will be affected with time.[61]

Adrenoleukodystrophy

Iinuma et al. found no FVEP or PVEP in an 8-year-old patient. Severe alterations were also found by Mabin et al. and Gastaut et al.[62-64]

Phenylketonuria

A significant prolongation of the P100 during pattern reversal stimulation was seen in adolescents with classical phenylketonuria (PKU). The VEP changes correlated significantly with the quality of treatment during the first 10 years of life but not with the serum phenylalanine level in the second decade or at the time of the investigation.[65] This is in line with a study in eight children by Landi et al.[66] It may be caused by the fact that in adolescence the brain is not longer sensitive to the neurotoxic effects of hyperphenylalanemia. In PKU, anomalous metabolism of neurotransmitters as well as incomplete myelination is described; both can be responsible for the observed PVEP abnormalities.[67, 68]

Hepatic Encephalopathy

Although several studies mentioned changes in the FVEP and PVEP in patients with hepatic encephalopathy, VEPs are not a reliable tool for the diagnosis or grading of the severity of the encephalopathy in the individual patient. Psychometric tests are more sensitive for the follow-up of individual patients.[69, 70]

Wilson's Disease

Satischandra et al. found a prolonged P100 latency of the PVEP in 7 of 13 patients. The site of the dysfunction is unknown, but neuropathologic studies of the optic nerve did not show abnormalities.[71]

Sjögren's Syndrome

PVEPs were abnormal in 3 of 24 patients with primary Sjögren's syndrome; 1 patient had papilledema and 2 others had a polyneuropathy. PVEP latencies were prolonged probably due to demyelination.[72]

Behçet's Syndrome

Rizzo et al. reported a longitudinal study in two patients with Behçet's syndrome. Both had abnormal PVEPs and optic disk atrophy.[73] In Behçet's syndrome, demyelination is a prominent feature.

Human Immunodeficiency Virus Infection

Malessa et al. studied multimodality evoked potentials in 31 men infected with human immunodeficiency virus (HIV) who did not have acquired immunodeficiency syndrome or associated clinical abnormalities. Foveal checkerboard stimulation revealed a prolonged VEP latency in 37%. Men with HIV and a pathologic VEP latency showed a significant reduction of the absolute number of peripheral T-helper cells. Demyelination of the central nervous system due to the HIV infection seems the cause of the delay.[74]

REFERENCES

1. Tan CB, King PJL, Chiappa KH: Pattern ERG: Effects of reference electrode site, stimulus mode and check size. *Electroencephalogr Clin Neurophysiol* 1989; 74:11–18.

2. Shih PY, Aminoff MJ, Gooding DS, Mantle MM: Effect of reference point on visual evoked potentials: Clinical relevance. *Electromyog Clin Neurophysiol* 1988; 71:319–322.

3. Keyser de M, Vissenberg I, Neetens A: Are visual evoked potentials (VEP) useful for determination of visual acuity? A clinical trial. *Neuro Ophthalmol* 1990; 10:153–163.

4. Pryds O, Greisen G, Trojaborg W: Visual evoked potentials in preterm infants during the first hours of life. *Electroencephalogr Clin Neurophysiol* 1988; 71:257–265.

5. Harding GFA, Grose J, Wilton A, et al: The pattern reversal VEP in short gestation infants. *Electroencephalogr Clin Neurophysiol* 1989; 74:76–80.

6. Sola P, Scarpa M, Faglioni P, et al: Diagnostic investigations in MS: Which is the most sensitive? *Acta Neurol Scand* 1989; 80:394–399.

7. Rossini PM, Zarola F, Floris R, et al: Sensory (VEP, BAEP, SEP) and motor-evoked potentials, liquoral and magnetic resonance findings in multiple sclerosis. *Eur Neurol* 1989; 29:41–47.

8. Müller FAJ, Hänny PE, Wichmann W, et al: Cerebrospinal fluid immunoglobulins and multiple sclerosis. Correspondence with magnetic resonance imaging and visually evoked potential changes. *Arch Neurol* 1989; 46:367–371.

9. Rigolet MH, Lubetzki C, Penet C, et al: Lésions rétrochiasmatiques dans la sclérose en plaques mise en évidence par les potentiels évoqués visuels corrélations avec l'imagerie par résonance magnétique. *Rev Neurol (Paris)* 1989; 145:378–383.

10. Guérit JM, Monje Argiles A: The sensitivity of multimodal evoked potentials in multiple sclerosis. A comparison with magnetic resonance imaging and cerebrospinal fluid analysis. *Electroencephalogr Clin Neurophysiol* 1988; 70:230–238.

11. Cutler JR, Amimoff MJ, Brandt-Zawadski M: Evaluation of patients with multiple sclerosis by evoked potentials and magnetic resonance imaging: A comparative study. *Ann Neurol* 1986; 20:645–648.

12. Hänny P, Müller F: VEP als Verlaufsparameter bei multipler Sklerose. *Schweiz Rundschau Med Prax* 1989; 36:956–959.

13. Gilmore RL, Kasarskis EJ, Allen Carr W, et al: Comparative impact of paraclinical studies in establishing the diagnosis of multiple sclerosis. *Electroencephalogr Clin Neurophysiol* 1989; 73:433–442.

14. Friedli WG, Fuhr P: Electrocutaneous reflexes and multimodality evoked potentials in multiple sclerosis. *J Neurol Neurosurg Psychiatry* 1990; 53:391–397.

15. Davies HD, Caroll WM, Mastaglia FL: Effects of hyperventilation on pattern-reversal visual evoked potentials in patients with demyelination. *J Neurol Neurosurg Psychiatry* 1986; 49:1392–1396.

16. Bednarik J, Novotny O: Value of hyperventilation in pattern-reversal visual evoked potentials. *J Neurol Neurosurg Psychiatry* 1989; 52:1107–1109.

17. MacFadyen DJ, Drance SM, Douglas GR, et al: The retinal nerve fiber layer, neuroretinal rim area and visual evoked potentials in MS. *Neurology* 1988; 38:1353–1358.

18. Papakostopoulos D, Fotiou F, Hart JCD, et al: The electroretinogram in multiple sclerosis and demyelinating optic neuritis. *Electroencephalogr Clin Neurophysiol* 1989; 74:1–10.

19. Milanese C, La Mantia L, Salmaggi A, et al: Double-blind randomized trial of ACTH versus dexamethasone versus methylprednisolone in multiple sclerosis bouts. Clinical, cerebrospinal fluid and neurophysiological results. *Eur Neurol* 1989; 29:10–14.

20. Austims Research Group: Interferon-alpha and transfer factor in the treatment of multiple sclerosis: A double-blind, placebo-controlled trial. *J Neurol Neurosurg Psychiatry* 1989; 52:566–574.

21. Heun R, Emser W, Schimrigk K: Evozierte Potenziale unter intrathekaler und systemischer Kortikosteroid-Therapie bei Multipler Sklerose. *Z EEG EMG* 1989; 20:88–91.

22. Halliday AM, Halliday F, Kriss A, et al: The pattern-evoked potentials in compression of the anterior visual pathways. *Brain* 1976; 99:357–374.

23. Holder GE, Bullock PR: Visual evoked potentials in the assesment of patients with non-functioning chromophobe adenomas. *J Neurol Neurosurg Psychiatry* 1989; 52:31–37.

24. Mahaptra AK, Bhatia R: Predictive value of visual evoked potentials in unilateral optic nerve injury. *Surg Neurol* 1989; 31:339–342.

25. Kaufman DI, Lorance RW, Woods M, et al: The pattern electroretinogram: A long-term study in acute optic neuropathy. *Neurology* 1988; 38:1767–1774.

26. Ryan S, Arden GB: Electrophysiological discrimination between retinal and optic nerve disorders. *Doc Ophthalmol* 1988; 68:247–255.

27. Holder GE: Pattern electroretinography in patients with delayed pattern visual evoked potentials due to distal anterior visual pathway dysfunction. *J Neurol Neurosurg Psychiatry* 1989; 52:1364–1368.

28. Holder GE: Significance of abnormal pattern electroretinography in anterior visual pathway dysfunction. *Br J Ophthalmol* 1987; 71:166–171.

29. Bagolini B, Porciatti V, Falsini B, et al: Simultaneous foveal and parafoveal electroretinograms in hereditary degeneration of the central retina. *Doc Ophthalmol* 1989; 71:435–443.

30. Gigli GL, Carlesimo A, Valente M, et al: Evoked potentials suggest cranial nerves and CNS involvement in chronic relapsing polyradiculopathy. *Eur Neurol* 1989; 29:145–149.

31. Thomas PK, Walker RWH, Rudge P, et al: Chronic demyelinating peripheral neuropathy associated with multifocal central nervous system demyelination. *Brain* 1987; 110:53–76.

32. Pakalnis A, Drake ME, Barohn RJ, et al: Evoked potentials in chronic inflammatory demyelinating polyneuropathy. *Arch Neurol* 1988; 45:1014–1016.

33. Ohtake T, Komori T, Hirose K, et al: CNS involvement in Japanese patients with chronic inflammatory demyelinating polyradiculoneuropathy. *Acta Neurol Scand* 1990; 81:108–112.

34. Collier A, Reid W, McInnes A, et al: Somatosensory and visual evoked potentials in insulin-dependent diabetics with mild peripheral neuropathy. *Diabetes Res Clin Pract* 1988; 5:171–175.

35. Yaltkaya K, Balkan S, Baysal AI: Visual evoked potentials in diabetes mellitus. *Acta Neurol Scand* 1988; 77:239–241.

36. Cosi V, Lombardi M, Zandrini C, et al: Somatosensory evoked potentials in Charcot-Marie-Tooth disease. *Neurophysiol Clin* 1989; 19:359–365.

37. Triantafyllou N, Rombos A, Athanasopoulou H, et al: Electrophysiological study (EEG, VEPs, BAEPs) in patients with Charcot-Marie-Tooth (type HMSN I) disease. *Electromyogr Clin Neurophysiol* 1989; 29:259–263.

38. Bodis-Wollner I, Yahr MD: Measurements of visual evoked potentials in Parkinson's disease. *Brain* 1978; 101:661–671.

39. Nightingale S, Mitchell KW, Howe JW: Visual evoked cortical potentials and pattern electroretinograms in Parkinson's disease and control subjects. *J Neurol Neurosurg Psychiatry* 1986; 49:1280–1287.

40. Gottlob I, Schneider E, Heider W, et al: Alteration of visual evoked potentials and electroretinograms in Parkinson's disease. *Electroencephalogr Clin Neurophysiol* 1987; 66:349–357.

41. Calzetti S, Franchi A, Taratufolo G, et al: Simultaneuos VEP and PERG investigations in early Parkinson's disease. *J Neurol Neurosurg Psychiatry* 1990; 53:114–117.

42. Bodis-Wollner I: Visual deficits related to dopamine deficiency in experimental animals and Parkinson's disease. *TINS* 1990; 13:296–302.

43. Tartaglione A, Pizio N, Bino G, et al: VEP changes in Parkinson's disease are stimulus dependent. *J Neurol Neurosurg Psychiatry* 1984; 47:305–307.

44. Harnois C, Di Paolo T, Marcotte G, et al: Retinal dopamine content in parkinsonian patients. *Invest Ophthalmol Vis Sci* 1988; 29:200.

45. Jaffe MJ, Bruno G, Campbell G, et al: Ganzfeld electroretinographic findings in parkinsonism: Untreated patients and the effect of levodopa intravenous infusion. *J Neurol Neurosurg Psychiatry* 1987; 50:847–852.

46. Bodis-Wollner I, Yahr MD, Mylin L, et al: Dopaminergic deficiency and delayed visual evoked potentials in humans. *Ann Neurol* 1982; 11:478–483.

47. Gottlob I, Weghaupt H, Vass C, et al: Effect of levodopa on the human pattern electroretinogram and pattern reversal visual evoked potentials. *Graefe's Arch Clin Exp Ophthalmol* 1989; 227: 421–427.

48. Drake ME, Pakalnis A, Hietter SA, et al: Visual and auditory evoked potentials in migraine. *Electromyogr Clin Neurophysiol* 1990; 30:77–81.

49. Nyrrke T, Kangasniemi P, Lang AH: Transient asymmetries of steady-state visual evoked potentials in classic migraine. *Headache* 1990; 30:133–137.

50. Diener HC, Scholz E, Dichgans J, et al: Central effects of drugs used in migraine prophylaxis evaluated by visual evoked potentials. *Ann Neurol* 1989; 25:125–130.

51. Katz B, Rimmer S, Iragui V, et al: Abnormal pattern electroretinogram in Alzheimer's disease: Evidence for retinal ganglion cell degeneration? *Ann Neurol* 1989; 26:221–225.

52. Visser SL, Stam FC, van Tilburg W, et al: Visual evoked response in senile and presenile dementia. *Electroencephalogr Clin Neurophysiol* 1976; 40:385–392.

53. Harding GFA, Doggett CE, Orwin A, et al: Visual evoked potentials in presenile dementia. *Doc Ophthalmol Proc Ser* 1981; 27:193–202.

54. Wright CE, Harding GFA, Orwin A: Presenile dementia: The use of the flash and pattern VEP in diagnosis. *Electroencephalogr Clin Neurophysiol* 1984; 57:405–415.

55. Wright CE, Drasdo M, Harding GFA: Pathology of the optic nerve and visual association areas. Information given by the flash and pattern visual evoked potentials, and the temporal and spatial contrast sensitivity function. *Brain* 1987; 110:107–120.

56. Hinton DR, Sadun AA, Blanks JC, et al: Optic nerve degeneration in Alzheimer's disease. *N Engl J Med* 1986; 315:485–487.

57. Ganes T, Kerty E: Multimodal evoked potentials, EEG and electroretinography in patients with dystrophia myotonica. *Acta Neurol Scand* 1988; 78:436–442.

58. Pinto F, Amantini A, de Sisciolo G: Electrophysiological studies of the visual system in myotonic dystrophy. *Acta Neurol Scand* 1987; 76:351–358.

59. Ghezzi A, Mazzalovo E, Locatelli C, et al: Multimodality evoked potentials in amyotrophic lateral sclerosis. *Acta Neurol Scand* 1989; 79:353–356.

60. Matheson JK, Harrington HJ, Hallett M: Abnormality of multimodality evoked potentials in amyotrophic lateral sclerosis. *Arch Neurol* 1986; 43:338–340.

61. Kostić VS, Drulović B, Todorović D: Visual evoked potentials in families with Friedreich's ataxia. *Electromyogr Clin Neurophysiol* 1988; 28:89–92.

62. Iinuma K, Haginoya K, Handa I, et al: Computed tomography, magnetic resonance imaging, positron emission tomography and evoked potentials at early stage of adrenoleukodystrophy. *Tohoku J Exp Med* 1989; 59:195–203.

63. Mabin D, Borsotti JP, Bercovici JP, et al: Adrenoleucodystrophie de l'enfant et adrenomyeloneuropathie. Etude de deux familles. *Neurophysiol Clin* 1989; 19:311–325.

64. Gastaut JL, Pellissier JF, Pfister B, et al: Adrénoleucomyeloneuropathie. Un cas familial. *Rev Neurol* 1988; 144:338–346.

65. Korinthenberg R, Ullrich K, Füllenkemper F: Evoked potentials and electroencephalography in adolescents with phenylketonuria. *Neuropediatrics* 1988; 19:175–178.

66. Landi A, Ducati A, Villani R: Pattern-reversal visual evoked potentials in phenylketonuric children. *Child Nerv Syst* 1987; 3:278–281.

67. McKean CM: The effects of high phenylalanine concentrations on serotonin and catecholamine metabolism in the human brain. *Brain Res* 1972; 4:469–476.

68. Shah SN, Peterson A, McKean CM: Lipid composition of human cerebral white matter and myelin in PKU. *J Neurochem* 1972; 19:2369–2376.

69. Sandford NL, Saul RE: Assessment of hepatic encephalopathy with visual evoked potentials compared with conventional methods. *Hepatology* 1988; 8:1094–1098.

70. Johansson U, Andersson T, Persson A, et al: Visual evoked potentials—a tool in the diagnosis of hepatic encephalopathy? *J Hepatol* 1989; 9:227–233.

71. Satischandra P, Sathyanaraya H: Visual and brain auditory evoked responses in Wilson's disease. *Acta Neurol Scand* 1989; 79:108–113.

72. Hietaharju A, Yli-Kerttula U, Häkkinen V, et al: Nervous system manifestations in Sjögren's syndrome. *Acta Neurol Scand* 1990; 81:144–152.

73. Rizzo PA, Valle E, Mollica A, et al: Multimodal evoked potentials in neuro-Behçet: A longitudinal study of two cases. *Acta Neurol Scand* 1989; 79:18–22.

74. Mallessa R, Heuser-Link M, Goos M, et al: Evozierte Potentiale bei neurologisch asymptomatischen Personen in frühen Stadien der HIV-Infektion. *Z EEG EMG* 1989; 20:257–266.

CHAPTER 20

Orbital Computed Tomography

Martin L. Leib, M.D.

Assistant Clinical Professor of Ophthalmology, Columbia University College of Physicians and Surgeons; Director, Orbit and Ophthalmic Plastic Surgery Service, The Edward S. Harkness Eye Institute, Columbia-Presbyterian Medical Center, New York, New York.

Peter Michalos, M.D.

Teaching Fellow, Columbia University College of Physicians and Surgeons; Clinical Fellow, Orbit and Ophthalmic Plastic Surgery, The Edward S. Harkness Eye Institute, Columbia-Presbyterian Medical Center, New York, New York.

Computed tomography (CT) still maintains its position as the near-definitive diagnostic modality in the evaluation of orbital disease.[1] Needless to say, the advent of high-resolution magnetic resonance imaging (MRI) with the increasing sensitivity of surface coils may complement or supplant CT in certain areas of orbital investigation.[2–4]

In reviewing the literature since 1988, one is struck by several observations: (1) the proliferation of sophisticated equipment at most medical centers throughout the world; (2) the extent to which CT has become the mainstay in the general diagnostic studies of orbital disorders; (3) the paucity of review articles on orbital CT as compared with previous years[5]; and (4) The increased use of MRI in the assessment of orbital pathologic conditions.

TECHNIQUE

Several technical advances have occurred over the past 2 years. Though introduced in vitro as early as 1982,[6] high-resolution CT, quantitative digital image analysis, and volume algorithms have facilitated a fairly accurate measurement of the volumes of the orbital contents in vivo.[7-11] Murase et al. have presented a computer-based simulation program to assess the usefulness of various attenuation correction algorithms and data acquisition methods in single photon emission computed tomography (SPECT) in a unified approach. Though in it's infancy, this modality may prove immensely useful in a mathematical dissection of the orbit.[12] In addition, there have been further advances in sagittal imaging[13, 14] and sequential dynamic CT.[18, 19]

Forbes et al.[7-9] devised a method of volume measurement by summing pixels (which have a known area) of a given radiodensity. Algorithms requiring separate computer hardware and software are used to determine the boundaries of isodense regions in the sections. Total orbital volume, fat, muscle, and total soft-tissue volume have been measured with an accuracy of 7% to 8%.[8] The authors have also demonstrated increased volume of the various tissue compartments in clinically apparent and inapparent Graves' disease[9] and increased volume of the bony orbit in a series of patients with enophthalmos.[9] Proptosis caused by excessive fat volume has also been demonstrated in Graves' disease, Cushing's disease, and obesity.[12] These methods advance a mathematical understanding of these structures in vivo. More attention should be paid to the orbital apex to elucidate the critical factors at play in compressive optic neuropathy. One must, however, recognize that there is artifact built into any system when patient movement is a consideration.

A simpler, but less revealing, quantitative approach taken by Mafee et al.[10] was to measure the linear distance between the medial orbital walls. This does have clinical importance in the diagnosis of craniofacial anomalies. A large series of patients with craniofacial clefts was studied with CT and three-dimensional reconstruction supporting some while contradicting other hypotheses and speculations presented by Tessier.[15]

Sagittal imaging with direct methods[13, 14] and multiplanar reformatting techniques[13] have been advocated for viewing the optic nerve, vertical rectus muscles, and orbital floor. Difficulty in positioning the patient, particularly if there is an acute injury, is the main problem with direct sagittal imaging. The quality of reformatted images is good, provided that a high-resolution instrument is used, and thin (1.5-mm), closely spaced sections are obtained. Although multiplanar reformations spare the patient additional ionizing radiation exposure, the best reformation images are inferior to those obtained directly.

ANATOMIC STUDIES

The volumes of the various orbital tissues have been measured by Forbes' group as described.[8] Upper limits for the volumes of the bony orbit, soft tissue exclusive of the globe, fat, and muscle are 30.1 mL, 20 mL, 14.4 mL, and 6.5 mL, respectively. Certain assumptions are made in establishing these values as normal standards. Tiny neurovascular channels are isodense in CT, and thus are averaged into muscle bundles in volume measurements. In addition, because the anterior border of the orbit is open, it is subject to various boundary definitions. The differences between men and women is small, and the left and right orbits are essentially equal in the same person. Racial variation has not been studied, though differences are well known in the anthropology literature. The separation between the medial orbit walls has been measured, the average being 2.67 cm in men and 2.56 in women.[6]

High-resolution, 1.5-mm coronal CT scans of the orbital apex were compared with corresponding anatomic thin sections by Daniels et al.[16] The amount of detail elucidated in this study could not have been possible with an earlier generation scanner. In the anatomic sections and CT scans of cadaver heads and patients, the optic nerve, annulus of Zinn, cranial nerves III to VI, and the ophthalmic vein were identified at the orbital apex by consulting anatomic and CT references. A similar investigation of the lacrimal drainage system has also been reported,[17] but without the gross anatomic correlation. Dacryocystography is superior to CT in elucidating the site of obstruction in classical dacryostenosis, whereas CT can assist in locating fracture fragments most often associated with post-traumatic epiphora. CT is more helpful than MRI in demonstrating bone changes involving the bony nasolacrimal canal.[18] In approaching the surgical management of orbital hypertelorism, CT has been found helpful in elucidating the spatial relationship of the orbits to the midline facial structures.[19]

NONNEOPLASTIC INFLAMMATION

The term pseudotumor formerly referred to this entire group of conditions; now they are generally subdivided according to the specific orbital tissue that is inflamed: orbital myositis, perineuritis, dacryoadenitis, trochleitis, scleritis, and lymphoid hyperplasia. This classification has only been possible because of CT. Recent studies have examined in detail the changes in the extraocular muscles as seen in CT scans[20, 21] and have led to the conclusion that accurate diagnosis requires integration of clinical and tomographic findings. Classically, in orbital myositis, the tendinous insertions of the muscles are involved along with the body of the muscle, as opposed to the fusiform enlargement, or "hamburger" appearance on coronal scans, with normal insertions as seen in Graves' disease. However, the insertion, or even the entire muscle, may appear normal in the CT scan. CT evidence of orbital myositis has been demonstrated in a patient with Lyme disease. CT continues to be very helpful in evaluating orbital myositis and determining whether or not there is tendon involvement.[22]

Sarcoidosis

This idiopathic systemic inflammation commonly affects the conjunctiva and orbital structure and is a common cause of dacryoadenitis. The CT scan cannot depict with certainty sarcoidosis of the lacrimal gland, and biopsy may occasionally be necessary for the diagnosis. Generally, a meticulous systemic investigation, including chest roentgenogram, and determinations of serum lysozyme and angiotensin-converting enzyme levels support the diagnosis. However, CT delineates the extent of the disease, and recent reports have indicated bilateral orbital sarcoidosis may be more common than was thought previously,[23, 24] and bone destruction can occur.[25]

A high level of suspicion for sarcoidosis, benign mixed tumor, and malignant lacrimal gland tumors must always be maintained, even in the context of classic roentgenographic findings.

Graves' Orbitopathy

Computed tomography is appropriate in the management of patients with undiagnosed proptosis, and in those with moderately severe to severe Graves' disease where therapeutic intervention may be indicated, especially when clinical optic neuropathy is present. In the management of Graves' orbitopathy, CT should be used either to elucidate the mechanical forces at play in tailoring therapeutic goals, or to establish the coexistence of a suspected neoplasm. The anatomic pathophysiology of thyroid orbitopathy, that enlargement of the extraocular muscle bellies is responsible for orbital congestion and its sequelae, was delineated previously with CT. More recently, efforts have been made to quantify the change in muscle volume.[9] CT continues to be a valuable tool in the diagnosis and treatment of dysthyroid compression optic neuropathy.[26] Warren et al. have proposed a muscular index that expresses the percentage of orbital width occupied by the extraocular muscles with a coronal CT scan that transects the optic nerve halfway between the posterior aspect of the eyeball and orbital apex. According to these authors, an index of more than 67% in a patient who has symptoms of optic nerve dysfunction is an indication for surgical decompression of the orbit.[26] CT continues to be very valuable in the management of Graves' ophthalmopathy, as far as depicting the extent of disease, choice and timing of treatment, radiation therapy, planning, and posttreatment follow-up.[27] CT continues to be an excellent tool in evaluating the distribution of rectus muscle involvement in Graves' ophthalmopathy,[28] though ultrasonography of the medial rectus width may provide an accurate, simple, and noninvasive means of evaluating orbits.[29]

Orbital Infection

The role of CT in the diagnosis of orbital infections is well established. The location (subperiosteal, extraconal, intraconal) and type (inflammatory edema, cellulitis, abscess) of the infectious process are well delineated with CT. The CT findings and their clinical associations have been restudied and confirmed.[30, 31] It has been suggested that in children with orbital cellulitis, CT should be used as an ancillary guide for surgical exploration of the orbit in patients who do not respond rapidly to medical treatment.[32]

Trauma

In the simple orbital floor blowout fracture, CT scanning plays a small role in clinical decision-making. Usually, the fracture can be demonstrated with plain x-rays,[33] and indeed, CT has been reported to give misleading impressions.[5, 34] Although Gilbard et al.[35] believe that the details of inferior rectus pathologic processes as seen on coronal CT scans (such as the presence of entrapment and the volume of herniated soft tissue) are prognostic indicators, the decision for surgical intervention must still be made on clinical grounds.[5] Although suggested by Forrest et al., CT cannot absolutely facilitate distinction between edema, hematoma, or entrapment of an extraocular muscle.[36] The direct coronal projection is superior to the standard axial view, which frequently misses orbital floor fractures.

CT is far superior to plain x-rays and conventional tomography in the roentgenographic assessment of complex fractures. The involvement of intraorbital soft tissues, the extent of complex fractures, and the precise localization of foreign bodies are in the domain of CT. Comminuted fractures, and details such as rotational displacement of the frontal process of the maxilla[37] are seen only with difficulty with conventional radiography, but are analyzed easily with CT.

The role of CT in trauma to the orbital apex and optic canal is growing. Only with modern, high-resolution instruments can such a compact region, with numerous vital structures coursing through a narrow passageway, be adequately analyzed.[16] Early efforts have now been made to correlate various clinical syndromes with the pathologic anatomy as revealed by CT in orbital apex fractures.[38] CT performed on a patient with progressive pulsatile proptosis after head trauma demonstrated an isolated blowin fracture of the orbital roof, with herniation of the left frontal lobe into the orbit. CT greatly enhanced the surgical planning of the repair.[39] Fractures of the orbital roof are more common in childhood and are frequently overlooked. CT has been able to demonstrate whether the fractures were isolated or associated with more extensive damage of the skull.[40] In one recent study, axial CT scans revealed only 70% of all orbital floor fractures. Thus coronal scans are especially necessary for evaluating the orbital floor and roof. CT is necessary for evaluating the medial wall since conventional radiology only shows 15% of all medial orbital wall fracture.[41] Recently there has been a report of intraorbital wooden foreign bodies not seen with CT but readily demonstrated with MRI.[42]

VASCULAR DISEASE

In large studies investigating orbital anomalies, venous malformations are the most common vascular abnormality encountered. Diffuse or discrete mass change associated with phleboliths affecting both the intraconal and extraconal space are commonly seen.[5]

Jugular compression may reveal an orbital varix that cannot be detected with conventional CT scans,[43, 44] but negative CT scans have been reported even with this manuever. Orbital phlebography, though imperfect, is superior to CT in the detection and elaboration of varices. CT and phlebography were helpful in depicting an orbital varix that arose from the superior ophthalmic vein.[45]

NEOPLASTIC PROCESSES

CT is indispensible in the management of orbital tumors because of the large number of tumor characteristics it reveals. Orbital tumor images can be classified in the following ways: location, size, shape, boundary, characteristics, radiation density, contrast enhancement, dynamic contrast enhancement, attachments to other intraorbital structures, presence of calcification, presence of cystic spaces, effect on bone (none, expansion, erosion), and involvement of adjacent structures (globe, sinuses, cranium). Assessment of all of these factors, when combined with clinical information (age, visual function, proptosis, time course, etc.) frequently allows a relatively secure diagnosis to be made.

However, these features are not present often enough to permit definitive diagnosis based solely on CT scanning, and thus CT does not replace biopsy. When a tissue specimen is necessary, CT plays an essential role in the biopsy of orbital lesions. It is rare to obtain a biopsy specimen of anything but the most superficial orbital tumor without CT guidance. The alternative, fine-needle aspiration biopsy, is only possible because of the availability of high-resolution CT guidance. Needle biopsy has been criticized because some clinicians have found that the biopsy specimen is inadequate for diagnosis. In cases of metastasis in which the primary was not known, CT facilitated guidance of the fine-needle aspiration biopsy, which provided the diagnosis.[46] CT is an excellent modality for evaluation of most orbital and intracranial tumors and strokes. As MRI improves speed and resolution, the trends to use CT may change in the future.[47] CT is not always reliable in depicting extension of paranasal sinus malignant neoplasms into the orbit in patients without ophthalmic symptoms.[48]

BENIGN NEOPLASMS

The most common benign neoplasm of the orbit in adults is the cavernous hemangioma, and its clinical and radiologic features have been reviewed. These tumors are well circumscribed, without attachments to other orbital structures, are enhanced with contrast, and are usually intraconal, although exceptions can occur.[49] Contrast enhancment is less than that of the extraocular muscles,[50] a finding that correlates with the absence of a discrete vascular pedicle observed surgically and pathologically. Few cases in the literature describing the clinical course of incompletely removed cavernous hemangiomas exist. Serial CT recently has shown a long period of slow growth, followed by a shorter interval of arrest, with eventual involution of tumor and relief of proptosis.[48]

In a recent description of two cases of orbital teratomas, CT was found to be virtually diagnostic, showing a variegated orbital mass with solid and cystic components.[51]

MALIGNANT NEOPLASMS

CT characteristics that are indicative of, but far from pathognomonic of, malignancy in orbital tumors are: violation of anatomic boundaries, such as the orbital walls or the sclera; and bone destruction. These same features can be present in other conditions. Bacterial and fungal infections of the sinuses can invade the orbit. Primary orbit inflammation,[52] including sarcoidosis,[25] and benign tumors such as spindle cell lipoma,[53] can cause bone destruction.

In any case, tissue diagnosis of malignancies is essential, since the tumor type determines therapy. Lymphoma[54] and leukemic infiltration[55] respond well to radiation therapy, whereas primary lacrimal gland tumors are best excised. Orbital melanoma may require exenteration and radiation therapy.[56]

CT can facilitate delineation of the retro-orbital extent and optic nerve involvement of histologically proven retinoblastoma.[57] Recently, plasmacytoma of the lateral orbital wall not seen with plain radiographs was seen accurately as an osteolytic bone lesion on CT and its evolution during therapy as followed up with CT.[58]

CT VS. MRI

The inevitable comparisons between CT and MRI have continued. Certain fundamental advantages and disadvantages persist. CT is rapid, readily available, and offers high resolution, but entails the use of ionizing radiation, and multiplanar imaging requires compromises (difficulty of head positioning in direct methods, and loss of resolution in reformatting). MRI, on the other hand, is slower, has limited availability to most patients and has relatively low resolution except in the most up-to-date instruments.[59] However, it offers far greater sensitivity to differences in soft tissues, and multiplanar imaging is straightforward. Significant technologic advances include the use of higher magnetic fields (1.5T), which improves the resolution and sensitivity, and surface coils, which concentrate the imaging power in a defined area of interest. The latter method is exceptionally useful in the orbit because of the small volume involved.[60]

Specific drawbacks of MRI are its inability to image bone and calcifications, the latter being an important clue in tumor diagnoses.[60, 61] In addition, orbital hemorrhage can be missed with MRI.[60]

SUMMARY

CT is a highly sophisticated diagnostic instrument of great speed, resolution, and flexibility. The introduction of MRI with surface coils in the examination of orbital disease will help to redefine the indications for and limitations of CT. MRI is likely to complement rather than supplant CT and will serve as an impetus to even higher refinement of resolution.

REFERENCES

1. Leib ML, Trokel SL: Orbital computer-assisted tomography, in Lessell S, van Dalen JTW (eds): *Neuro-Ophthalmology*, vol 3. Amsterdam, Elsevier, 1984, pp 389–398.
2. Sullivan JA, Harms SE: Surface-coil MR imaging of orbital neoplasms. *Am J Neuroradiol* 1986; 7:29–34.
3. Schenck JF, Hart JR Jr., Foster TH, et al: Improved imaging of the orbit at 1.5 T with surface coils. *Am J Radiol* 1985; 144:1033–1036.
4. Edwards JH, Hyman RA, Vacirca SJ, et al: 0.6 T magnetic resonance imaging of the orbit. *Am J Radiol* 1985; 144:1015–1025.
5. Leib ML: Computerized tomography of the orbits, in Haik B (ed): *Advanced Imaging Techniques in Ophthalmology*, vol 26. *In Ophthalmol Clin* Boston, Little Brown & Co, 1986, pp 113–118.
6. Leib ML, Cooper WC, Wai PM, et al: Volume determination of the orbit with high resolution CT scans and quantitative digital image analysis. *Orbit* 1982; 1:150.
7. Forbes G, Gehring DG, Gorman CA, et al: Volume of normal orbital structures by computerized tomographic analysis. *Am J Neuroradiol* 1985; 6:419–424.
8. Forbes G, Gehring DG, Gorman CA, et al: Volume measurements of normal orbital structures by computed tomographic analysis. *Am J Radiol* 1984; 145:149–159.

9. Bite U, Jackson IT, Forbes GS, et al: Orbital volume measurements using three-dimensional CT imaging. *Plast Reconstr Surg* 1985; 75:502–508.

10. Mafee MF, Pruzansky S, Corrales MM, et al: CT in the evaluation of the orbit and the bony interorbital distance. *Am J Neuroradiol* 1986; 7:265–269.

11. Hemmy DC, Tessier PL: CT of dry skulls with craniofacial deformities: Accuracy of three-dimensional reconstruction. *Radiology* 1985; 157:113–116.

12. Murase K, Tanada S, Higashimo H, et al: A unified computer program for assessment of attenuation correction and data acquisition methods in single photon emission computed tomography (SPECT). *Eur J Nucl Med* 1989; 15:248–253.

13. Gaetani P, Silvani V, Butti G, et al: Usefulness of sagittal computer tomography in neurosurgery. *J Neurosurg Sci* 1984; 28:67–73.

14. Zooneveld FW, Koorneef L: Patient positioning for direct sagittal CT of the orbit parallel to the optic nerve. *Radiology* 1986; 158:547–549.

15. David DJ, Moore MH, Cooter RD: Tessier clefts revisited with a third dimension. *Cleft Palate J* 1989; 26:163–184.

16. Daniels DL, Pech P, Kay MC, et al: Orbital apex: Correlative anatomic and CT study. *Am J Radiol* 1985; 145:1141–1146.

17. Russell EJ, Czervionke J, Huckman M, et al: CT of the inferomedial orbit and the lacrimal drainage apparatus: Normal and pathologic anatomy. *Am J Radiol* 1985; 145:1147–1154.

18. Menestrina LE, Osborn RE: Congenital dacryocystocele with intranasal extension: Correlation of CT and MRI imaging. *J Am Osteopath Assoc* 1990; 3:264–268.

19. Hoffman WY, McCarthy JG, Cutting CB, et al: Computerized tomographic analysis of orbital hypertelorism repair, spatial relationship of the globe and the bony orbit. *Ann Plast Surg* 1990; 2:124–131.

20. Dresner SC, Rothfus WE, Slamovits TL, et al: Computed tomography of orbital myositis. *Am J Radiol* 1984; 143:671–674.

21. Rothfus, WE, Curtin, HD: Extraocular muscle enlargement: A CT review. *Radiology* 1984; 151:677–681.

22. Seidenberg KB, Leib ML: Orbital myositis with lyme disease. *Am J Ophthalmol* 1990; 109:13–16.

23. Sacher M, Lanzieri CF, Sobel LL, et al: Computer tomography of bilateral lacrimal gland sarcoidosis. *J Comput Assist Tomogr* 1984; 8:213–215.

24. Signorini E, Cianciulli E, Ciorba E, et al: Rare multiple orbital localizations of sarcoidosis: A case report. *Neuroradiology* 1984; 26:145–147.

25. Wolk RB: Sarcoidosis of the orbit with bone destruction. *AJNR* 1984; 5:204–205.

26. Warren JD, Spector JG, Burde R: Long-term follow-up and recent observations on 305 cases of orbital decompression for dysthyroid obitopathy. *Laryngoscope* 1989; 1:35–40.

27. Shah KJ, Dasher BJ, Brooks B: CT of Graves ophthalmopathy. Bigghos's management and post-therapeutic evaluation. *Clin Imaging* 1989; 1:58–61.

28. Wiersinga WM, Smith T, Van der Gaas R, et al: Clinical presentation of Graves ophthalmopathy. *Ophthalmic Res* 1989; 21:73–82.

29. Given-Wilson R, Pope RM, Michell MJ, et al: The use of real-time orbital ultrasound in Graves' ophthalmopathy: A comparison with computed tomography. *Br J Radiol* 1989; 62:705–709.

30. Bergin DJ, Wright JE: Orbital cellulitis. *Ophthalmology* 1986; 70:174–178.

31. Towbin R, Han BK, Kaufman RA, et al: Postseptal cellulitis: CT in diagnosis and management. *Radiology* 1986; 158:735–737.

32. Noel LP, Clarke WW, MacDonald N: Clinical management of orbital cellulitis in children. *Can J Ophthalmol* 1990; 1:11–16.

33. Kenne J, Doris PE: A simple radiographic diagnosis of occult blow-out fractures. *Emerg Med* 1985; 14:335–338.

34. McArdle CB, Amparo EG, Mirfakhraee M: MR imaging of orbital blow-out fractures. *J Comput Assist Tomogr* 1986; 10:116–119.

35. Gilbard SM, Mafee MF, Lagouros PA, et al: Orbital blowout fractures: The prognostic significance of computed tomography. *Ophthalmology* 1985; 92:1523–1528.

36. Forrest AL, Schuller DE, Strauss RH: Management of orbital blow-out fracture. *Am J Sports Med* 1989; 17:217–220.

37. Johnson DH Jr, Colman M, Larsson S, et al: Computed tomography in medial maxilla-orbital fractures. *J Comput Assist Tomogr* 1984; 8:416–419.

38. Unger JM: Orbital apex fractures: The contribution of computed tomography. *Radiology* 1984; 150:713–717.

39. Antworth MV, Bech RW: Traumatic orbital encephalocele. *Can J Ophthalmol* 1989; 24:129–131.

40. Greenwald MJ, Boston D, Pensler JM, et al: Orbital roof fractures in childhood. *Ophthalmology* 1989; 96:491–496.

41. Langen HJ, Dans HJ, Boharfk, et al: *ROFO* 1989; 150:582–587.

42. Green BF, Kraft SP, Carter KD, et al: Intraorbital wood detection by magnetic resonance imaging. *Ophthalmology* 1990; 97:608–611.

43. Wu EH, Bai RJ, Zhang YT, et al: CT with pressure on neck veins in the diagnosis of primary orbital varices. *Chin Med J* 1985; 98:287–288.

44. Shields JA, Dolinskas C, Augsburger JJ, et al: Demonstration of orbital varix with computed tomography and valsalva maneuver. *Am J Ophthalmol* 1984; 97:108–110.

45. Kubota T, Kuroda E, Jujii T, Kawano H, et al: Orbital varix with phlebolith (case report). *J Neurosurg* 1990; 73:291–295.

46. Capone A Jr, Slamovitz TL: Discrete metastasis of solid tumors to extraocular muscles (review). *Arch Ophthalmol* 1990; 108:237–243.

47. Slamovitz TL, Gardner TA: Neuroimaging in neuro-ophthalmology. *Ophthalmology* 1989; 96:555–568.

48. Graamans K, Slootweg PJ: Orbital exenteration in surgery of malignant neoplasms of the paranasal sinus. The value of preoperative CT. *Arch Otolaryngol Head Neck Surg* 1989; 115:977–978.

49. Costa E, Silva I, Symon L: Cavernous hemangioma of the optic canal: Report of two cases. *J Neurosurg* 1984; 60:838–841.

50. Sklar EL, Quencer RM, Byrne SF, et al: Correlative study of the computed tomographic, ultrasonographic, and pathological characteristics of cavernous versus capillary hemangiomas of the orbit. *J Clin Neuro Ophthalmol* 1986; 6:14–21.

51. Weiss AH, Greenwald MJ, Margo CE, et al: Primary and secondary orbital teratomas. *J Pediatric Ophthalmol Strabismus* 1989; 26:44–49.

52. Frohman LP, Kupersmith MJ, Lang J, et al: Intracranial extension and bone destruction in orbital pseudotumor. *Arch Ophthalmol* 1986; 104:380–384.

53. Bartley GB, Yeats RP, Garrity JA, et al: Spindle cell lipoma of the orbit. *Am J Ophthalmol* 1985; 100:605–609.

54. Font RL, Shields J: Large cell lymphoma of the orbit with microvillous projections ('porcupine lymphoma'). *Arch Ophthalmol* 1985; 103:1715–1719.

55. Skinnider LF, Romanchuk KG: Orbital involvement in chronic lymphocytic leukemia. *Can J Ophthalmol* 1984; 19:142–144.

56. Shields JA, Augsburger JJ, Dougherty MJ: Orbital recurrence of choroidal melanoma 20 years after enucleation. *Am J Ophthalmol* 1984; 97:767–770.

57. John-Mikolajewski V, Messmer E, Sauerwein W, et al: Orbital computed tomography. Does it

help in diagnosing the infiltration of choroid, sclera and/or optic nerve in retinoblastoma. *Ophthalmic Paediatr Genet* 1987; 8:101–104.

58. Morlion J, Vanneste F, Lemachieu SF, et al: Two cases of bulky plasmacytoma of the lateral orbital wall. *J Belge Radiol* 1990; 73:211–213.

59. Sobel DR, Kelly W, Kjos BO, et al: MR imaging of orbital and ocular disease. *Am J Neuroradiol* 1985; 6:259–264.

60. Bilaniuk JT, Schenck JF, Zimmerman RA, et al: Ocular and orbital lesions: Surface coil MR imaging. *Radiology* 1985; 156:669–674.

61. Edwards JH, Hyman RA, Bacirca SJ, et al: 0.6 T MRI of the orbits. *Am J Neuroradiol* 1985; 6:253–258.

CHAPTER 21

MRI of the Visual System

Raymond F. Carmody, M.D.
Associate Professor of Radiology, University of Arizona College of Medicine, University of Arizona Health Sciences Center; Attending Neuroradiologist, University Medical Center, Tucson, Arizona

Mark T. Yoshino, M.D.
Assistant Clinical Professor of Radiology, Section of Neuroradiology, University of Arizona College of Medicine, University of Arizona Health Sciences Center, Tucson, Arizona

J.T.W. van Dalen, M.D., Ph.D.
Associate Professor, Department of Ophthalmology, University of Arizona College of Medicine, University of Arizona Health Sciences Center, Tucson, Arizona

While only minor improvements in high-resolution computed tomography (CT) scanning have been made in recent years, magnetic resonance imaging (MRI) has undergone rapid advances, both in instrumentation and software design. High-field-strength (1.5 T) superconductive units are still the most versatile systems; however, newer, less expensive intermediate-field-strength units with permanent magnets are now available. These units not only produce excellent images, but also make MRI affordable at smaller hospitals. Additionally, even smaller (0.05 T) units designed for emergency room or intensive care unit use are now under investigation. Location costs and maintenance on these units are significantly reduced. Innovations in surface coil design have also improved image quality. New pulse sequences such as short inversion time inversion recovery (STIR) and chop-

Reprinted from *Current Neuro-ophthalmology*®, vol. 3.
Copyright 1991, Mosby–Year Book, Inc.

per have increased the utility of MRI. Moreover, as our clinical experience with MRI grows, its strengths and weaknesses become more clearly defined. This chapter is a discussion of the recent MRI literature as it pertains to the visual apparatus. The role of CT vis à vis MRI is also covered, where relevant.

OPTIC NERVE

Optic Neuritis

STIR pulse sequences have been developed and shown to be effective in imaging optic neuritis.[1, 2] These new magnetic resonsance (MR) pulse sequences are important because in contrast to CT, in which orbital fat facilitates visualization of the optic nerves because of its low density, on older MRI sequences this same fat is so bright that it obscures detail on T1-weighted images. STIR pulse sequences overcome this problem by suppressing the MR signal from fat, thus making the optic nerve more visible. The drawbacks of STIR imaging are that pictures take roughly twice as long to acquire and have a lower signal-to-noise ratio. These factors make STIR images appear more grainy and less visually pleasing; nonetheless, they are better for detecting optic neuritis because they increase lesion conspicuity.[3] However, it should be noted that for other orbital applications, some investigators think that standard spin-echo sequences are preferable to STIR.[4] Thus pulse sequence selection must be based on the clinical indications for the examination.

Other MR pulse sequences have recently been designed to enhance optic nerve visualization by suppressing signal from orbital fat. The chopper sequence, which is a modification of an older fat suppression technique known as the Dixon method,[5] shows promise for orbital imaging.[6] This technique can be used for a wide range of repetition times (TR) and echo times (TE) does not significantly lengthen imaging time, and eliminates much of the chemical shift artifact inherent in standard spin-echo sequences. Disadvantages of the chopper sequence are its increased sensitivity to patient motion and its lower signal-to-noise ratio. Another technique, chemical shift selective imaging, has been applied to the optic nerve for optic neuritis with limited success.[7]

The ability of MRI to demonstrate the location and extent of optic neuritis may have prognostic significance, since it has been shown that involvement of the intracanalicular portion of the optic nerve has a worse prognosis.[2] Others have speculated that this might predict which patients could benefit from steroid treatment.[8] A major advantage of using MRI in the diagnosis of optic neuritis is that intracranial lesions of multiple sclerosis can be demonstrated at the same time (Fig 1).

Guy and his colleagues used gadolinium-diethylenetriamine pentaacetic acid (Gd-DTPA)–enhanced MRI to investigate optic neuritis and found enhancement of the optic nerve in 7 of 13 patients with acute optic neuritis.[9] Involvement of the intracranial portion of the optic nerve was readily seen, but orbital fat interfered

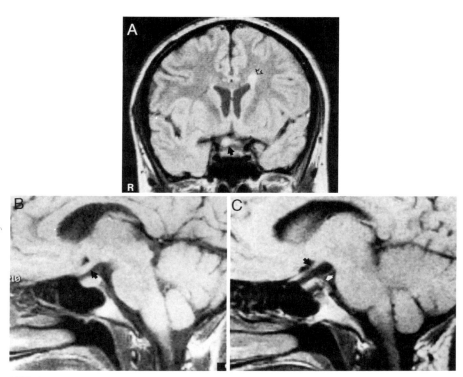

FIG 1.
Multiple sclerosis with optic nerve involvement. Thirty-six-year-old woman with 1-month history of fatigue, clumsiness, and decreased vision OD. **A,** intermediate weighted coronal image shows enlargement and increased signal intensity in right side of optic chiasm *(solid arrow).* An MS plaque is also visible in left periventricular white matter *(open arrow).* **B,** T1-weighted sagittal image through right optic tract shows enlargement of tract *(arrow).* Normal left optic tract is shown in **C** *(black arrow).* Left third nerve is also visible *(white arrow).*

with the visualization of the intraorbital segment. Two patients with radiation-induced optic neuropathy also showed gadolinium enhancement of the intracranial optic nerves. Experimentally induced optic neuritis in guinea pigs has also been successfully demonstrated with Gd-DTPA.[10] The enhancement pattern of the optic nerves and chiasm was thought to be the result of early blood-optic nerve-barrier breakdown as a manifestation of demyelination.

Optic Nerve Tumors

CT and MRI are complementary procedures for demonstrating tumors of the optic nerve or sheath. CT is preferable for suspected nerve sheath meningiomas, since the calcifications often present in these tumors are unlikely to be seen with MRI. However, MRI is superior in demonstrating intracranial extension of orbital meningiomas.[11, 12] The use of Gd-DTPA enhancement has increased the diagnostic accuracy of MRI for intracanalicular meningiomas.[13, 14] Moreover, Hendrix et al.[15] found that a combination of Gd-DTPA enhancement and fat suppression improves MRI of optic nerve lesions and may be helpful in differentiating nerve sheath meningiomas from optic nerve gliomas.

Intraorbital optic nerve gliomas can be readily demonstrated by either CT or MRI. However, MRI may show chiasmal involvement not visible with CT, as was discussed in a nice review article by Zimmerman et al.[16] MRI has the added advantage of depicting images in all three planes. The clinical course of optic nerve gliomas in 31 children was recently studied by Wright and colleagues.[17] They found that in about half of these patients, the tumors were stable over many years, and the other half had progressive enlargement of the tumor. Patients with neurofibromatosis were more likely to have stable tumors. Hemorrhage into an intraorbital optic nerve glioma has been shown with MRI.[18] The importance of obtaining neuroimaging studies early in children with unexplained visual loss has been illustrated in a review of 18 cases of optic nerve glioma by Appleton and Jan.[19] Many of their cases had incorrect initial diagnoses and inordinately long delays in detecting the gliomas.

Other

Other lesions affecting the optic nerve include orbital lymphoma and pseudotumor, both of which may closely resemble perioptic meningioma. On MRI images, pseudotumor tends to be dark on T2-weighted images, whereas lymphoma or metastatic disease have bright T2 signal.[20] MRI was also used to investigate 13 cases of Leber's hereditary optic neuropathy.[21] Eight cases had STIR images of the optic nerves, all of which were abnormal. Unlike optic neuritis, however, no brain lesions were found in the patients with Leber's hereditary optic neuropathy.

Brain stem anesthesia with respiratory depression can occur as a rare complication of retrobulbar anesthetic injection if the anesthetic agent is inadvertently injected into the subarachnoid space surrounding the optic nerve. To determine the position of the optic nerve in the posterior orbit, Smiddy and his associates performed orbital MRI in various positions of gaze.[22] With the eye rotated superonasally, the retrobulbar optic nerve was taut and laterally displaced. In the primary position, the nerve was medially positioned and slack. They concluded that the injection should be given in the inferotemporal quadrant with the eye in the primary position.

OPTIC CHIASM AND JUXTASELLAR REGION

The ability of MRI to directly image in all three orthogonal planes has made it the procedure of choice for evaluating the optic chiasm. Not only are intrinsic optic chiasm lesions such as gliomas better shown, but the relationship of the optic chiasm to adjacent lesions can be visualized better.

Chiasmal Lesions

The association of neurofibromatosis (NF) with optic nerve and optic chiasm gliomas is well known. In a review of 53 patients with NF who had MR images, Boganno et al. found 8 optic chiasm and 2 optic nerve gliomas.[23] Brown and his colleagues studied the MR images of 21 patients with NF and found 13 optic pathway gliomas.[24] Pomerantz et al. studied 6 patients with NF to determine which pulse sequences best delineated the prechiasmatic, chiasmatic, and retrochiasmatic visual system at 0.35 T.[25] They found that the orbital and intracanalicular optic nerves were seen best on axial and coronal T1 sequences (TR, 300 ms; TE, 35 ms), the optic chiasm with intermediate T2-weighted coronal images (TR, 1,500 ms; TE, 35 ms), and the retrochiasmal pathway with T2-weighted images (TR, 1,500 ms; TE, 70 ms). All of these investigators concluded that while CT could adequately define optic nerve and optic chiasm lesions, MRI was far superior in depicting optic tract and optic radiation involvement.

The National Institutes of Health has recently recognized neurofibromatosis as two distinct entities: NF1 (von Recklinghausen's disease), and NF2 (bilateral acoustic neurofibromatosis).[26] NF1 is related to chromosome 17 and NF2 to chromosome 22. Aoki and collaborators studied 53 patients with NF1 and 11 patients with NF2 by MRI. In the NF1 group, 19 patients had optic gliomas and eight had parenchymal gliomas.[27] Many of their patients also had hamartomatous malformations of the basal ganglia, thalamus, midbrain, or cerebellar peduncles (Fig 2). In the NF2 group, all 11 had acoustic schwannomas, six had meningiomas, and eight had other cranial nerve tumors. No optic gliomas or hamartomas were found in the NF2 group. Listernick et al. found a 15% incidence of optic gliomas in children with NF1 who had routine CT scanning.[28] The hamartomatous malformations and areas of heterotopia that MRI quite often demonstrates in the basal ganglia and brain stem are not visible on CT scans.[29, 30]

Besides defining the presence and extent of optic chiasm gliomas, MRI has provided additional information about the optic chiasm. For example, intrachiasmal hemorrhage resulting from head trauma has been described,[31] as has acute chiasmal syndrome resulting from hemorrhage into a suprasellar cavernous angioma.[32] Because cavernous angiomas are usually multiple and often familial, routine screening of family members has been suggested, a task best performed with MRI.

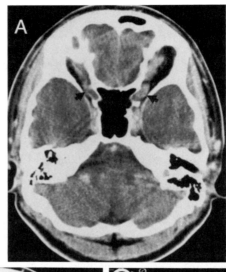

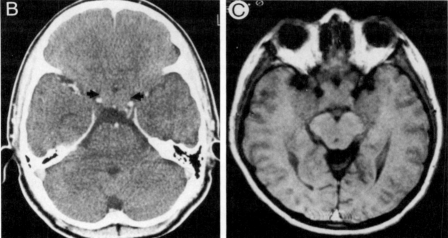

FIG 2.
Type I neurofibromatosis. Twelve-year-old girl with bilateral visual loss (20/200 O.U.) **A, B,** contrast-enhanced CT scans show enlargement of both optic nerves and chiasm *(arrows)* due to glioma. **C,** T1-weighted axial MRI confirms optic nerve, optic chiasm, and tract involvement. *(Continued.)*

The relationship of primary or secondary empty sellae to visual disturbances has long been a controversial subject. Primary empty sella is due to a congenital deficiency in the diaphragma sellae, whereas secondary empty sella is the result of prior surgery, pituitary infarction, infection, radiation, or some other cause. Kaufman and coworkers used MRI to study herniation of the suprasellar visual

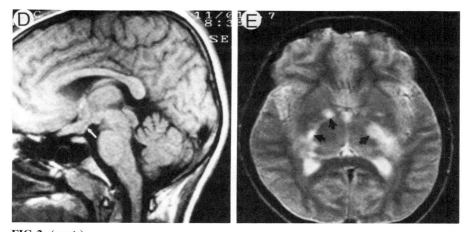

FIG 2. (cont.).
D, T1-weighted sagittal section shows marked tumor enlargement of optic tract *(arrow).* **E,** T2-weighted axial image shows increased signal intensity in basal ganglia, presumably due to hamartomas *(arrows).*

system (SVS) (optic nerve, optic chiasm, optic tract) into empty sellae . A total of 24 cases of enlarged primary empty sellae and eight cases of secondary empty sellae with SVS herniation were investigated.[33] Results were correlated with visual symptoms. Three patients with SVS herniation into primary empty sellae were found; two had visual disturbances. Roughly half of the patients with secondary empty sella had visual disturbances, mainly field abnormalities. However, no correlation between the degree of herniation and severity of symptoms in either group was found. Also, visual disturbances proved to be an unreliable indicator of herniation.

Pituitary Tumors

MRI is now accepted as the procedure of choice for imaging sellar and juxtasellar masses, and for this indication its advantages are well known and extensively documented. The multiplanar capabilities of MRI are extremely useful to the treating neurosurgeon or radiation therapist since the precise location, size, and relationship of the tumor to adjacent structures can be ascertained (Figs 3, 4). Alternatively, when these lesions are treated medically, subtle changes in tumor size are more easily detected. Furthermore, MRI is more sensitive for diagnosing hemorrhage into pituitary adenomas. Ostrov et al.[34] investigated 12 patients with MRI evidence of hemorrhage into pituitary adenoma. Clinically only 3 of these patients had apoplexy, while 7 had visual symptoms. CT was sensitive for demonstrating acute intratumoral hemorrhage, especially in the first 2 or 3 days, but MRI was

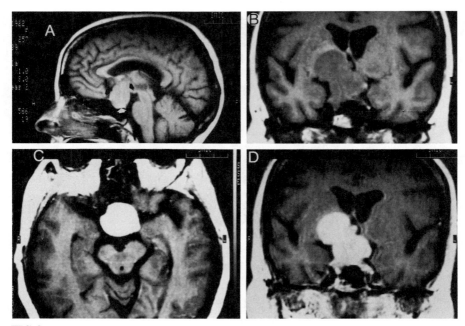

FIG 3.
Large pituitary adenoma. Sixty-six-year-old woman who presented with Foster-Kennedy syndrome (optic disk atrophy OD, optic disc edema OS), decreased vision OD, and bitemporal hemianopia. **A,** T1-weighted sagittal and **B** coronal nonenhanced images show a large sellar-suprasellar mass extending into third ventricle (*arrows,* **A**). **C,** axial and **D** coronal T1-weighted images after Gd-DTPA enhancement. Tumor is so large that optic chiasm and optic tracts are obscured.

more sensitive and specific for subacute or chronic hemorrhage. Seven of their 12 patients had visual symptoms.

The Cavernous Sinus

Since recent advances in neurosurgical techniques have made some cavernous sinus masses resectable, often with sparing of the internal carotid artery and preservation of cranial nerve function, accurate and detailed demonstration of the anatomy and pathology of this area is now of paramount importance. The need to reliably distinguish aneurysm from tumor and to delineate the relationship of mass to adjacent normal structures is obvious (Fig 5).

Daniels and coworkers investigated the MRI appearance of the cavernous sinus,[35] with special emphasis on the cavernous sinus-pituitary gland interface. They used T1-weighted spin-echo coronal images without and with Gd-DTPA, and gradient-re-

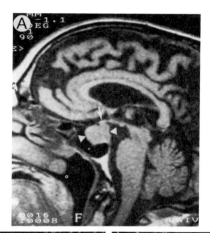

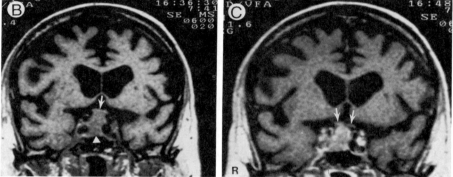

FIG 4.
Incidental pituitary adenoma in an elderly man being evaluated for memory loss. No visual symptoms. **A,** sagittal and **B** coronal T1-weighted images show isointense 1.8-cm mass in pituitary fossa *(arrowheads),* which is elevating the optic chiasm *(arrow).* **C,** coronal image after Gd-DTPA enhancement. *Arrows* indicate optic nerves near optic chiasm.

called echo images. A vertically oriented dural membrane was inconsistently shown between the pituitary gland and cavernous sinus. However, correlating T1-weighted spin-echo images with corresponding gradient-recalled images proved to be a reliable means of separating the pituitary gland from the adjacent cavernous venous spaces. Hirsch and associates compared the efficacy of MRI, CT, and angiography in the evaluation of the enlarged cavernous sinus.[36] Twenty-one of their patients underwent both MRI and CT, and 18 also underwent angiography. They found MRI to be superior to CT for differentiating parasellar aneurysms from tumors, and to be superior to both CT and angiography for defining the relationship of cavernous sinus tumors to adjacent structure such as the internal carotid artery, pituitary gland, and optic chiasm. Neither CT nor MRI could demonstrate the third, fourth, or sixth cranial nerves in the cavernous sinus if a mass were present. MRI was superior to angiogra-

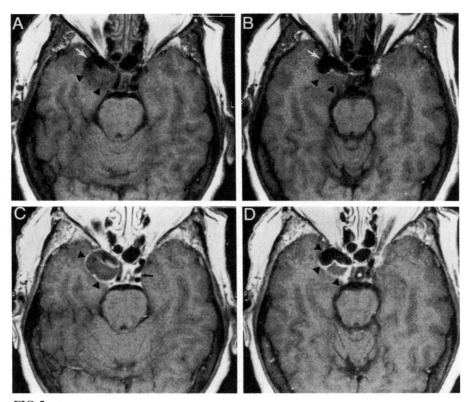

FIG 5.
Cavernous carotid aneurysm. Sixty-three-year-old woman with right sixth nerve palsy. **A, B,** contiguous T1-weighted axial sections through cavernous sinuses show dark structure *(white arrow),* which is caused by flow-void in aneurysm. Poorly defined isointense area outlined by *arrowheads* is thrombus within lumen of aneurysm. **C, D,** same sections after Gd-DTPA enhancement. Note peripheral enhancing rim around aneurysm *(arrowheads)* and normally enhancing left cavernous sinus *(arrow).*

phy in demonstrating carotid displacement by tumor since on coronal images both carotid arteries and the tumor could be simultaneously visualized. CT was superior to MRI for showing bony changes secondary to tumor, such as hyperostosis associated with sphenoid meningioma. Additional potential pitfalls in using MRI for evaluating sellar/parasellar lesions include difficulty in demonstrating small cavernous aneurysms in patients with tortuous carotid arteries, and the potential for confusing hemorrhagic neoplasms with aneurysms.

The Tolosa-Hunt syndrome (THS) consists of painful ophthalmoplegia due to nonspecific inflammatory changes in the cavernous sinus. Before the advent of CT and MRI, this condition was a diagnosis of exclusion, since cavernous sinus biopsy is hazardous. Yousem et al.[37] studied 11 patients with the clinical features of THS with MRI and found abnormalities in 9 of them. Eight had tissue in the cavernous sinus which, on short TR/TE images, had low signal intensity with respect to fat and was isointense to muscle. On long TR/TE sequences, the tissue was isointense to fat. Six of the 9 also had enlargement of the cavernous sinus. Extension into the orbital apex was seen in 8 cases, and 3 patients had internal carotid artery encasement. These investigators think that since THS and orbital pseudotumor have similar histologic findings and MRI signal characteristics, these diseases are related entities in different anatomic locations.

Goto and coworkers investigated three cases of THS with CT and MRI.[38] CT showed abnormal tissue in the orbital apex and optic nerve enlargement in one patient and no abnormalities in the other two. On T1-weighted or intermediately weighted images, MRI demonstrated abnormal soft tissue of intermediate to high signal intensity in the cavernous sinus in all three patients. After steroid therapy, MRI showed regression of the lesions.

POSTERIOR VISUAL PATHWAYS

Cerebral Ischemia and Infarction

It is well established that standard T2-weighted MRI can depict ischemic infarction consistently at 6 hours and, in some cases, as early as 1 to 2 hours postinfarction. In contrast, CT usually requires 12 to 24 hours to reliably demonstrate infarcts, although subtle findings can occasionally be seen after 4 hours. However, the diagnosis of cerebral infarction is usually made from the clinical picture, and the main role of imaging procedures is to distinguish between ischemic and hemorrhagic events (Fig 6). CT, being very sensitive for depicting acute hemorrhage, is well suited for this purpose. This will probably change as early interventional therapy for stroke becomes more efficacious, and the need for reliable imaging methods for ischemic damage will be more critical.

Recently a new MRI technique, diffusion-weighted imaging, has been shown to be effective in depicting early ischemic brain injury.[39–41] This technique detects the microscopic motion of water protons as they move from the extracellular to intracellular compartment in response to ischemic injury. With experimental middle cerebral artery occlusion in a cat model, cerebral infarction has been consistently demonstrated in less than 1 hour with diffusion-weighted MRI, whereas standard T2-weighted spin-echo MRI could not reliably demonstrate the infarcts at 2 to 3 hours.

The role of Gd-DTPA in the MRI evaluation of infarcts is continuing to evolve. Imakita et al. used Gd-DTPA–enhanced MRI to study 35 patients with infarcts ranging from 4 hours to 27 months old.[42, 43] They found that Gd-DTPA–enhanced MRI was more sensitive than enhanced CT, especially for small cortical infarcts near the inner table of the calvarium. Gd-DTPA enhancement was also helpful in detecting new foci of infarction in patients with multiple

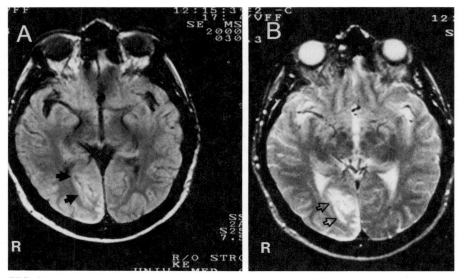

FIG 6.
Acute ischemic infarct, right calcarine cortex. Fifty-one-year-old man with sudden onset of left homonymous quadrantanopia. **A,** intermediate- and **B,** T2-weighted images obtained within 12 hours of event show increased signal intensity in right occipital lobe *(arrows).*

infarcts. Nearly all subacute infarcts enhanced, and a few lesions showed faint enhancement in as early as 24 hours. By 6 weeks postinfarction, enhancement had become faint or was absent. Cordes and coworkers also investigated Gd-DTPA enhancement in subacute and chronic cerebral infarctions[44] and found that the earliest enhancement was seen 5 days after infarction. They also found that Gd-DPTA facilitated differentiation of subacute from chronic infarcts. Additionally, a new MR contrast agent that causes T2 shortening, dysprosium DTPA-BMA (bis-methylamide), has also been recently developed. This adds sensitivity to T2-weighted spin-echo MRI for early stroke detection.[39]

Several reports have appeared recently on cortical blindness associated with severe preeclampsia or eclampsia.[45–49] MRI in these women usually shows areas of increased signal intensity in both occipital lobes, consistent with edema due to ischemic injury. The lesions are thought to be due to vasospasm and usually resolve clinically over a matter of hours or days. Follow-up MRI after 1 to 5 weeks is generally normal, unless there has been hemorrhage into the affected area.

Demyelinating Disease

Because of its high sensitivity to white matter change, MRI is the procedure of choice for imaging patients with multiple sclerosis (MS). Yet the white matter lesions seen on T2-weighted images in MS are in many cases nonspecific and are difficult to differentiate from deep white matter ischemic areas (DWMI), which are exceedingly common in older individuals. The latter condition is also known as white matter changes of the elderly, and subcortical arteriosclerotic encephalopathy (SAE). Various investigators have attempted to develop MRI criteria for distinguishing lesions of MS from DWMI. One promising observation is that MS plaques on T2-weighted images are frequently ovoid with the long axis of the oval perpendicular to the lateral ventricular wall and contiguous with the lateral ventricular margin. This reflects the perivascular distribution of the plaque, as has been demonstrated pathologically (Dawson's fingers).[50] Uhlenbrock and Sehlen have developed a list of criteria for distinguishing MS from SAE and stress the importance of T1-weighted sequences.[51] They found that MS lesions are often dark on T1-weighted images, whereas vascular white matter lesions are uncommonly seen on T1-weighted sequences. However, as Gebarski has pointed out, MRI findings are never *diagnostic* of MS.[52] New developments in pulse sequence design may improve the clarity of MS lesions on T2-weighted images and thus make these studies more specific. Runge and colleagues have developed a computer-optimized radio frequency pulse that offers increased lesion conspicuity when compared to the more customary truncated sinc pulses.[53] This resulted in 37% more lesions being found in ten patients with MS.

Gd-DTPA–enhanced MRI has been used in MS to distinguish active from inactive lesions. Active MS lesions that have perivenous inflammatory change and blood-brain barrier alterations usually enhance. Grossman et al. followed up 13 patients with MS for 2 years to determine the relationship of disease activity to Gd-DTPA enhancement.[54] They thought that Gd-DTPA–enhanced MRI was more sensitive than the clinical examination for assessing disease activity.

The clinical, MRI and CT features of MS in 12 adolescents were reported by Osborn and coworkers.[55] The adolescent patients showed a striking preponderance of affected girls (10/12), had more severe disease, and showed more frequent infratentorial involvement. Cortical atrophy was not seen in this group, presumably due to the shorter duration of the disease.

An unusual cause of demyelination is carbon monoxide (CO) poisoning. Victims who survive CO intoxication frequently have permanent neurologic sequelae. Attempts at predicting long-term outcome on the basis of the acute clinical picture or CT findings have not been successful. Some individuals will make an initial recovery, followed by a lucid interval, and then undergo progressive neurologic deterioration,[56] presumably due to progressive demyelination of subcortical white matter. Vieregge et al. used MRI findings to evaluate the white matter changes in CO victims and found it to be a better prognosticator of long-term outcome than CT findings.[57]

Neoplastic Disease

One of the more common indications for a neuroimaging procedure is to rule out intracranial metastases in a patient with a known primary tumor. To determine the most reliable test for this purpose, Sze et al. examined 50 consecutive patients for brain metastases with contrast-enhanced CT, noncontrast-enhanced MRI, and contrast-enhanced MRI.[58] Twenty-seven of the 50 patients had metastases. Of these, T1-weighted Gd-DTPA–enhanced MRI showed more lesions than did contrast-enhanced CT in eight cases. In no case, however, were CT findings completely normal when contrast-enhanced MRI showed metastases. Contrast-enhanced CT was never superior to contrast-enhanced MRI for intraparenchymal metastases. Contrast-enhanced MRI was superior to long TR noncontrast-enhanced images in most cases, although the T2-weighted images did provide useful ancillary information, especially with hemorrhagic metastases. The authors suggested a minimum screening examination of one long TR sequence and one short TR, Gd-DTPA–enhanced sequence.

BRAIN STEM AND CEREBELLUM

Vascular Disease

Top of the basilar syndrome is a clinical term that is used to describe a multitude of neurologic signs and symptoms resulting from occlusion or embolus involving the vascular territory supplied by the distal basilar artery and its branches.[59] Barkhoff and Valk described the clinical presentation and MRI findings in four patients with top of the basilar syndrome[60] and reviewed the pertinent vascular anatomy of this part of the brain. Oculomotor and behavioral disturbances were characteristically present in these patients. On MRI, thalamic and mesencephalic involvement were constant findings, and three of the four patients had cerebellar and posterior cerebral artery territory infarcts. They found MRI to be superior to CT for depicting the widespread lesions seen in this syndrome (Fig 7).

Trauma

The incidence of brain stem injury accompanying head trauma is unknown, with estimates varying widely. Gentry et al. compared CT and MRI in 87 patients with head trauma to determine the relative accuracies of these modalities for depicting brain stem injury.[61] Forty-eight traumatic lesions were found in 36 patients; 35 of these individuals had neurologic findings that supported the radiologic

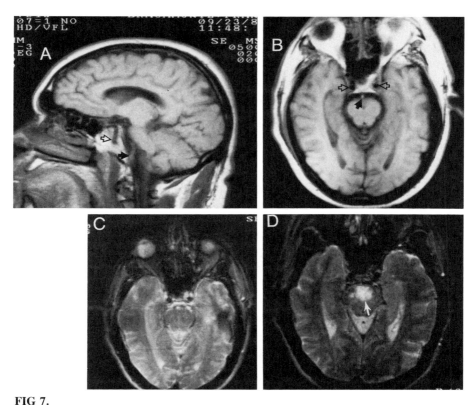

FIG 7.
Brain stem infarct due to basilar artery thrombosis. Fifty-three-year-old man who had two episodes of bilateral complete blindness, diplopia, and ataxia. **A,** sagittal and **B,** axial T1-weighted images show absence of flow void in basilar artery *(solid arrows),* indicating thrombosis. Normal flow void is seen in cavernous carotid artery *(open arrow).* **C,** T2-weighted axial image shows normal brain stem on day of event (9-23-88). **D,** follow-up MRI on 10-6-88, after clinical deterioration, now shows infarct in upper pons *(arrow).*

impression of brain stem injury. T1-weighted images showed 84.4% of the nonhemorrhagic lesions, while T2-weighted images depicted 96.9%, and CT scans demonstrated 21.9%. With hemorrhagic lesions, T2-weighted images showed 85.7%; T1-weighted sequences 57.1%; and CT scans, 71.4%. Thus, MRI was much more sensitive for nonhemorrhagic brain stem trauma.

The Cranial Nerves

MRI, being free of the beam hardening artifacts that degrade CT of the skull base and posterior fossa, has markedly improved imaging of the cranial nerves, their nuclei, tracts, and related structures. Three excellent review articles have appeared recently on MRI of the cranial nerves[62–64]; interested readers should find these rewarding.

Ocular motility problems are now being evaluated with MRI. Five cases of cryptogenic oculomotor palsy in children have been reported recently,[65] illustrating the need for repeated neuroimaging studies. After repeated evaluations, three of the five children were eventually found to have a small tumor, presumably schwannoma, compressing the oculomotor nerve. No surgical proof was available. The other two patients were being followed up with repeated neuroimaging procedures every 2 years, with the expectation that a mass will eventually be discovered.

A case of trochlear nerve palsy due to closed head trauma has recently been described.[66] CT was normal, but MRI showed a dorsal midbrain lesion on the contralateral side. Two cases of contralateral trochlear nerve paresis with ipsilateral Horner's syndrome have also been reported,[67] and the anatomic basis for these findings was discussed. Both patients had dorsal midbrain lesions in the location of the trochlear nucleus; one lesion was an arteriovenous malformation, and the other lesion was of unknown etiology.

CONGENITAL ANOMALIES

Tuberous Sclerosis

Both CT and MRI have been used to image the cortical tubers, subependymal nodules, and white matter heterotopias found in tuberous sclerosis.[68, 69] Inoue et al. compared the CT and MRI findings in ten patients with tuberous sclerosis and related these findings to the clinical severity of disease.[70] Since periventricular nodules are frequently calcified, they were better seen with CT. However, small peripheral lesions in the hemispheres, which were thought to be areas of demyelination, were well demonstrated by MRI and only occasionally seen with CT (Fig 8). The cortical tubers were not reliably seen with either method. More severely retarded patients tended to have more subcortical white matter lesions, but the number of subependymal nodules did not correlate with intelligence.

Neuronal Migration Disorders

MRI has been a major advance in the evaluation of these disorders because of its clear separation of gray and white matter as well as its ability to image in multiple planes. Anomalies usually considered in this group include schizencephaly, lissencephaly (agyria), pachygyria, heterotopias, and polymicrogyria. These disor-

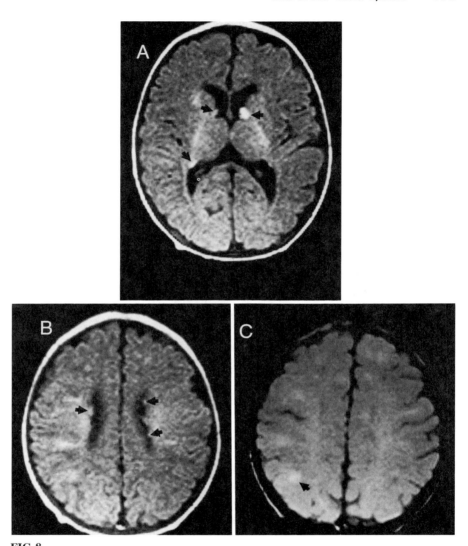

FIG 8.
Tuberous sclerosis. Two-month-old boy with delayed development and seizures. **A, B,** T1-weighted sagittal images show subependymal nodules *(arrows)*. **C,** white matter heterotopia is better seen on intermediately weighted images (TR, 2,000 ms; TE, 30 ms) *(arrow)*.

ders are discussed here because some of them have associated visual pathway abnormalities.

The anatomic abnormality in schizencephaly is a cleft, lined with gray matter, that extends from the ependymal surface of the ventricle to the pial surface of the brain.[71] The cleft may be an open cavity (open mouth schizencephaly) or fused (closed lip schizencephaly) (Fig 9). Clefts are usually bilateral, but may be unilateral. The gray matter–lined clefts of fused schizencephaly are seen better with MRI because of its superior gray-white matter differentiation.[72] Dysmorphic brain tissue, usually consisting of gray matter heterotopias and areas of polymicrogyria, are frequently found in or near the cleft.[73]

Several reports have appeared recently on the association of schizencephaly and septo-optic dysplasia. In an analysis of 6 cases of schizencephaly, Barkovich and Norman found 2 patients with optic nerve hypoplasia and an absent septum pellu-

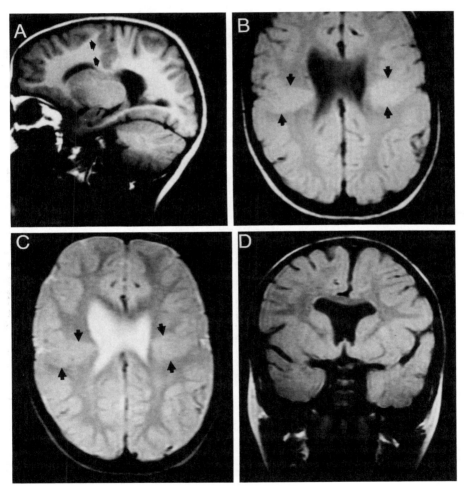

FIG 9.
Schizencephaly and absent septum pellucidum in a 6-year-old girl (case courtesy of Todd Burt, M.D.). **A,** T1-weighted sagittal image shows closed-lip cleft from pial surface to ventricle *(arrows)*. **B,** intermediate- and **C,** T2-weighted images show bilateral closed clefts *(arrows)*. **D,** coronal, intermediately weighted image shows absence of septum pellucidum.

cidum.[73] Both of these were in association with the open-mouthed type. In a follow-up report, they found that of 11 patients with septo-optic dysplasia, 5 had schizencephaly.[74] These 5 individuals had normal ventricular size, normal-appearing optic radiations, and a remnant of the septum pellucidum. They usually presented with seizures or visual disturbances. The remaining 6 patients with septo-optic dysplasia and no schizencephaly had diffuse white matter hypoplasia, enlarged ventricles, complete absence of the septum pellucidum, and presented with symptoms of hypothalamic-pituitary gland dysfunction. The authors propose that these two fairly distinct subsets of patients with septo-optic dysplasia result from different types of intrauterine insults. Kaufman et al. recently found pituitary stalk hypoplasia on MRI images of 2 children with septo-optic dysplasia.[75] Both of these patients had laboratory evidence of pituitary insufficiency. In a retrospective review of 9 cases of agenesis of the septum pellucidum diagnosed with CT or ultrasonography, 5 cases also had optic nerve hypoplasia, and 4 had schizencephaly; of the 4 cases of schizencephaly, 3 had optic nerve hypoplasia.[76] Schizencephaly may cause localized thinning of the corpus callosum due to absence of transcallosal fibers but is not associated with agenesis of the corpus callosum.[77]

Lissencephaly is the most severe neuronal migration disorder, with most infants dying in the first 6 to 18 months of life.[78] In MRI, these patients have an abnormally thick, small cortex, with thin, poorly arborized underlying white matter.[72] Clinically, lissencephaly can be divided into three types, and only type II has associated ocular abnormalities. These include retinal dysplasia, microphthalmia, colobomas, leukomas, optic nerve hypoplasia, and gliosis.[78] For a discussion of pachygyria, nodular heterotopia, and polymicrogyria, the reader is referred to the articles by Byrd and Smith.[71, 72, 78]

Aicardi Syndrome

This syndrome has been discussed recently in the MRI literature, often in articles on callosal dysgenesis.[77, 79-82] It is seen only in girls, and clinical features include agenesis or dysgenesis of the corpus callosum, seizures, and choroidal lacunae. Microphthalmia, colobomas, cerebral asymmetry, and heterotopias have also been found. Hall-Craggs and her collaborators used MRI to study the pattern of myelination in three infants with Aicardi syndrome and found delayed asymmetric myelination in two of them.[82]

MR ANGIOGRAPHY

MR angiography has significantly improved in the past 2 years, and vascular imaging packages are now available on many commercial scanners. However, ultrasound remains the noninvasive method of choice in evaluating the carotid bifurcation, while intraarterial angiography is still needed for evaluation of the smaller intracranial vessels.

In experienced hands, ultrasound has an accuracy of 90% to 95% in the evaluation of carotid bifurcation stenoses[83] and is comparatively inexpensive. Additionally, ultrasound gives information about internal plaque morphology that helps to predict which lesions will progress and are likely to ulcerate.[84] MR angiography is still limited by a lack of spatial resolution and artifacts produced by turbulent flow and thereby tends to overestimate the degree of stenosis.[85] Intracranial MR angiography currently does not have sufficient spatial resolution to evaluate the 1 to 2 mm ophthalmic artery (maximum spatial resolution of MR angiography at this time being 0.5 to 1.0 mm),[86] although it is a satisfactory screening test for arteriovenous malformations[87, 88] and is rapidly approaching that status for intracranial aneurysms.[89]

The field of MR angiography is developing rapidly. Currently many centers are working on technologic advances that promise great improvement in image quality and thus clinical utility. These improvements include more sophisticated flow compensation gradients, reduction in echo times, utilization of saturation pulses, exploitation of flow-related enhancement, and implementation of more accurate post-processing algorithms and subtraction techniques.[86] Detailed description of MR angiography is beyond the scope of this chapter. For interested readers, Edelman's review article is recommended for a practical, non-mathematical overview of the techniques currently utilized for MR angiography.[90]

CONCLUSION

MRI of the visual system has undergone marked advances in the past 2 years and is now the imaging modality of choice in most circumstances. New pulse sequences allow detection of optic neuritis. Combined unit/software improvements have increased MRI resolution and contrast to the point where it is the single best imaging modality for tumors, ischemia, posttraumatic changes, and congenital abnormalities of the visual system. CT is still useful as a complementary modality and is the procedure of choice in patients who are unable to undergo MRI scanning (for example, individuals who have metallic intraocular foreign bodies, aneurysm clips, pacemakers or other contraindications for MRI) and in those patients suspected of having calcified or acutely hemorrhagic lesions, such as optic nerve sheath meningiomas or hemorrhagic infarction.

REFERENCES

1. Johnson G, Miller DH, MacManus D, et al: STIR sequences in NMR imaging of the optic nerve. *Neuroradiology* 1987; 29:238–245.
2. Miller DH, Newton MR, van der Poel JC, et al: Magnetic resonance imaging of the optic nerve in optic neuritis. *Neurology* 1988; 38:175–179.

3. Smith RR, Edwards MK, Farlow MR, et al: Imaging of optic neuritis utilizing STIR MR (abstract). *AJNR* 1989; 10:905.

4. Atlas SW, Grossman RI, Hackney DB, et la: STIR MR imaging of the orbit. *AJNR* 1988; 51:1025–1030.

5. Dixon WT: Simple proton spectroscopic imaging. *Radiology* 1984; 153:189–194.

6. Simon J, Szumowski J, Totterman S, et al: Fat-suppression MR imaging of the orbit. *AJNR* 1988; 9:961–968.

7. Larsson HBW, Thomsen C, Frederiksen J, et al: Chemical shift selective magnetic resonance imaging of the optic nerve in patients with acute optic neuritis. *Acta Radiol* 1988; 29:629–632.

8. Blackwell CL: MRI in optic neuritis. *Arch Ophthalmol* 1989; 107:789.

9. Guy J, Mancuso A, Quisling RG, et al: Gadolinium-DTPA-enhanced magnetic resonance imaging in optic neuropathies. *Ophthalmology* 1990; 97:592–600.

10. Guy J, Fitzsimmons J, Ellis EA, et al: Gadolinium-DTPA-enhanced magnetic resonance imaging in experimental optic neuritis. *Ophthalmology* 1990; 97:601–607.

11. Azar-Kia B, Mafee MF, Horowitz SW, et al: CT and MRI of the optic nerve and sheath. *Semin Ultrasound, CT, MRI* 1988; 9:443–454.

12. Castillo M, Davis PC, Ross WK, et al: Meningioma of the chiasm and optic nerves: CT and MR findings. *J Comput Assist Tomogr* 1989; 13:679–681.

13. Zimmerman CF, Schatz NJ, Glaser JS: Magnetic resonance imaging of optic nerve meningiomas. *Ophthalmology* 1990; 97:586–591.

14. Haik BG, Zimmerman R, Saint Louis L: Gadolinium-DTPA enhancement of an optic nerve and chiasmal meningioma. *J Clin Neuro-opthalmol* 1989; 9:122–125.

15. Hendrix LE, Kneeland JB, Haughton VM, et al: MR Imaging of optic nerve lesions: Value of gadopentetate dimeglumine and fat-suppression technique. *AJNR* 1990; 11:749–754.

16. Zimmerman RA, Savino PJ, Armington WG, et al: MRI of visual field defects. *MRI Decis* 1989; 3:2–12.

17. Wright JE, McNab AA, McDonald WI: Optic nerve glioma and the management of optic nerve tumours in the young. *Br J Ophthalmol* 1989; 73:967–974.

18. Applegate LJ, Pribram HFW: Hematoma of optic nerve glioma—a cause for sudden proptosis. Magnetic resonance imaging findings. *J Clin Neuro-ophthalmol* 1989; 9:15–19.

19. Appleton RE, Jan JE: Delayed diagnosis of optic nerve glioma: A preventable cause of visual loss. *Pediatr Neurol* 1989; 5:226–228.

20. Sullivan JA, Harris SE: Characterization of orbital lesions by surface coil MR imaging. *Radio-Graphics* 1987; 7:9–28.

21. Kermode AG, Moseley IF, Kendall BE, et al: Magnetic resonance imaging in Leber's optic neuropathy. *J Neurol Neurosurg Psychiatry* 1989; 52:671–674.

22. Smiddy WE, Michaels RG, Kumar AG: Magnetic resonance imaging of retrobulbar changes in optic nerve position with eye movement. *Am J Ophthalmol* 1989; 107:82–83.

23. Bognanno JR, Edward MK, Lee TA, et al: Cranial MR imaging in neurofibromatosis. *AJR* 1988; 151:381–388.

24. Brown EW, Riccardi VM, Mawad M, et al: MR Imaging of optic pathways in patients with neurofibromatosis. *AJNR* 1987; 8:1031–1036.

25. Pomeranz SJ, Shelton JJ, Tobias J, et al: MR of visual pathways in patients with neurofibromatosis. *AJNR* 1987; 8:831–836.

26. National Institutes of Health Consensus Development: Neurofibromatosis. *Arch Neurol* 1988; 45:565–578.

27. Aoki S, Barkovich AJ, Nishimura K, et al: Neurofibromatosis types 1 and 2: Cranial MR findings. *Radiology* 1989; 172:527–534.

28. Listernick R, Charrow J, Greenwald MJ, et al: Optic gliomas in children with neurofibromatosis type 1. *J Pediatr* 1989; 114:788–792.

29. Hurst RW, Newman SA, Cail WS: Multifocal intracranial MR abnormalities in neurofibromatosis. *AJNR* 1988; 9:293–296.

30. Mirowitz SA, Sartor K, Gado M: High-intensity basal ganglia lesions on T1-weighted MR images in neurofibromatosis. *AJNR* 1989; 10:1159–1163.

31. Crowe NW, Nickles TP, Troost BT, et al: Intrachiasmal hemorrhage: A cause of delayed post-traumatic blindness. *Neurology* 1989; 39:863–865.

32. Corboy JR, Galetta SL: Familial cavernous angiomas manifesting with an acute chiasmal syndrome. *Am J Ophthalmol* 1989; 108:245–250.

33. Kaufman B, Tomsak RL, Kaufman BA, et al: Herniation of the suprasellar visual system and third ventricle in empty sellae: Morphologic and clinical considerations. *AJR* 1989; 152:597–608.

34. Ostrov SG, Quencer RM, Hoffman JC, et al: Hemorrhage within pituitary adenomas–How often associated with pituitary apoplexy syndrome? *AJR* 1989; 153:163–160.

35. Daniels DL, Czervionke LF, Bonneville JF, et al: MR imaging of the cavernous sinus: value of spin echo and gradient recalled echo images. *AJR* 1988; 151:1009–1014.

36. Hirsch WL, Hryshko FG, Sekhar LN, et al: Comparison of MR imaging, CT, and angiography in the evaluation of the enlarged cavernous sinus. *AJR* 1988; 151:1015–1023.

37. Yousem DM, Atlas SW, Grossman RI, et al: MR Imaging of Tolosa-Hunt syndrome. *AJNR* 1989; 10:1181–1184.

38. Goto Y, Hosokawa S, Goto I, et al: Abnormality in the cavernous sinus in three patients with Tolosa-Hunt syndrome: MRI and CT findings. *J Neurol Neurosurg Psychiatry* 1990; 53:231–234.

39. Moseley ME, Kucharczyk J, Mintorovitch J, et al: Diffusion-weighted MR imaging of acute stroke: Correlation with T2-weighted and magnetic susceptibility-enhanced MR in cats. *AJNR* 1990; 11:423–429.

40. Le Bihan D, Breton E, Lallemand D, et al: Separation of diffusion and perfusion in intravoxel incoherent motion MR imaging. *Radiology* 1988; 168:497–505.

41. Moseley ME, Cohen Y, Kucharczyk J, et al: Diffusion-weighted MR imaging of anisotropic water diffusion in cat central nervous system. *Radiology* 1990; 176:439–445.

42. Imakita S, Nishimura T, Naito H, et al: Magnetic resonance imaging of human cerebral infarction: Enhancement with Gd-DTPA. *Neuroradiology* 1987; 29:422–429.

43. Imakita S, Nishimura T, Yamada N, et al: Magnetic resonance imaging of cerebral infarction: Time course of Gd-DTPA enhancement and CT comparison. *Neuroradiology* 1988; 30:372–378.

44. Cordes M, Henkes H, Roll D, et al: Subacute and chronic cerebral infarctions: SPECT and gadolinium-DTPA enhanced MR imaging. *J Comput Assist Tomogr* 1989; 13:567–571.

45. Coughlin WF, McMurdo SK, Reeves T: MR imaging of postpartum cortical blindness. *J Comput Assist Tomogr* 1989; 13:572–576.

46. Duncan R, Hadley D, Bone I, et al: Blindness in eclampsia: CT and MR imaging. *J Neurol Neurosurg Psychiatry* 1989; 52:899–902.

47. Nalliah S, Thavarashah AS: Transient blindness in pregnancy induced hypertension. *Int J Gynecol Obstet* 1989; 29:249–251.

48. Seaward GR, England MJ, Nagar AK, et al: Transient postpartum amaurosis. A report of four cases. *J Reprod Med* 1989; 34:253–257.

49. Beg MF, Dempsey PJ, Marsland TG: Transient cortical blindness in a severe preeclamptic. *NZ Med J* 1990; 103:52.

50. Horowitz AL, Kaplan RD, Grewe G, et al: The ovoid lesion: A new MR observation in patients with multiple sclerosis. *AJNR* 1989; 10:303–305.

51. Uhlenbrock D, Sehlen S: The value of T1-weighted images in the differentiation between MS,

white matter lesions, and subcortical arteriosclerotic encephalopathy (SAE). *Neuroradiology* 1989; 31:203–212.

52. Gebarski SS: The passionate man plays his part: Neuroimaging and multiple sclerosis. *Radiology* 1988; 169:275–276.

53. Runge VM, Wood ML, Kaufman DM, et al: MR imaging section profile optimization: Improved contrast and detection of lesions. *Radiology* 1988; 167:831–834.

54. Grossman RI, Braffman BH, Brorson JR, et al: Multiple sclerosis: Serial study of gadolinium-enhanced MR imaging. *Radiology* 1988; 169:117–122.

55. Osborn AG, Harnsberger HR, Smoker WRK, et al: Multiple sclerosis in adolescents: CT and MR findings. *AJNR* 1990; 11:489–494.

56. Horowitz AL, Kaplan R, Sarpel G: Carbon monoxide toxicity: MR imaging in the brain. *Radiology* 1987; 162:787–788.

57. Vieregge P, Klostermann W, Blumm RG, et al: Carbon monoxide poisoning: Clinical, neurophysiological, and brain imaging observations in acute disease and follow-up. *J Neurol* 1989; 236:478–481.

58. Sze G, Milano E, Johnson C, et al: Detection of brain metastases: Comparison of contrast-enhanced MR with unenhanced MR and enhanced CT. *AJNR* 1990; 11:785–791.

59. Sato M, Tanaka S, Kohama A: "Top of the basilar" syndrome: Clinico radiological-evaluation. *Neuroradiology* 1987; 29:354–359.

60. Barkhof F, Valk J: "Top of the basilar" syndrome: A comparison of clinical and MR findings. *Neuroradiology* 1988; 30:293–298.

61. Gentry LR, Godersky JC, Thompson BH: Traumatic brain stem injury: MR imaging. *Radiology* 1989; 171:177–187.

62. Lanzieri CF: MR imaging of the cranial nerves. *AJR* 1990; 154:1263–1267.

63. Osborn AG, Harnsberger HR: MRI of cranial nerves. Part 1: Upper cranial nerves (I-IV). *MRI Decis* 1990; 4:2–11.

64. Osborn AG, Harnsberger HR: MRI of cranial nerves. Part 2: Lower cranial nerves (VII-XII). *MRI Decis* 1990; 4:2–15.

65. Abdul-Rahim AS, Savino PJ, Zimmermann RA, et al: Cryptogenic oculomotor nerve palsy. The need for repeated neuroimaging studies. *Arch Opthalmol* 1989; 107:387–390.

66. Burgerman RS, Wolf AL, Kelman SE, et al: Traumatic trochlear nerve palsy diagnosed by magnetic resonance imaging: Case report and review of the literature. *Neurosurgery* 1989; 25:978–981.

67. Guy J, Day AL, Mickle JP, et al: Contralateral trochlear nerve paresis and ipsilateral Honer's syndrome. *Am J Ophthalmol* 1989; 107:73–76.

68. McMurdo SK, Moore SG, Brant-Zawadzki, et al: MR imaging of intracranial tuberous sclerosis. *AJNR* 1987; 8:22–82.

69. Roach ES, Williams DP, Laster DW: Magnetic resonance imaging in tuberous sclerosis. *Arch Neurol* 1987; 44:301–303.

70. Inoue Y, Nakajima S, Fukuda T, et al: Magnetic resonance images of tuberous sclerosis: Further observations and clinical correlations. *Neuroradiology* 1988; 30:379–384.

71. Byrd SE, Osborn RE, Bohan TP, et al: The CT and MR evaluation of migrational disorders of the brain: Part II. Schizencephaly, heterotopia and polymicrogyria. *Pediatr Radiol* 1989; 19:219–222.

72. Smith AS, Blaser SI, Ross JS, et al: Magnetic resonance imaging of disturbances in neuronal migration: Illustration of an embrylogic process. *RadioGraphics* 1989; 9:509–522.

73. Barkovich AJ, Norman D: MR imaging of schizencephaly. *AJR* 1988; 150:1391–1396.

74. Barkovich AJ, Fram EK, Norman D: Septo-optic dysplasia: MR imaging. *Radiology* 1989; 171:189–192.

75. Kaufman LM, Miller MT, Mafee MF: Magnetic resonance imaging of pituitary stalk hypoplasia: A discrete midline anomaly associated with endocrine abnormalities in septo-optic dysplasia. *Arch Ophthalmol* 1989; 107:1485–1489.

76. Kuban KCK, Teele RL, Wallman J: Septo-optic-dysplasia-schizencephaly: Radiographic and clinical features. *Pediatr Radiol* 1989; 19:145–150.

77. Barkovich JA, Norman D: Anomalies of the corpus callosum: Correlation with further anomalies of the brain. *AJR* 1988; 151:171–179.

78. Byrd SE, Osborn RE, Bohan TP, et al: The CT and MR evaluation of migrational disorders of the brain: Part I. Lissencephaly and pachygyria. *Pediatr Radiol* 1989; 19:151–156.

79. Curnes JT, Laster DW, Koubek TD, et al: MRI of corpus callosal syndromes. *AJNR* 1986; 7:617–622.

80. Igidbashian V, Mahboubi S, Zimmerman RA: CT and MR findings in Aicardi syndrome. *J Comput Assist Tomogr* 1987; 11:357–358.

81. Baieri P, Markl A, Thelen M, et al: MR imaging in Aicardi syndrome. *AJNR* 1988; 9:805–806.

82. Hall-Craggs MA, Harbord MG, Finn JP, et al: Aicardi syndrome: MR assessment of brain structure and myelination. *AJNR* 1990; 11:532–536.

83. O'Leary DH, Polak JF: High-resolution carotid sonography: Past, present and future. *AJR* 1989; 153:699–704.

84. Langsfeld M, Gidy-Weale A, Lusby RJ: The role of plaque morphology and diameter reduction in the development of new symptoms in asymptomatic carotid arteries. *J Vasc Surg* 1989; 9:548–557.

85. Anderson CM, Saloner D, Tsuruda J, et al: Artifacts in maximum-intensity-projection display of MR angiograms. *AJR* 1990; 154:623–629.

86. Haacke EM, Masaryk TJ: The salient features of MR angiography. *Radiology* 1989; 173:611–612.

87. Marchal G, Bosmans H, Vanfraeyenhoven L, et al: Intracranial vascular lesions: Optimization and clinical evaluation of three-dimensional time-of-flight MR angiography. *Radiology* 1990; 175:443–448.

88. Edelman R, Wentz KU, Mattle HP, et al: Intracerebral arteriovenous malformations: Evaluation with selective MR angiography and venography. *Radiology* 1989; 173:831–837.

89. Ross JS, Masaryk TJ, Modic MT, et al: Intracranial aneurysms: Evaluaion by MR angiography. *AJNR* 1990; 11:449–456.

90. Edelman RR, Mattle HP, Atkinson DJ: MR angiography. *AJR* 1990; 154:937–946.

Index

413